Scars

Sebastian P. Nischwitz
Lars-Peter Kamolz • Ludwik K. Branski
Editors

Scars

A Practical Guide for Scar Therapy

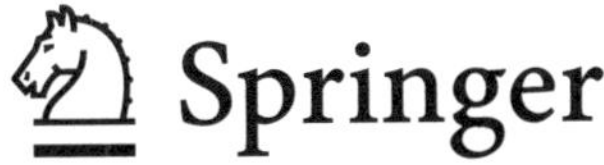

Springer

Editors
Sebastian P. Nischwitz
Division of Plastic, Aesthetic and
Reconstructive Surgery, Department of
Surgery
Medical University of Graz
Graz, Steiermark, Austria

Ludwik K. Branski
Division of Plastic Surgery, Department
of Surgery
The University of Texas Medical
Branch, Shriners Hospital for Children
Galveston, TX, USA

Lars-Peter Kamolz
Division of Plastic, Aesthetic and
Reconstructive Surgery, Department of
Surgery
Medical University of Graz
Graz, Steiermark, Austria

COREMED-Cooperative Centre for
Regenerative Medicine
JOANNEUM RESEARCH
Forschungsgesellschaft mbH
Graz, Steiermark, Austria

ISBN 978-3-031-24139-0   ISBN 978-3-031-24137-6   (eBook)
https://doi.org/10.1007/978-3-031-24137-6

This Springer imprint is published by the registered company Springer Nature Switzerland AG
The registered company address is: Gewerbestrasse 11, 6330 Cham, Switzerland

Contents

Part III Scar Treatment

Part IV Scar Rehabilitation

Part I

Skin, Wounds and Scars

Anatomy and Physiology of the Skin

Johann Zwirner and Niels Hammer

Core Messages

- The five-layered epidermis is a constantly renewing protection layer against physical, chemical and biochemical influences on the human body.
- The epidermal-dermal junction is a highly organized transition zone that can be considered an independent anatomical unit.
- The two-layered dermis contains the bulk of the extracellular matrix of the skin, which makes it the key layer for the biomechanical characteristics of the skin as a composite tissue.
- Highly specialized receptors enable the skin to detect and mediate mechanical, thermal, nociceptive and potentially chemical stimuli.

J. Zwirner
Institute of Legal Medicine, University Medical Center Hamburg-Eppendorf, Hamburg, Germany

Department of Oral Sciences, University of Otago, Dunedin, New Zealand
e-mail: j.zwirner@uke.de

N. Hammer (✉)
Division of Macroscopic and Clinical Anatomy, Gottfried Schatz Research Center, Medical University of Graz, Graz, Austria

Department of Orthopaedic and Trauma Surgery, University of Leipzig, Leipzig, Germany

Division of Biomechatronics, Fraunhofer Institute for Machine Tools and Forming Technology, Dresden, Germany
e-mail: niels.hammer@medunigraz.at

Introduction

The skin forms the outermost and largest organ of the human body [1]. It makes up between 6 and 16% of the entire body weight depending on whether subcutaneous fat is included in this calculation [2]. Strictly speaking, skin is composed of two layers, the superficial epidermis and the deeper dermis even though the subcutaneous fat is frequently included as a third layer [1, 3]. Both epidermis and dermis are composed of several sub-layers. Studying the anatomy of the skin forms the basis to understand why the epidermis is predominantly a physical, chemical and biochemical protective barrier for the body and the dermis is mostly responsible for the biomechanical characteristics of the skin [4, 5]. The detailed anatomy including the thickness and development of the specific sub-layers of the skin varies depending on several factors such as age, sex as well as the respective anatomical site with its specific functional requirements and challenges [6]. As an example, the thin skin of the eyelid covers the eye to prevent it from dehydration and protect it from foreign bodies. It moves every time we blink and is, therefore, a dynamic tissue. On the contrary, the skin at the soles of our feet is oftentimes stressed by a multiple of the body weight. This functional difference directly reflects on the morphology and the thicknesses of the various layers involved in load distribution. The eyelid is considerably thinner compared to the soles of our feet, which is potentially both the least sophisticated as well as the most comprehensible way to emphasize the relationship between the form and function of the skin. Consequently, summarizing the anatomy and physiology of 'the skin' as a whole can be misleading. However, studying the general anatomical and physiological characteristics of the skin is an essential starting point to gain a basic understanding of this fascinating organ. Basically, two different classes of skin can be distinguished: thin hirsute (hairy) skin covering most of the body and glabrous (hairless) skin covering the palmar and plantar regions extending to the digits [7].

Anatomy of the Skin

Epidermis

The epidermis forms the most superficial layer of the skin that completely renews itself within the time frame of 52–75 days [8]. It is composed of the following five layers (or 'strata') from superficial to deep: stratum corneum, stratum lucidum, stratum granulosum, stratum spinosum and stratum basale [9]. The epidermal cell renewal takes place from the basal layer towards the stratum corneum, so the layers are most logically studied in this order. The **basal cell layer** (derived from the Greek word 'basis' as 'ground' or 'bottom'; Fig. 1) is also called stratum germinativum and consists of a single layer of columnar nucleated basal cells and melanocytes [1]. The basal cells form the earliest developmental stage of the later keratinocytes and are comprised of two different proliferative cells: stem cells with an unlimited capacity of self-renewal and transit amplifying cells, which withdraw from the cell cycle to enter a transitional state between stem cells and a cell that eventually differentiates following numerous divisions [10]. Basal cells are connected to one another and to the superficial squamous cells via desmosomes and attached to the underlying basal membrane via hemidesmosomes [1, 11]. These cell-cell and cell-extracellular matrix links are of key importance for the integrity and homeostasis of the epidermis [12]. Melanocytes are present in

the basal layer of the epidermis and in hair follicles [13]. Throughout life, the ratio of melanocytes and keratinocytes stays constant at 1:10; however, the reason for this is unknown [14]. The spinous layer (derived from the Latin word 'spīnōsus' meaning 'thorny'), also known as the **prickle cell layer** (Fig. 1), is the next and thickest epidermal layer the keratinocytes have to proceed through on their way to the surface. In this layer, the keratinocytes increase in size and establish strong intercellular connections through desmosomes [11, 15]. The strong interdigitation by means of spinous extensions between the keratinocytes is what gives this layer its characteristic name. Cells that are close to the basal layer remain mitotically active and hence are similar to the basal layer but are less basophilic [3]. The term 'Malpighian layer' summarizes the structural and functional similarity between the two [3]. The predominantly polyhedral-shaped keratinocytes flatten towards the granular layer and their cytoplasm becomes acidophilic [3]. Two types of bone marrow-derived antigen-presenting dendritic cells, the Langerhans cells, can be found in the spinous layer with dendritic processes that can reach up to the stratum corneum [16]. Type 1 is of a classic dendritic shape with numerous 'tennis racket-shaped' granules, also called Birbeck bodies, and small numbers of lysosomes and mitochondria [16, 17]. Type 2 describes a less dendritic cell that can be found supra-basally or even in the basal layer, which contains more mitochondria, fewer Birbeck bodies and a more electron-dense cytoplasm compared to the Type 1 cells [17]. The **granular layer** (derived from the Latin word 'granum' meaning 'grain'; Fig. 1) comprises multiple layers of nucleated keratinocytes of a polygonal shape without a limiting membrane [3]. Lamellar membrane-bound lipid granules are the characteristic cytoplasmatic feature that gave this layer its name [3]. These keratohyalin granules synthesize profilaggrin, which after proteolytic processing to filaggrin aggregates filaments of keratin into dense bundles [4, 18]. This is the reason for the progressive flattening of the keratinocytes towards the surface [4]. High levels of lysosomal enzymes are present in the granular

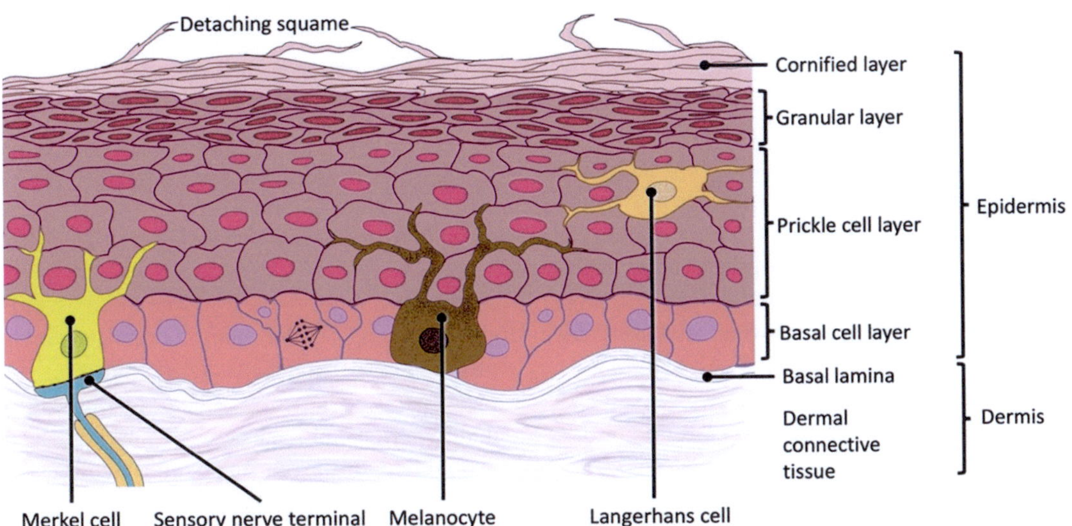

Fig. 1 Fine structure of the epidermis and dermis. Layers, features and characteristic cell types are depicted. (Adapted from [7])

layer, which are required for the elimination of cell components of the resilient anuclear corneocytes as the terminally differentiated keratinocytes [1, 18]. The **lucid layer** (derived from the Latin word 'lūcidus' meaning 'clear') is only present in thick skin areas such as the palm of the hand or the sole of the foot [3]. The keratinocytes of the lucid layer are non-vital and contain the clear intracellular protein eleidin as opposed to the keratin in deeper layers [19]. The **cornified layer** (derived from the Latin word 'cornu' meaning 'horn'; Fig. 1) forms the outermost epidermal layer and consists of flattened anucleated cells that are filled with keratin [3]. The extracellular matrix of the corneal layer contains mainly lipids that are organized within characteristic lamellar bilayers but also enzymes, antimicrobial peptides and structural proteins [20]. Superficial corneocytes are continuously shed off and replaced through an ongoing supply of corneocytes from the granular or lucid layer [3, 9]. This lines up with the fact that corneocytes of deeper layers are more tightly interconnected with desmosomes compared to superficial layers as desmosomes are subjected to proteolytic degradation towards the surface [1].

The Epidermal-Dermal Junction

The epidermal-dermal junction is a transitional zone that anchors the epidermis onto the dermis and can be considered an independent anatomical unit [21]. From superficial to deep, it consists of the following four components:

1. *The dermal surface of the plasma membrane of the epidermal basal cells:* Hemidesmosomes, which describe multiprotein complexes that link the epidermal basal cells to the basal lamina, are the most significant structures of this layer [21, 22].
2. *The lamina lucida as an intermembranous space:* This layer is not to be confused with the epidermal lucid layer. The similar name originates from common microscopic features between the two. In electron microscopy, light can pass through this layer but the space does not occur completely transparent as fine filaments from hemidesmosomes cross on their course between the epidermal basal cells and the basal membrane [21, 23].
3. *The basal lamina:* It is a continuous band of type IV collagen, laminin, nidogen, and per-

lecan [21, 24]. The basal lamina varies in density and is thicker in areas of attaching hemidesmosomes [21]. The basal lamina is of epidermal origin [25].

4. *Fibrous elements of the sub-basal lamina:* Anchoring fibrils connect the basal lamina to the epidermis [21]. They can form a meshwork within the dermis as well as reattach to the basal lamina after looping around collagens [21]. Microfibril bundles can run over considerable distances between the basal lamina and the deep dermis [21]. Also, randomly oriented single collagen fibres with no attachment to the basal lamina can be found in this compartment.

Dermis

The dermis makes up the main body of the skin consisting of dense connective tissue organized in two layers: a superficial thin papillary layer that is tightly connected to the epidermis via the epidermal-dermal junction and a thick deep reticular layer that connects to the hypodermis [3]. The dermal thickness depends on the body site and sex. It is thicker in palms and soles compared to the eyelid and thicker in males compared to females [3]. The **papillary layer** (derived from the Latin word 'papilla' meaning 'nipple') is named after the finger-like elongations that extend towards the epidermis. Thin type I and III collagen fibres can be found in this layer, which are organized in a loose meshwork [26]. Also, fibroblasts, elastic fibres, looped capillaries and tactile corpuscles are located in the papillary layer [3, 27, 28]. The **reticular layer** (derived from the Latin word 'rete' meaning 'network') is composed of dense connective tissue [3]. The main feature of this layer is the presence of thick, coarse type I collagen bundles [26]. Moreover, the reticular dermis contains cells such as fibroblasts and immune cells, elastic fibres, hair follicles, sebaceous and sweat glands, vessels, nerves and sensory receptors such as Pacinian corpuscles and Ruffini corpuscles [1, 3, 27, 29] (Fig. 2). Collagens and elastic fibres of the reticular dermis create tension lines called Langer's lines that are relevant to surgery and wound healing [30]. The boundary between the reticular dermis and the hypodermis is unclear in contrast to the distinct epidermal-dermal junction [3].

Hypodermis

The hypodermis (derived from the Greek words 'hypo' meaning 'under' and 'dérma' meaning 'skin') is located beneath the dermis and describes a layer of loose connective tissue, blood vessels including a rich capillary network and nerves [1, 3]. Simplified, this layer is also referred to as subcutaneous fat as this is the predominant component of this layer, which connects the dermis to the deep fascia, aponeurosis or periosteum [3].

Vascular Supply

The skin has the capacity to alter the regional blood flow almost 20-fold. This vast increase in supply is owing to the thermoregulatory function of the skin. Three sources of supply exist, one direct to the cutaneous tissue, one to underlying musculature and one to the fascio-cutaneous system. The latter two deviate either as muscle perforators under the investing fascia or superficial to it, respectively. A total of six vascular plexus can be found in the dermal layers. Arteriovenous shunts exist especially in the deeper skin layers, which are under autonomic nerve control. Blood supply is influenced by thermal needs and also by emotions. The lymphatics originate in the papillary dermis and receive the interstitial fluid via small vessels into subcutaneous channels. They help transport macrophages, Langerhans cells and lymphocytes to regional lymph nodes [7].

Innervation

The skin forms a major sensory organ, and regional differences exist for both the types and densities of innervation. A number of receptors can be distinguished throughout the layers, which help mediate mechanical, thermal, nociceptive and potentially chemical stimuli. Figure 2 summarizes the locations of these receptors.

- Free nerve endings detect thermal (heat and cold), mechanical stretch or pain and can be found in most of the layers of the skin.
- Meissner [tactile] corpuscles exist in the dermal papillae close to the dermo-epidermal junction. They are rapidly adapting sensors important for the sensation of touch.
- Merkel nerve endings are situated in the epidermis (basal cell layer) and are characterized as slow-adapting mechanoreceptors, detecting continuous pressure. Moreover, they are important for object discrimination.
- Pacinian corpuscles are situated in the dermis or hypodermis predominantly in the digits. They primarily detect vibration and deep pressure.
- Ruffini [Bulbous] corpuscles can be found in the dermis (reticular layer) and are slow-adapting mechanoreceptors responding to ongoing pressure with low capacity to adapt.

Biomechanics of the Skin

Determinants of Biomechanical Properties of Human Skin

Based on the description in the section 'Anatomy of the Skin', it can be concluded that the skin is a composite material of several layers, which are organized into sub-layers with characteristic structural components. That poses the question of which components are responsible for the characteristic biomechanical (load-deformation) behaviour of the skin. Irrespective of the layer, the following two components determine the biomechanics of the skin: cellular components and the extracellular matrix. Tensile tests have demonstrated that predominantly the extracellular matrix forms the mechanical backbone of skin [31, 32]. The epidermis seems less relevant with regard to elasticity and load-bearing of the skin when stretched [32]. However, cells play a role in the strain behaviour of human skin. Following cell removal, skin samples can be strained to a further extent, indicating that cells limit the straining of skin in the native state [32]. The main extracellular matrix components of the skin are collagen, elastin and ground substance [5]. The

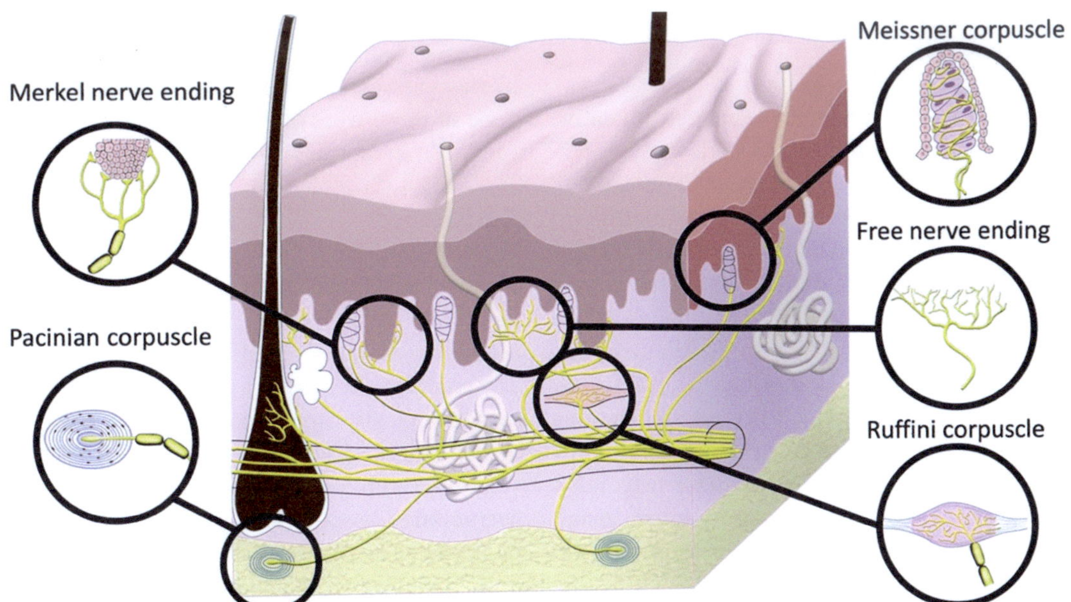

Fig. 2 Skin mechanoreceptor types. Receptor locations are depicted within the layered skin. Each receptor presents unique features, allowing for a broad range of mechanical, thermal and chemical stimuli being transduced

collagen network in the dermis makes up approximately 77% of the dry weight of the skin, forming its key component [1, 5]. Collagen-rich tissues are well known for their mechanical robustness and generally determine the strength of human tissues. Hence, dermal types I and III collagens almost exclusively determine the mechanical strength of human skin under strain [33]. Elastin, which accounts for approximately 4% of the human skin, is predominantly responsible for the recoiling of skin after being stretched with no significant contribution to its strength [34]. Overstretching [5] or mechanical wear of elastic fibres induces a lack of recoiling, which negatively affects the capacity of the skin to regain its initial condition. Ground substance summarizes the physicochemical linkage of the glycosaminoglycans chondroitin, keratin, heparin, dermatan and hyaluronic acid to a protein, which results in so-called proteoglycans [5]. The ground substance likely contributes to the (time-dependent) viscoelastic property of human skin. The ground substance also plays a role in the lubrication of collagens and elastin during movements as well as in the direction of collagen fibre formation [5].

Effects of Ageing on Skin Biomechanics

With age, the skin undergoes changes indicative of mechanical ageing. Eye wrinkles are a common sign of this phenomenon. The section 'Determinants of Biomechanical Properties of Human Skin' outlined that the dermis is the key layer for the mechanical behaviour of the human skin. Thus, age-related structural changes of the dermis will strongly reflect on the biomechanical behaviour of the skin with age. Ageing of the skin can be subdivided into two categories that describe characteristic structural alterations of the skin related to whether these originated within or outside the human body: intrinsic and extrinsic ageing [5]. Intrinsic ageing of the skin describes the atrophy of the dermis that results from a degeneration of collagen and elastin and

a decreased tissue hydration with age [5]. Extrinsic ageing, also called 'photoageing', is mainly caused by (types A and B) ultraviolet light and results in an excessive accumulation of abnormal elastin material within the upper and mid-portion of the dermis [5]. This ageing is considered premature. Also, extrinsic ageing of the skin appears to cause an increased collagen degeneration compared to intrinsic ageing [5]. The following characteristic age-related changes in the mechanical properties of the human skin can be observed: Firstly, the skin progressively loses its ability to elastically recover in areas of small stresses, which is related to the elastin network changes in the dermis [35]. Secondly, the time for viscoelastic recovery from larger stresses progressively increases with age, which is thought to be related to changes in the dermal ground substance rather than the proteins [35]. Thirdly, dermal collagen degeneration results in decreased tensile strength of the skin [5]. It has to be noted that the biomechanical behaviour of human skin is complex and might be influenced by other factors such as sex or the way the experimental data was obtained. Therefore, generalizations should be handled with care. For example, a study on human scalp conducted on samples with an age range between 6 and 94 years observed strong age-related decreases in elasticity and tensile strength in females, but none of these were observed in males [33].

Conclusion

The human skin is a composite tissue that is organized into several layers and sub-layers. These are highly adapted to fulfil complex functions. The epidermis is mainly a protective layer that is morphologically structured in different developmental stages of keratinocytes on their progression to the surface. Apart from the protection of deeper body tissues, the collagen-rich dermis is of importance for the thermoregulation, sensation, immune system and biomechanical characteristics of the skin.

References

1. Kolarsick PAJ, Kolarsick MA, Goodwin C. Anatomy and physiology of the skin. J Dermatol Nurses Assoc. 2011;3(4):203–13.
2. Leider M. On the weight of the skin. J Invest Dermatol. 1949;12(3):187–91.
3. Arda O, Goksugur N, Tuzun Y. Basic histological structure and functions of facial skin. Clin Dermatol. 2014;32(1):3–13.
4. Baroni A, Buommino E, De Gregorio V, Ruocco E, Ruocco V, Wolf R. Structure and function of the epidermis related to barrier properties. Clin Dermatol. 2012;30(3):257–62.
5. Hussain SH, Limthongkul B, Humphreys TR. The biomechanical properties of the skin. Dermatol Surg. 2013;39(2):193–203.
6. Firooz A, Rajabi-Estarabadi A, Zartab H, Pazhohi N, Fanian F, Janani L. The influence of gender and age on the thickness and echo-density of skin. Skin Res Technol. 2017;23(1):13–20.
7. Standring S, Borley NR, Gray H. Gray's anatomy: the anatomical basis of clinical practice. 14th ed. Amsterdam: Elsevier; 2020. p. 1551.
8. Halprin KM. Epidermal "turnover time"—a re-examination. Br J Dermatol. 1972;86(1):14–9.
9. Wickett RR, Visscher MO. Structure and function of the epidermal barrier. Am J Infect Control. 2006;34(10):S98–S110.
10. Watt FM. Epidermal stem cells: markers, patterning and the control of stem cell fate. Philos Trans R Soc Lond Ser B Biol Sci. 1998;353(1370):831–7.
11. Peltonen S, Raiko L, Peltonen J. Desmosomes in developing human epidermis. Dermatol Res Pract. 2010;2010:698761.
12. Walko G, Castanon MJ, Wiche G. Molecular architecture and function of the hemidesmosome. Cell Tissue Res. 2015;360(3):529–44.
13. Cichorek M, Wachulska M, Stasiewicz A, Tyminska A. Skin melanocytes: biology and development. Postepy Dermatol Alergol. 2013;30(1):30–41.
14. Haass NK, Herlyn M. Normal human melanocyte homeostasis as a paradigm for understanding melanoma. J Investig Dermatol Symp Proc. 2005;10(2):153–63.
15. Roger M, Fullard N, Costello L, Bradbury S, Markiewicz E, O'Reilly S, et al. Bioengineering the microanatomy of human skin. J Anat. 2019;234(4):438–55.
16. Jaitley S, Saraswathi T. Pathophysiology of Langerhans cells. J Oral Maxillofac Pathol. 2012;16(2):239–44.
17. Breathnach AS. Variations in ultrastructural appearance of Langerhans cells of normal human epidermis. Br J Dermatol. 1977;97(15):14.
18. Matoltsy AG. Keratinization. J Invest Dermatol. 1976;67(1):20–5.
19. Nguyen AV, Soulika AM. The dynamics of the skin's immune system. Int J Mol Sci. 2019;20(8):1811.
20. Elias PM. Structure and function of the stratum corneum extracellular matrix. J Invest Dermatol. 2012;132(9):2131–3.
21. Briggaman RA, Wheeler CE Jr. The epidermal–dermal junction. J Investig Dermatol. 1975;65(1):71–84.
22. Borradori L, Sonnenberg A. Structure and function of hemidesmosomes: more than simple adhesion complexes. J Invest Dermatol. 1999;112(4):411–8.
23. Kobayasi T. An electron microscope study on the dermo-epidermal junction. Acta Derm Venereol. 1961;41:481–91.
24. Mak KM, Mei R. Basement membrane type IV collagen and laminin: an overview of their biology and value as fibrosis biomarkers of liver disease. Anat Rec (Hoboken). 2017;300(8):1371–90.
25. Briggaman RA, Dalldorf FG, Wheeler CE Jr. Formation and origin of basal lamina and anchoring fibrils in adult human skin. J Cell Biol. 1971;51(21):384–95.
26. Meigel WN, Gay S, Weber L. Dermal architecture and collagen type distribution. Arch Dermatol Res. 1977;259(1):1–10.
27. Driskell RR, Lichtenberger BM, Hoste E, Kretzschmar K, Simons BD, Charalambous M, et al. Distinct fibroblast lineages determine dermal architecture in skin development and repair. Nature. 2013;504(7479):277–81.
28. Garcia-Piqueras J, Cobo R, Carcaba L, Garcia-Mesa Y, Feito J, Cobo J, et al. The capsule of human Meissner corpuscles: immunohistochemical evidence. J Anat. 2020;236(5):854–61.
29. Uitto J, Li Q, Urban Z. The complexity of elastic fibre biogenesis in the skin—a perspective to the clinical heterogeneity of cutis laxa. Exp Dermatol. 2013;22(2):88–92.
30. Pierard GE, Lapiere CM. Microanatomy of the dermis in relation to relaxed skin tension lines and Langer's lines. Am J Dermatopathol. 1987;9(3):219–24.
31. Schleifenbaum S, Prietzel T, Aust G, Boldt A, Fritsch S, Keil I, et al. Acellularization-induced changes in tensile properties are organ specific—an in-vitro mechanical and structural analysis of porcine soft tissues. PLoS One. 2016;11(3):e0151223.
32. Zwirner J, Ondruschka B, Scholze M, Schulze-Tanzil G, Hammer N. Load-deformation characteristics of acellular human scalp: assessing tissue grafts from a material testing perspective. Sci Rep. 2020;10(1):19243.
33. Falland-Cheung L, Scholze M, Lozano PF, Ondruschka B, Tong DC, Brunton PA, et al. Mechanical properties of the human scalp in tension. J Mech Behav Biomed Mater. 2018;84:188–97.
34. Wilkes GL, Brown IA, Wildnauer RH. The biomechanical properties of skin. CRC Crit Rev Bioeng. 1973;1(4):453–95.
35. Daly CH, Odland GF. Age-related changes in the mechanical properties of human skin. J Invest Dermatol. 1979;73(1):84–7.

From Wound to Scar: Scarring Explained—Pathophysiology of Wound Healing

Thomas Wild, Ahmed A. Aljowder, A. Aljawder, Joerg Marotz, and Frank Siemers

Abbreviations

b-FGF	Basic fibroblast growth factor
ECM	Extracellular matrix
EGF	Epidermal growth factor
FGF	Fibroblast growth factor
HSI	Hyperspectral imaging
IGF-1	Insulin-like growth factor-1
IL-1	Interleukin-1
IL-6	Interleukin-6
KGF	Keratinocyte growth factor
MMPs	Matrix metalloproteinases
NFG	Nerve growth factor
PDGF	Platelet-derived growth factor
TGF-α	Transforming growth factor α
TGF-β 1	Transforming growth factor-β 1
TIMPS	Tissue inhibitors of metalloproteinases
TNF-α	Tumor necrosis factor-α
TNF-β	Tumor necrosis factor β
VEGF	Vascular endothelial growth factor

T. Wild (✉)
University of Applied Science, Institute of Bioscience and Process Management, University of Applied Science Anhalt, Anhalt, Germany

Clinic of Plastic, Hand and Aesthetic Surgery, Burn Center, BG Clinic Bergmannstrost, Halle, Germany

Outpatient Operating Center, MVZ Saale Klinik, Martin Luther University, Medical University, Halle, Germany
e-mail: thomas.wild@woundconsulting.com

A. A. Aljowder
Regenerative Medicine, Arabian Gulf University, Manama, Bahrain

Department of Dermatology, King Hamad University Hospital, Al Sayh, Bahrain
e-mail: Ahmed.Aljowder@khuh.org.bh

A. Aljawder
Clinic of Pathology, King Hamad University Hospital, Al Sayh, Bahrain

The Department of Anatomical and Cellular Pathology at Prince of Wales Hospital, The Chinese University Hong Kong, Hong Kong, China
e-mail: aysha.aljawder@khuh.org.bh

J. Marotz
University of Applied Science, Institute of Bioscience and Process Management, University of Applied Science Anhalt, Anhalt, Germany

Clinic of Plastic, Hand and Aesthetic Surgery, Burn Center, BG Clinic Bergmannstrost, Halle, Germany
e-mail: joerg.marotz@ipross.de

F. Siemers
Clinic of Plastic, Hand and Aesthetic Surgery, Burn Center, BG Clinic Bergmannstrost, Halle, Germany
e-mail: frank.siemers@bergmannstrost.de

Introduction

The human body is encased in a protective mantle by the skin, the biggest organ with an average surface area of 1.8 m². It is important for maintaining water and electrolyte balance, as well as thermoregulation and serving as a secure barrier against harmful elements from the outside world, such as germs and other pathogens. Large sections of skin can be destroyed by trauma (e.g., burns) or skin illnesses (e.g., toxic epidermal necrolysis) and result in long-term significant damage or death. Chronic skin defects are also a significant burden for people who are affected: chronic leg ulcers caused by venous and arterial circulation diseases affect around 1% of the European population, and up to 10% of bedridden patients develop decubital ulcers.

The primary goal in the treatment of wounds is a rapid, functionally and aesthetically satisfactory wound closure. A prerequisite for this is an understanding of the basic wound-healing processes.

Wound healing is an extremely complex and dynamic repair process: blood cells, connective tissue cells, epidermal cells, the extracellular matrix (ECM), and countless cytokines and growth factors play an essential role and interact in complex ways [1–3].

Definition: Wound—Ulcer Wounds are acute substance defects that are traumatic (e.g., injuries, surgical procedures, interventions, etc.) and occur in primarily healthy, non-pre-damaged skin. They have a good healing tendency [4, 5]. Surgical wounds heal within 1–3 weeks.

Ulcers, on the other hand, are deep defects extending into the dermis or subcutis ("full-thickness-depth") in previously damaged skin. They are characterized by poor healing tendency [4, 5]. The successful healing process of ulcers requires the elimination of the causes and any interfering factors [6, 7]. The most common causes include venous and arterial circulatory disorders, diabetic neuropathy, and pressure. The most important confounding factors are hypoxia, malnutrition, certain drugs (e.g., corti-costeroids, immunosuppressants, and cytotoxic drugs), and certain diseases (e.g., diabetes mellitus) [8–11]. The course of wound healing can be divided into several coordinated and interacting processes:

- Initial processes
- Inflammatory phase
- Proliferation phase: formation of granulation tissue and angiogenesis
- Remodeling phase

Multilayered, extremely finely tuned processes take place: chemotaxis and phagocytosis, new connective tissue formation with synthesis, degradation and remodeling of collagen, angiogenesis, production of new glycosaminoglycans and proteoglycans, and, last but not least, epithelialization. The result of wound healing, as soon as the stratum reticular or deeper skin layers are damaged, is always a scar in the post-fetal individual [12].

The Physiology of Wound Healing

Initial Processes

Hemostasis and Temporary Wound Closure

A fresh wound quickly fills with blood, which immediately clots and closes the defect for the time being. The injured blood and lymph vessels react initially with vasoconstriction lasting a few minutes [13]. Platelets immediately attach to the walls of the damaged vessels and, losing their disc shape and forming fine pseudopodia, fuse into ever larger platelet aggregates. At the same time, they initiate the actual blood coagulation by releasing platelet factors. At the end of the coagulation cascade, the enzyme thrombin catalyzes the synthesis of long-chain fibrin polymers from water-soluble fibrinogen peptides. The platelets are literally woven into a three-dimensional fibrin network, into which other blood cells (e.g., erythrocytes, neutrophils, and monocytes/macrophages) are also incorporated [14].

The resulting blood clot eventually fills the entire wound gap and forms a provisional matrix for subsequent adhesion, migration, and proliferation of cells at the beginning of the reparative process. The main components of the provisional matrix are primarily the high molecular weight non-water-soluble protein fibrin and to a lesser extent the glycoproteins fibronectin, vitronectin, and thrombospondin [14]. As the surface dries out, a firm scab is formed, which acts as a provisional "biological dressing" to adhere to and protect the wound [15].

Vasodilation and Increased Vascular Permeability

The initial vasoconstriction is followed by vasodilatation, which peaks after about 10 min and lasts for about an hour. Reddening and overheating of the skin are the consequences. The simultaneous increase in vascular permeability causes blood plasma to leak into the interstitium and leads climatically to wound edema [16, 17]. These reactions are triggered, among other things, by prostaglandins from the destroyed tissue, by histamine release from mast cells, and by the release of vasoactive amines (e.g., serotonin) from the activated thrombocytes.

Chemotactic Factors

Platelets within the blood clot are not only responsible for hemostasis, but they also secern numerous wound healing mediators [e.g., platelet-derived growth factor (PDGF), insulin-like growth factor-1 (IGF-1), epidermal growth factor (EGF), and transforming growth factor-β 1 (TGF-β 1)]. These cytokines initiate the wound-healing cascade by directing and activating macrophages, fibroblasts, and vascular cells into the wound area [18, 19]. Similarly, fibrinopeptides A and B, which are produced during the conversion of fibrinogen to fibrin, attract inflammatory cells to the wound bed. Complement components (e.g., C5a), leukotrienes, and bacterial products (e.g., formyl methionyl peptides) also play a role, as do certain degradation products of the ECM (e.g., collagen and elastin fragments) [20].

Inflammatory Phase

Immigration of Leukocytes

Attracted by chemotactic signals, leukocytes infiltrate the wound. The passage of leukocytes from blood vessels into the wound area (leukocyte diapedesis) is mediated by certain adhesion molecules. Selectins and integrins—stimulated by inflammatory mediators—are ex-primed at the vascular endothelia of the venules around the wound area. The intraluminal passing leukocytes have corresponding ligands on their cell surface. The interlocking of the adhesion molecules with their ligands slows down the intraluminal cell flow, stops the leukocytes, and ultimately enables them to actively exit the vascular lumen into the wound area [21, 22].

Neutrophilic granulocytes are found in the wound as early as a few hours after injury. The peak of their migration is passed after 2 days and decreases over the following days, provided that no infection takes place. With a few days delay, the immigration of monocytes (and their transformation into tissue macrophages) reaches its peak (days 4–5). Finally, lymphocytes follow (day 6).

Wound Cleansing by Leukocytes

The main temporal function of neutrophils is thought to be the prevention of wound infection: they phagocytose and eliminate bacteria and degrade foreign material and devitalized tissue. Neutrophils synthesize and release inflammatory mediators such as tumor necrosis factor-α (TNF-α) and interleukin-1 (IL-1), which in turn activate fibroblasts and epithelial cells. Furthermore, they produce and store large amounts of aggressive proteins and oxygen-free radicals, which they use to digest phagocytized material. After cell death, these noxious substances enter the wound area, damage the tissue and possibly prolong the inflammation. Ultimately, they are deposited on the wound surface with the exudate and debris or phagocytosed by macrophages [23–25].

In the wound, monocytes bind to collagen or fibronectin fragments via integrin receptors, change phenotype and function, and eventually differentiate into tissue macrophages. Macrophages perform a dual function. As phagocytes, they eliminate microorganisms and debris as well as stalled neutrophils. The release of proteolytic enzymes (e.g., collagenases and elastases) supports the degradation of devitalized tissue and contributes significantly to wound cleansing. By also producing inhibitors of the released proteolytic enzymes, macrophages can precisely regulate enzymatic tissue degradation in the wound [26].

Macrophages—Key Cells in Wound Healing

Macrophages also play a key role in wound repair and mediate the transition from the inflammatory phase to the proliferative phase [27]. They produce numerous cytokines and growth factors, e.g., TNF-α, PDGF, vascular endothelial growth factor (VEGF), TGF-α, -β, IL-1, IL-6, IGF-1, and fibroblast growth factor (FGF). These factors lead to the orderly recruitment and proliferation of fibroblasts and endothelial cells and the regular formation of granular tissue. Macrophages thus play an essential role in wound healing [28]. Two different types of macrophages (M1 and M2) with different functions are known. Depletion of monocytes and tissue macrophages causes wound healing disorders and results in poor wound debridement and delayed connective tissue proliferation [29].

Because of the vascular damage, there is oxygen depletion in the wound area immediately after injury. This undoubtedly threatening situation also has beneficial effects: hypoxia stimulates migration of keratinocytes, angiogenesis, and proliferation of fibroblasts. The synthesis of critical growth factors and cytokines including PDGF, VEGF, and TGF-β 1 is also stimulated.

Proliferation Phase

After 4–5 days of injury, reparative refilling of the tissue defect begins with fresh connective tissue from sprouting vessels, fibroblasts, and newly formed ECM. Over the course of the following days to weeks, the initial provisional wound plug of clotted blood is completely penetrated and replaced by this granulation tissue. Finally, a new epithelial rim restores the final integrity of the skin [30, 31].

Granulation

The proliferative phase begins approximately 3 days after tissue injury and continues for approximately 2 weeks. It is characterized by the replacement of the provisory fibrin/fibronectin matrix with new formed granulation tissue. Macrophages, fibroblasts, and blood vessels migrate together from the surrounding tissue into the wound. The macrophages continuously release growth factors, and in this way regulate and stimulate the complex process of fibroplasia and angiogenesis [32].

Initially, the provisional matrix of fibrin, fibronectin, and vitronectin serves as an anchor for the sprouting cells during cell division and as a track for cell migration. However, the provisional matrix is more than an inert guide structure where mere scar tissue is deposited. It is an important reservoir for the myriad growth factors and cytokines that cells synthesize and release from the wound and wound environment to stimulate and guide the complex healing process. In addition, fibroblasts, endothelial cells, and keratinocytes receive important signals for activation, cell division, migration, and differentiation from the provisory matrix via the integrin receptors on the cell surface.

Fibroblast migration is essentially controlled by PDGF, TGF-β, and basic fibroblast growth factor (b-FGF). Furthermore, nerve growth factor (NFG) from peripheral nerves of the wound area also appears to play an important role [33, 34]. The direction of migration is determined by the concentration gradients of chemotactic factors and the orientation of the fibrillar structures of provisional matrix and newly formed ECM [35].

The integrin receptors on the cell surface serve as adhesion structures during migration on the matrix of collagen, fibronectin, vitronectin, and fibrin. While one part of the cell remains attached to the matrix, cytoplasmic extensions at the other cell pole reach out for new binding sites. As soon as the cell has found a new hold, the old attachment sites are released enzymatically. The enzymes that accomplish this are grouped as matrix metalloproteinases (MMPs), which are essential for cell migration across and through the ECM. Active forward movement is mediated by constant reorganization and redistribution of actin filaments inside the cell [35].

The most important MMPs are collagenases (MMP-1), which denature native collagen; gelatinases (MMP-2 and MMP-9), which degrade partially denatured collagen (gelatin); stromelysin (MMP-3), which attacks numerous protein substrates (including proteoglycans) of the ECM. MMPs have not only an important function in cell migration, but they are also essential in the degradation and remodeling of the ECM as part of the remodeling process [35].

Under physiological conditions, the activity of these MMPs is tightly regulated by MMP inhibitors (TIMPS), which are also present in the tissue. Disturbance of this critical balance can cause excessive degradation of matrix proteins, degradation of growth factors and their receptors, and result in a chronic wound healing disorder. A second family of proteolytic enzymes of prominent importance in wound healing are the serine proteinases. One important representative, neutrophil elastase, can cleave almost all types of protein molecules. The activity of the serine proteinases is also kept in check by enzyme inhibitors under physiological wound-healing conditions [33–35].

After immigration into the wound, the proliferating fibroblasts begin to produce matrix proteins and thus gradually replace the provisional matrix. The synthesis of collagen is now the main process. A critical step in collagen synthesis is the hydroxylation of proline and lysin residues. Important cofactors for this are oxygen, iron, and vitamin C. A deficiency of these cofactors can lead to wound-healing disorders [30] (Table 1).

In addition to the predominant protein, type III collagen, fibroblasts produce adhesion matrix proteins (e.g., fibronectin, vitronectin) and other important components of the ECM such as glycosaminoglycans (e.g., hyaluronic acid) and glycoproteins (Figs. 1–3).

Angiogenesis, Neovascularization

New blood vessel formation is also induced by growth factors (e.g., b-FGF, TGF-β, VEGF). The local wound environment including hypoxia, acidic pH, and high lactate levels also stimulate angiogenesis. Endothelial cells migrate, proliferate, form new blood vessels, and grow through the fibrin matrix with a richly branched meshwork. The young blood vessels thus ensure the supply of oxygen and nutrients needed for the reparative processes.

The dense agglomeration of vascular loops gives the granulation tissue its typical velvety granular appearance. The granulation tissue consists mainly of pro-life fibroblasts, capillaries, and tissue macrophages surrounded by a matrix of collagen, glycosaminoglycans (hyaluronic acid), and glycoproteins (fibronectin, tenascin) [33–36].

Table 1 Influence of different substances on healing process and optimal blood level concentrations

Substrate	Pathophysiology	Result	Normal blood level
Vitamin C	Lack of vitamin C decreased transcription of pro-collagen, leads to epigenetic DNA hypermethylation, and inhibits various types of collagen as well in skin, blood vessels and in tissue	Instable scar formation	0.6–2 mg/dL
Protein	Decreased collagen synthesis	Instable scar formation and fibroblast metabolism	60–83 g/L
Zinc	Central ion for collagen synthesis	Lead to an insufficient drilling of collagen helix	0.66–1.0 mcg/mL
Arginine	Decrease of prostaglandin E1 based on failing NO donator	Inhibition of neoangiogenesis leads to hypoxia	81–113 ymol/L

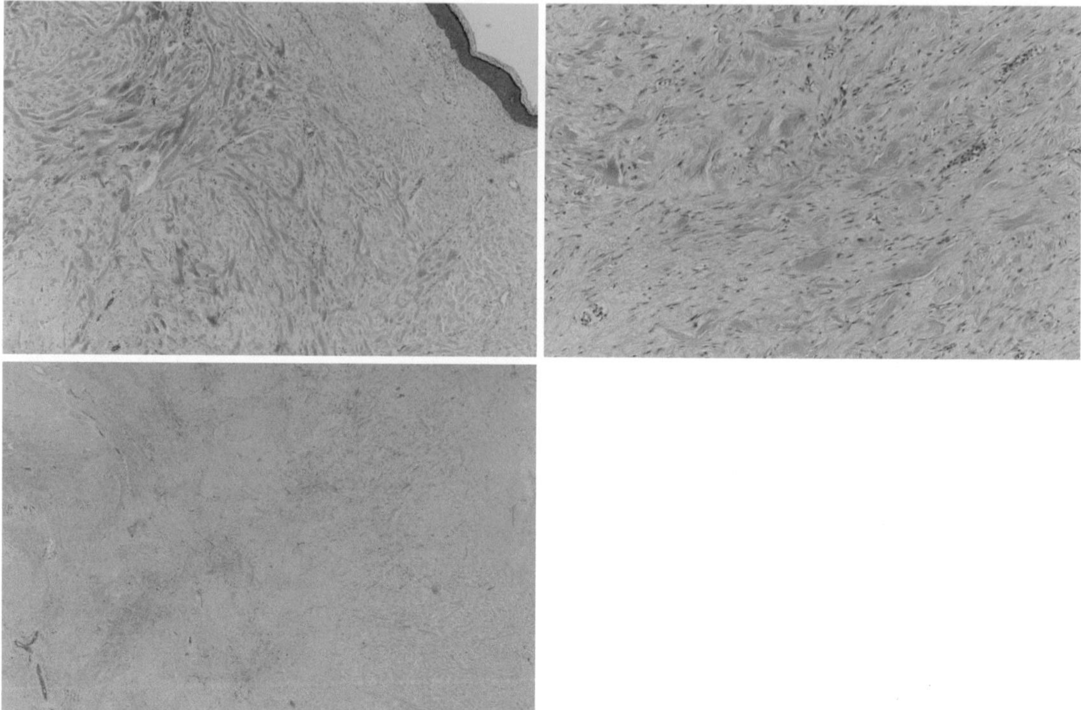

Figs. 1–3 The histologic appearances are typified by a nodular fibroblastic proliferation and the presence of glassy, eosinophilic, thick hyalinized collagen fibers in the dermis (refer to the figures). Reference Mckees pathology of the skin with clinical correlation fifth edition. (Figures taken from collection of cases reported by Dr. A. Aljawder during her training in Prince of Wales Hospital)

TGF-β plays a key role in the formation of granular tissue: it stimulates not only angiogenesis and the proliferation of fibroblasts but also the differentiation of myofibroblasts and the production of ECM [36, 37] (Figs. 1–3).

Wound Contraction

Wound contraction is a powerful process that considerably accelerates wound closure. The defect is not filled with new tissue, but the healthy wound edges are actively brought closer together. Wound contraction begins—simultaneously with the remodeling phase—already a few days after the injury.

Overall, wound contraction requires an incredibly complex interplay of cells, ECM, and cytokines. Wound contraction is made possible by myofibroblasts, i.e., modified fibroblasts with contractile properties. Myofibroblasts possess actin-containing contractile filaments that give them smooth muscle cell properties. The contraction of the myofibroblasts, which run through the granulation tissue like a meshwork, eventually leads to shrinkage and reduction of the wound volume. Cell–cell bonds between the myofibroblasts, intertwining of the myofibroblasts with the collagen fibers and bundles of the ECM, and cross-linking of the branched collagen bundles with each other form the necessary mechanical conditions [38].

Wound contraction is stimulated by TGF-β and PDGF, among others. The extent of wound contraction is critically influenced by all important healing factors such as general condition, nutrition, infection, and etiology of the wound. The geometric shape of the wound also strongly influences wound contraction. While it is rapid in narrow, line-shaped wounds, it naturally takes longer in wide and round-configured wounds. As soon as the wound is closed, the growth factor receptors of the fibroblasts are downregulated, and some of the fibroblasts undergo apoptosis (especially the fibroblast cells).

Re-epithelialization

Re-epithelialization of the wound begins within a few hours after injury. Starting from the skin appendages (e.g., hair follicles) and the wound margins, epidermal keratinocytes gradually cover the wound surface with an epithelial turf, thus closing the wound surface [41, 42].

Migration, proliferation, and differentiation of keratinocytes are crucial steps. The otherwise very grounded keratinocytes change their appearance and function. Cohesion among keratinocytes is lost as retraction of tonofilaments occurs and intercellular desmosomes are dissolved. Finally, the epithelial cells also lose their adhesion to the basement membrane because the hemidesmosomes of the basal keratinocytes are also dissolved. The keratinocytes flatten, form foot-like projections, and actively migrate laterally toward the wound matrix [43].

A prerequisite for the migration of keratinocytes is the formation of new adhesion molecules for attachment to the provisional matrix or wound dermis. Fibronectin/tenascin, vitronectin, and collagen receptors ensure the necessary adhesion and alignment to the corresponding matrix proteins during keratinocyte locomotion. The amoeboid locomotion of keratinocytes is enabled by intracellular contractile actinomyosin filaments, which alternately contract and redistribute accordingly in the newly formed lamellipodia [25, 34, 43]. The keratinocytes migrate horizontally individually or in cell assemblies. They typically glide over the newly formed epidermal cell seam.

Migration and proliferation of keratinocytes from the wound edge are induced by the lack of contact with (destroyed) neighboring cells ("free edge effect") and stimulated by local release of growth factors (e.g., EGF, TGF-α, and -β) and expression of growth factor receptors-β, keratinocyte growth factor (KGF). As soon as epithelial cell fronts meet, keratocyte migration is halted by contact inhibition. Parallel to progressive re-epithelialization, the basement membrane—fundamental connection and separating layer between epidermis and dermis—is also restored. The final step is the fixation of the basal lamina by the anchoring fibrils. In the end, keratinocyte proliferation and differentiation lead to the formation of a regular keratinizing epidermis [10, 15, 22].

Epithelialization proceeds most rapidly with a clean wound bed, intact basal lamina, and moist wound conditions. Necrotic tissue, debris, or crusts slow down epithelialization. The advancing epithelial front undermines wound coatings and forces its way between the necrosis zone and the granulation tissue. To enable this penetration, keratinocytes release plasminogen activator for fibrinolysis using plasmin present in the coagulum and MMPs for lysis of collagen [15, 30, 32].

Remodeling Phase

The remodeling phase includes the transformation from granulation tissue to scar. It begins at the same time as the granulation phase, lasts up to 2 years, and completes wound healing. In this phase, a slow remodeling of the connective tissue takes place, during which the scar acquires its final properties such as function, strength, and appearance. The remodeling phase is characterized by the coexistence of collagen degradation and collagen synthesis: type 3 collagen, which was synthesized during the first weeks of wound healing, is now continuously replaced by stable type 1 collagen [40, 41].

Collagen fibers are dissolved by specific MMPs released into the extracellular space by macrophages, granulocytes, epidermal cells, endothelial cells, and fibroblasts in the wound area. While remodeling, the activity of MMPs steadily decreases, while the activity of inhibitors increases. The presence of TIMPs protects against excessive proteolysis. A balanced ratio of MMPs and their inhibitors in the wound is thus an absolute prerequisite for trouble-free healing.

The ongoing synthesis of stable collagen, its consolidation with the formation of cross-links, the interweaving into thicker bundles, and their proper alignment contribute to the increasing strength of the healing wound. The orientation of the collagen bundles is adapted to local and functional requirements. Nevertheless, scar tissue never becomes as strong as healthy tissue. Two weeks after an injury, the healing wound has on average only regained 5% of its original resilience, 3 weeks later about 20%, and 1 month later about 40%. Even after an optimal healing process, the tensile strength of the scar tissue always remains below 80% of its initial state [41].

At the end of the remodeling phase, the scar is poor in cells and vessels, with loss of skin appendages. The density of the collagen fibers increases, and the originally complex interwoven collagen is replaced by dense parallel bundles. The connective tissue becomes cell depleted as macrophages and fibroblasts are reduced by apoptosis. Capillary growth stops and blood vessels are reduced; the reddish color of the friable vascular scars gives way to the pale discoloration of the vascular-poor old scar.

Chronic Wounds

In western industrialized nations, about 1–2% of the population suffers from chronic wounds. The incidence increases with age and reaches 4–5% after the age of 80 [11]. Especially arterial, venous, and diabetic ulcers, as well as decubital ulcers, occur more frequently in older than in younger people. The main causes are certainly the numerous comorbidities of the elderly, consumptive diseases, prolonged administration of drugs with negative influence on healing such as steroids, antiphlogistic, or cytostatic, limited mobility, malnutrition, and finally cellular and biochemical changes in the aging skin.

Although most wound specialists have very concrete ideas of what a chronic wound is, there is yet no binding definition of it. Some already speak of a chronic wound at a healing time of >4 weeks, others only at a healing time of >12 weeks. In the documents of World Union of Wound Healing Societies, 6 weeks is a critical time to define a wound as a chronic wound. However, time limits alone can only reflect the actual wound condition to a limited extent. A chronic wound is characterized above all by the fact that, despite intensive therapy, healing does not occur within a reasonable period. According to the guidelines of the German Society for Phlebology, a leg ulcer is considered chronic if it shows no healing tendency within 3 months or has not healed within 12 months [14, 16, 22, 28].

Biology of Chronic Wounds

In chronic wounds, physiologic phasic healing is disrupted, and the process is "stuck," usually in the inflammatory or proliferative phase. Growth factors, cytokines, proteases, cells, and ECM are the main components of healing; alterations and disturbances of individual elements can severely slow down wound healing. Wound healing is also significantly impaired by excessive inflammation, tissue damage by free oxygen radicals, cell aging, disease-specific factors such as metabolic disorders (e.g., diabetes mellitus), hypoxia of various origins, or nutritional deficiencies. Necrotic tissue, exudate, and infection also hinder healing in the long term [4, 5, 12, 23, 36, 43, 48].

In chronic venous leg ulcers, for example, increased neutrophils and macrophages can be detected in the tissue. These are activated and release more reactive oxygen species and various proteases. The inflammatory phase with neutrophils and macrophages persists and severely affects the subsequent phases of matrix deposition and re-epithelialization [40].

The main characteristics of a chronic wound are essentially
- An increased activity of matrix metalloproteinases (MMPs).
- A decreased response to growth factors.
- Senescence of cells (cell aging).

In undisturbed healing of acute wounds, there is a balance between catabolic and anabolic processes, and production and activity of tissue proteinases are under tight and effective control. In chronic ulcers, however, the enzymatic activity of MMPs is increased. At the same time, the activity of MMP inhibitors in the tissue is decreased. This leads to a sustained and excessive degradation of ECM proteins (e.g., collagen, fibronectin, and vitronectin). Since the latter are invisible guiding structures for the proliferation, migration and spatial orientation of fibroblasts, endothelial cells, and keratinocytes, their continuous destruction results in a wound-healing arrest [18, 23, 29].

However, it is not only the permanent degradation of matrix proteins that leads to a halt in cell proliferation and cell migration in the chronic wound. Cytokines and growth factors cannot exert their healing-promoting effects in the wound area, as they are also enzymatically degraded and inactivated by MMPs [24]. In addition, there is evidence that MMPs in chronic wounds can also inactivate receptor proteins for cytokines and growth factors, further enhancing their anti-healing effects [7, 9, 16, 21, 23]. This "aggressive microenvironment" may explain the widespread failure of locally applied recombinant growth factors in the therapy of chronic wounds [40].

Chronic wounds are usually characterized by excessive inflammation. Indeed, the exudate of chronic wounds is rich in pro-inflammatory cytokines such as TNF-α and IL-1 β. These cytokine levels correlate closely with the clinical course and decrease with the onset of wound healing. Approximately 100-fold higher concentrations of TNF-α and IL-1 β were measured in wound fluid from chronic wounds than in acute wound fluid after mastectomy [23]. In cell cultures of healthy fibroblasts, endothelial cells, and keratinocytes, the addition of exudate from chronic wounds causes growth inhibition [6], whereas exudate from acute wounds increases proliferation.

The cellular inflammatory response is also altered; neutrophilic leukocytes from patients with chronic venous ulcers are more active and produce more oxygen-free radicals than from healthy control subjects [39, 40]. In contrast, macrophages from patients with chronic venous

ulcers are insufficiently activated and the release of healing-promoting cytokines and growth factors is unsuppressed [12].

The so-called replicative senescence ("aging") of fibroblasts is also to blame for the poor healing tendency of chronic wounds [17]: physiologically, all cells have a limited proliferative capacity, i.e., the number of possible cell divisions is limited. At the end of their proliferative lifespan, fibroblasts change their phenotype, become resistant to apoptotic cell death, and lose their proliferative capacity [28, 37, 39, 41].

In chronic venous ulcers with poor healing tendency, more fibroblasts can be detected in the stage of senescence [17]. They divide more slowly than fibroblasts from healthy tissue and can only generate a limited number of daughter cells [33, 40].

On the one hand, pro-inflammatory cytokines, oxidative stress, or bacterial toxins probably cause the phenomenon of premature cell aging in the chronic wound environment. Experimental evidence suggests that chronic wound fluid inhibits DNA synthesis and fibroblast growth [6, 32]. On the other hand, prolonged excessive and uncoordinated cell divisions may deplete proliferative capacity in chronic wounds [1, 16].

Senescent fibroblasts produce increased amounts of proteolytic enzymes such as collagenase, elastase, and stromelysin and decreased TIMP-1 and TIMP-9 compared to healthy cells. The accumulation of senescent fibroblasts in the wound area thus probably contributes decisively to the chronic course [17]. Table 2 summarizes several factors influencing wound healing (Table 2).

Table 2 Extrinsic and intrinsic factors with influence in wound healing

Extrinsic factor	Intrinsic factor
Radiation	Indirect gen defects
Mechanical stress	Collagen diseases
Nutrition	Ethnicity
Thermal damage	Metabolic stress
Medication (e.g., cyclooxygenase inhibitor)	Chronic inflammation

Wound Healing in Old Age

Aging skin is more vulnerable overall and wound healing is delayed [12]. Certain diseases (e.g., chronic venous insufficiency, arterial perfusion disorders), comorbidities (e.g., cardiovascular insufficiency, diabetes mellitus), medication (e.g., anti-inflammatory drugs), and the manifold structural and functional changes in aging skin increase the risk of developing chronic ulcers. The skin of the elderly is thinned in all layers, has fewer cells, and is rarefied at the function-bearing structures. There is a slower turnover of epidermis, the mitotic rate is reduced, and the re-epithelization of wounds takes about twice as long. The sawtooth profile of the dermo-epidermal junctional zone is leveled, and the rete cones flatten or disappear. This leads to increased mechanical vulnerability to shear trauma, tendency to blistering, and poorer nutritional conditions of the epidermis. Parallel to the general weakening of immune competence, the Langerhans cells of the epidermis decrease by about 50% with age. Inflammatory and immune-mediated reactions are slower and milder. Rarefaction of all components also occurs in the dermis. The percentage of senescent fibroblasts with low proliferation increases. In addition, there is an altered composition and reduced quality of ECM proteins. Reduced tissue turgor and lower tensile strength are the consequences. The vascular system is also massively affected by the aging process: Dilatation and wall rigidity of postcapillary venules lead to telangiectasias and hemorrhages after trivial trauma. The number of capillaries dwindles and there is a loss of up to 30% of the cumulative cross-section [15].

Hyperspectral Imaging as a Measurement Method for Skin, Tissue Wounds, and Scars

Compared to other optical measurement methods, hyperspectral imaging (HSI) simultaneously enables the acquisition of information about biochemical, structural, and physiological functional properties of the measured volume. This is limited in the usual spectral range of 400–1000 nm in skin and similar perfused tissue to a depth of approx. 5–8 mm [44, 45]. However, HSI, as a non-contact measurement method, allows relatively large-area imaging in a relatively short time (a few seconds), so that not only highly localized samples can be measured, but also, for example, the blood flow quality of larger areas can be determined.

The measurement of biochemical properties is essentially based on the different absorption behavior of different components. The strongest shape imprinting is given to the remission spectrum by the absorption of hemoglobin [39, 45, 46].

Structural features, such as the different layers of the skin, are essentially imprinted in the remission spectrum by the scattering of the incident light and the different penetration depths depending on the wavelength.

Physiological-functional properties, primarily blood flow, can be recorded and evaluated via the absorption of hemoglobin in conjunction with the structural features [46].

The remission spectra show a complicated nonlinear dependence on the system structure and the system parameters due to the different volume fractions of various components (melanin, collagen, hemoglobin, etc.) depending on the depth (layer structure of the skin) and the paths of the light through the layers to remission caused by scattering. The spectra are heterogeneous depending on the wavelength, i.e., spectral components of different wavelengths refer to different measurement volumes. This dependence prevents almost in principle an unambiguous solution of the inverse problem, i.e., the computation of system parameters from the spectra [46–48].

In practice, mostly simple system models are assumed, which allow the calculation of parameters from the spectra, but which, with respect to the real structure, represent more or less strongly averaged and only very limited comparable values.

Models based on Monte Carlo simulations of the remission by more realistic structures are in principle more appropriate, but the inverse determination of the model parameters is also here a process that cannot be solved unambiguously, since an adjustment to the current actual structure is hardly possible.

An alternative method is based on a description of the remission process by a reasonably realistic skin model (six layers with all relevant components) and a modeling based on a 3D cablelike description supported by MC simulations.

Again, the model imposes a limitation on the determination of real physiological parameters, but the advantage is the consistency of the transformation of the spectral information into the model parameters, which allow a complete reproduction of the actual spectra by the model.

This practically does not mean a physically strictly correct solution of the inverse problem, but a consistent transformation of the information content of the spectra into a parameter space, which at least allows an interpretation of the parameters much closer to physiology (example: Perfusion profiles charts).

From the modeling, so-called perfusion profiles (depth profiles) for the relative volume frac-tion of hemoglobin (vHb) and oxygen saturation ($xHbO_2$) can be displayed to assess the perfusion conditions corresponding to the six layers of the skin model. The depth axis does not correspond to an actual depth or the layer thicknesses; the relative scaling of the vHb values against each other is globally fixed. In addition, the relative volume fraction of water (vH_2O) is also deter-mined [46–49].

vHb as an index parameter is scaled from 0 to 2.5; $xHbO_2$ means the percentage of oxygen (0.0.100%) and ranges from [0.0.1] (Figs. 4, 5, and 6).

Microcirculation

Due to its limited penetration depth, HSI mea-sures properties of the skin's microcirculatory system in the 400–1000 nm spectral range.

The microcirculation is the area where the metabolism between the blood and the surround-ing tissue takes place. Thus, for the supply of the tissue, this is crucial. The macrocirculation, of

Fig. 4 Normal circulation

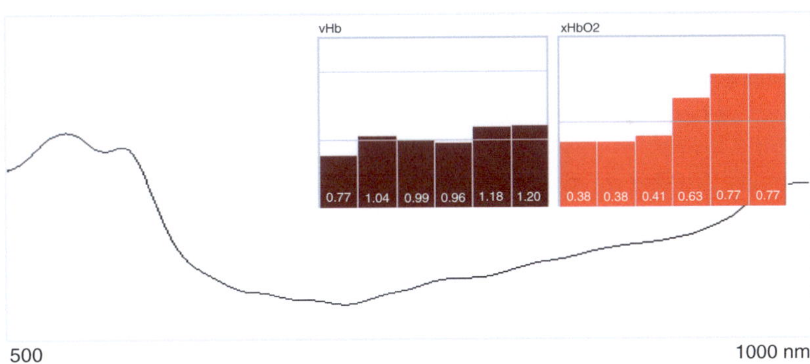

Fig. 5 Venous hyperten-sion: increased deep t-vHb, reduced $xHbO_2$

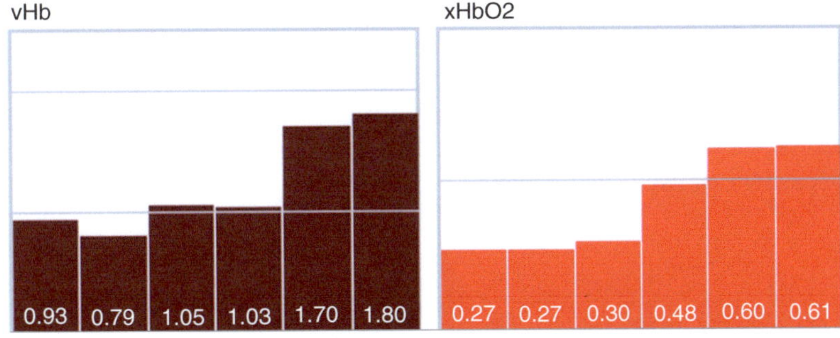

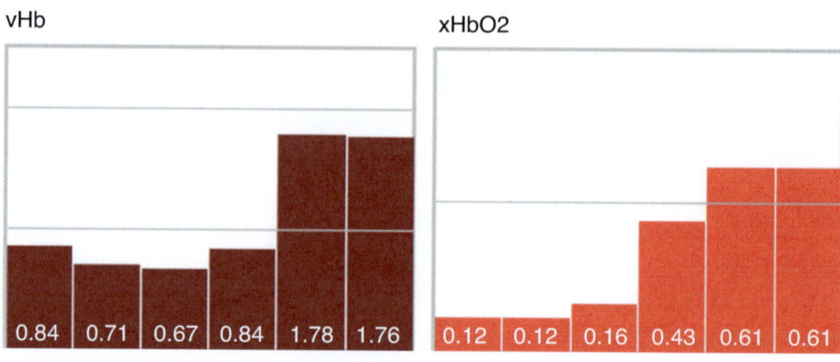

Fig. 6 Arterial hypertension: reduced superficial vHb, increased deep-vHb, esp. superficial severe reduced xHbO$_2$

course, ensures adequate inflow and outflow of blood. Essential for the assessment of tissue supply is thus the ratio of micro- to macrocirculation: how much blood/oxygen is brought in and is available in the capillary, arteriolar and venular systems, how much of it is consumed.

In general, it is important to detect microcirculatory disturbances even before the onset of tissue damage, e.g., due to a reduced oxygen supply.

Averaged oxygen saturations (tissue oximetry) or pure flow values (LDI) are inadequate or at least suboptimal for a differentiated assessment of microcirculation.

More adequate model-based evaluations (see above) allow a more advanced structural representation of perfusion properties, e.g., perfusion values (relative volume fraction and oxygen saturation of hemoglobin in a six-layer model of the skin). This results in so-called perfusion (depth) profiles, which can serve as an information-rich and specific basis for the analysis and evaluation of skin perfusion [48, 49].

Evaluation of the Measurement Results/Parameters

Global quantitative assessment of microcirculation at least of the skin is very difficult. Numerous adaptation and control mechanisms lead to a high variation of measured blood flow parameter values on the skin, both inter- and intrapersonally, dependent on time and situation. Globally, the range for "normal values" strongly overlaps with that of patients with "circulatory disorders."

Global parameters are also difficult to achieve because penetration depths or measurement volumes vary for different skin types and locations. Temporal singular measurements do not account for variation in blood flow due to vasomotion rhythms, for example, comparable and scalable parameters can be determined by spatial or temporal relativity, by response to provocations or to treatments [48–50].

Evaluation of heterogeneous spectra in terms of measurement depth with the determination of perfusion profiles allows at least evaluation of the relative ratio of depth to surface perfusion.

HSI Measurements on Chronic Wounds

Inadequate perfusion and tissue supply is a significant factor in the development of hard-to-heal chronic wounds. This is often due to a systemic or regional circulatory disorder, i.e., insufficient supply of arterial blood to certain areas and the resulting insufficient quality of microcirculatory perfusion and oxygen supply to the tissue, which favors wound development. In the wound that then develops, the same factors ensure a significantly impaired healing process.

In addition to the treatment and improvement of the basic blood circulation problem, the regular control of skin blood circulation in high-risk patients (diabetes, PAVK, nursing patients with low mobility) can help prevent the development of wounds, especially in the known localizations. For this purpose, HSI represents a simple measurement method that is not burdensome for the patient and that can reliably detect deterioration of the condition and preliminary stages of wound formation (via the formation of local edema and inflammation) by measuring large areas and observing the course of values over time [44–47, 49].

The HSI evaluation generates perfusion parameters of the upper skin layers, which are well comparable and meaningful, at least relatively over time. Increased vH_2O values (relative volume fraction of water in the tissue) are often also conspicuous in such patients [50].

In the treatment of already existing wounds that are difficult to heal, ensuring sufficient blood flow and oxygen supply, at least in the wound area and the wound environment, is an important factor among others. Here, too, the regular measurement of the wound area and the wound environment by means of HSI can generate decisive information on the current and temporal development of the blood flow quality.

In addition, evaluation of the shape characteristics of the remission spectra, which correlate with certain biochemical features, enables qualitative and, in some cases, quantitative determination of relevant wound components (various tissue types, such as necrosis, fibrin, critical, undersupplied tissue, granulation, epithelialization). Using these spectral features and imaging, an exact segmentation and classification of the wound area are possible, resulting in an overall comprehensive objective description of the wound and wound progression, which allows optimization of wound treatment and thus wound healing via analysis of the objectified and quantified response of the wound to various treatments. The advantage over the imprecise, individually different visual wound assessment by the physician is the availability of objective parameters which cannot be determined in a similar way with any other methods at present and which allow a much earlier assessment and evaluation of the wound process [45, 47, 48] (Figs. 7, 8, and 9).

Excessive scarring, consisting essentially of collagen structures, is characterized by low superficial perfusion values and the clear expression of collagen in the spectrum (Fig. 10). An improvement by treatment, which leads to the degradation or remodeling of the scar tissue with an increase in perfusion, can be observed and controlled by means of the perfusion profiles over time as well as the change in the individual collagen types.

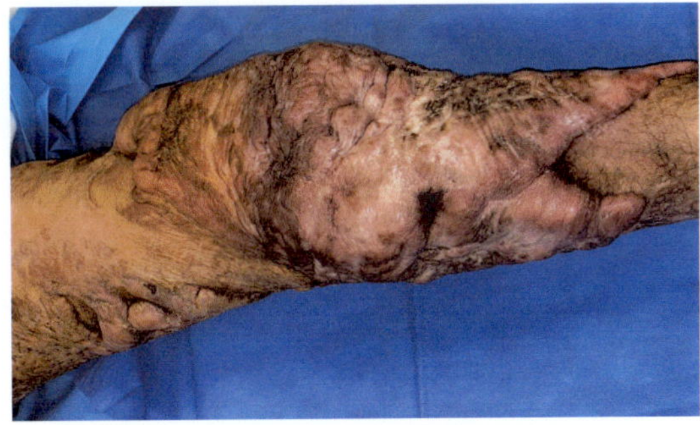

Fig. 7 Keloid after burn 15 years before with several fistula with infection

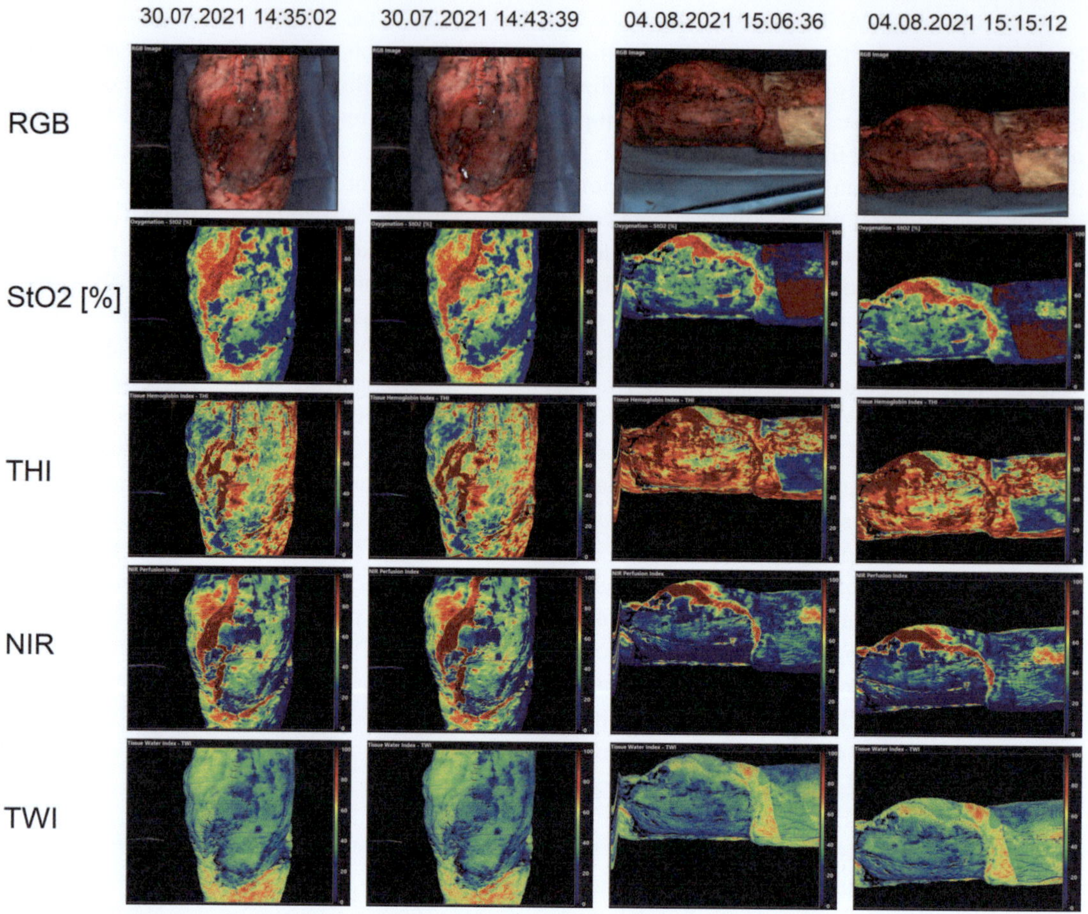

Fig. 8 HIS show the pathological perfusion and oxygenation, important for planning any kind of intervention and controlling the postinterventional effects in short time and long time follow up

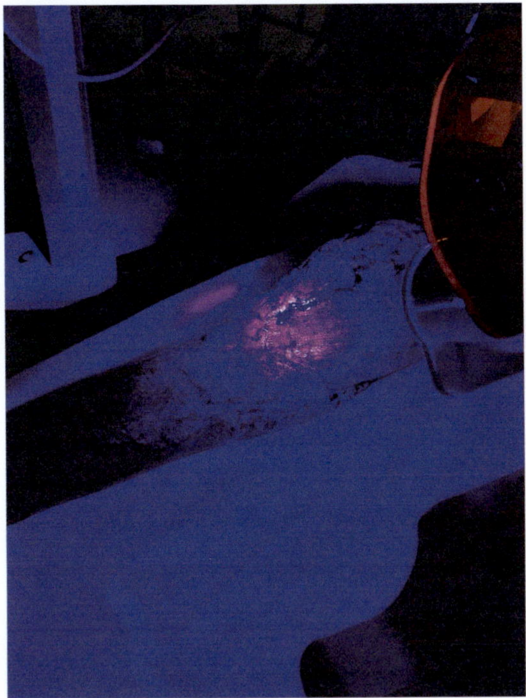

Fig. 9 Detection of microbiological burden in the spectrum from 390 to 430 nm, important for local removement and short time and longtime follow up

Fig. 10 Strong scar tissue: collagen input is essential in the front part of the spectrum, the determination of the blood flow is only possible below the scar tissue in the depth

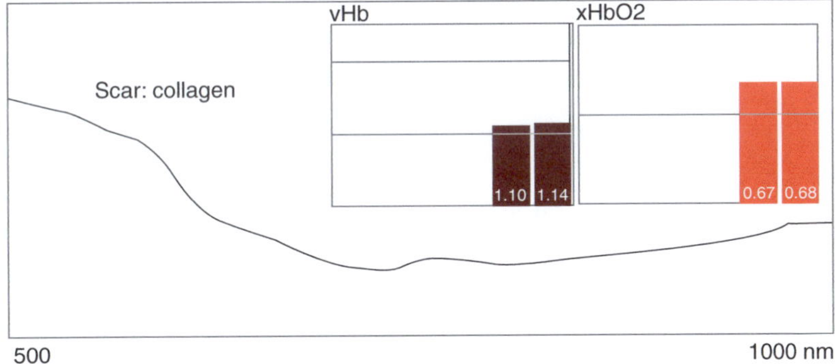

References

1. Werner S, Krieg T, Smola H. Keratinocyte-fibroblast interactions in wound healing. J Invest Dermatol. 2007;127(5):998–1008.
2. Zhu Z, Ding J, Tredget EE. The molecular basis of hypertrophic scars. Burns Trauma. 2016;4:2.
3. Tredget EE, Nedelec B, Scott PG, Ghahary A. Hypertrophic scars, keloids, and contractures. The cellular and molecular basis for therapy. Surg Clin N Am. 1997;77(3):701–30.
4. Wynn TA. Fibrotic disease and the T(H)1/T(H)2 paradigm. Nat Rev Immunol. 2004;4(8):583–94.
5. Ruzehaji N, Grose R, Krumbiegel D, Zola H, Dasari P, Wallace H, Stacey M, Fitridge R, Cowin AJ. Cytoskeletal protein flightless (Flii) is elevated in chronic and acute human wounds and wound fluid: neutralizing its activity in chronic but not acute wound fluid improves cellular proliferation. Eur J Dermatol. 2012;22(6):740–50. https://doi.org/10.1684/ejd.2012.1878.
6. Lu L, Saulis AS, Liu WR, Roy NK, Chao JD, Ledbetter S, Mustoe TA. The temporal effects of anti-TGF-beta1, 2, and 3 monoclonal antibody on wound healing and hypertrophic scar formation. J Am Coll Surg. 2005;201(3):391–7.
7. Lee TY, Chin GS, Kim WJ, Chau D, Gittes GK, Longaker MT. Expression of transforming growth factor beta 1, 2, and 3 proteins in keloids. Ann Plast Surg. 1999;43(2):179–84.
8. Rohani MG, Parks WC. Matrix remodeling by MMPs during wound repair. Matrix Biol. 2015;46:113–21.
9. Zhao B, Guan H, Liu JQ, Zheng Z, Zhou Q, Zhang J, Su LL, Hu DH. Hypoxia drives the transition of human dermal fibroblasts to a myofibroblast-like phenotype via the TGF-β1/Smad3 pathway. Int J Mol Med. 2017;39(1):153–9.
10. Wilkinson HN, Hardman MJ. Wound healing: cellular mechanisms and pathological outcomes. Open Biol. 2020;10(9):200223. https://doi.org/10.1098/rsob.200223.
11. Mujahid N, Shareef F, Maymone MBC, Vashi NA. Microneedling as a treatment for acne scarring: a systematic review. Dermatol Surg. 2020;46(1):86–92. https://doi.org/10.1097/DSS.0000000000002020.
12. Osman MA, Shokeir HA, Fawzy MM. Fractional erbium-doped yttrium Aluminum garnet laser versus microneedling in treatment of atrophic acne scars: a randomized split-face clinical study. Dermatol Surg. 2017;43(Suppl 1):S47–56. https://doi.org/10.1097/DSS.0000000000000951.
13. Lichtman MK, Otero-Vinas M, Falanga V. Transforming growth factor beta (TGF-β) isoforms in wound healing and fibrosis. Wound Repair Regen. 2016;24(2):215–22. https://doi.org/10.1111/wrr.12398.
14. Cowin AJ, Holmes TM, Brosnan P, Ferguson MW. Expression of TGF-beta and its receptors in murine fetal and adult dermal wounds. Eur J Dermatol. 2001;11(5):424–31.
15. Wild T, Rahbarnia A, Kellner M, Sobotka L, Eberlein T. Basics in nutrition and wound healing. Nutrition. 2010;26(9):862–6.
16. Agren MS, Steenfos HH, Dabelsteen S, et al. Proliferation and mitogenic response to PDGF-BB of fibroblasts isolated from chronic venous leg ulcers is ulcer-age dependent. J Invest Dermatol. 1999;112:463–9.
17. Baum CL, Arpey C. Normal cutaneous wound healing: clinical correlation with cellular and molecular events. Dermatol Surg. 2005;31:674–86.
18. Bello YM, Phillips TJ. Recent advances in wound healing. JAMA. 2000;283:716–8.
19. Braun Falco O, Plewig G, Wolff HH, Burgdorf WHC, Landthaler M. Dermatologie und venerologie. 5th ed. Heidelberg: Springer; 2005. p. 13.
20. Bucalo B, Eaglestein WH, Falanga V. Inhibition of cellular proliferation by chronic wound fluid. Wound Rep Reg. 1993;1:181–6.
21. Bullen EC, Longaker MT, Updike DL, et al. TIMP-1 is decreased and activated gelatinases are increased in chronic wounds. J Invest Dermatol. 1995;104:236–40.
22. Clark RAF. Cutaneous tissue repair. Basic biologic considerations. J Am Acad Dermatol. 1985;13:701–25.
23. Cowin AJ, Hatzirodos N, Holding CA, et al. Effect of healing on the expression of transforming growth factor βs and their receptors in chronic venous leg ulcers. J Invest Dermatol. 2001;117:1282–9.
24. Desmoulière A, Chaponnier C, Gabbiani G. Tissue repair, contraction, and the myofibroblast. Wound Rep Reg. 2005;13:7–12.
25. Dissemond J. Wann ist eine Wunde chronisch? Hautarzt. 2006;57:55.
26. Enoch S, Price P. Cellular, molecular and biochemical differences in the pathophysiology of healing between acute wounds, chronic wounds and wounds in the aged. World wide wounds. 2004. http://www.worldwidewounds.com/2004/august/enoch/pathophysiology-of-healing.html
27. Falanga V. Chap. 21: Mechanisms of cutaneous wound repair. In: Freedberg IM, Eisen AZ, Wolff K, Austen KF, Goldsmith LA, Katz SI, editors. Fitzpatrick's dermatology in general medicine. 6th ed. New York: McGraw-Hill Medical Publishing Division; 2003. p. 236–46.
28. Falanga V, Shen J. Growth factors, signal transduction and cellular responses. In: Falanga V, editor. Cutaneous wound healing. London: Martin Dunitz; 2001. p. 81–93.
29. Micera A, Vigneti E, Pickholtz D, et al. Nerve growth factor displays stimulatory effects on human skin and lung fibroblasts, demonstrating a direct role for this factor in tissue repair. Proc Natl Acad Sci U S A. 2001;98:6162–7.
30. Mitchison TJ, Cramer LP. Actin-based cell motility and cell locomotion. Cell. 1996;84:371–9.

31. Moseley R, Stewart JE, Stephens P, Waddington RJ, Thomas DW. Extracellular matrix metabolites as potential bio-markers of disease activity in wound fluid: lessons learned from other inflammatory diseases? Br J Dermatol. 2004;150:401–13.

32. Raffetto JD, Mendez MV, Phillips TJ, et al. The effect of passage number on fibroblast cellular senescence in patients with chronic venous insufficiency with and without ulcer. Am J Surg. 1999;178:107–12.

33. Santoro MM, Gaudino G. Cellular and molecular facets of keratinocyte reepithelization during wound healing. Exp Cell Res. 2005;304:274–86.

34. Schaffer CJ, Nanney LB. Cell biology of wound healing. Int Rev Cytol. 1996;169:151–81.

35. Stanley A, Osler T. Senescence and the healing rates of venous ulcers. J Vasc Surg. 2001;33:1206–11.

36. Tomasek JJ, Gabbiani G, Hinz B, et al. Myofibroblasts and mechano-regulation of connective tissue remodelling. Nat Rev Mol Cell Biol. 2002;3:349–63.

37. Chen W, Fu X, Ge S, Sun T, Zhou G, Jiang D, Sheng Z. Ontogeny of expression of transforming growth factor-beta and its receptors and their possible relationship with scarless healing in human fetal skin. Wound Repair Regen. 2005;13(1):68–75. https://doi.org/10.1111/j.1067-1927.2005.130109.x.

38. Wang PH, Huang BS, Horng HC, Yeh CC, Chen YJ. Wound healing. J Chin Med Assoc. 2018;81(2):94–101. https://doi.org/10.1016/j.jcma.2017.11.002.

39. Monavarian M, Kader S, Moeinzadeh S, Jabbari E. Regenerative scar-free skin wound healing. Tissue Eng Part B Rev. 2019;25(4):294–311. https://doi.org/10.1089/ten.TEB.2018.0350.

40. Hassanshahi A, Hassanshahi M, Khabbazi S, Hosseini-Khah Z, Peymanfar Y, Ghalamkari S, Su YW, Xian CJ. Adipose-derived stem cells for wound healing. J Cell Physiol. 2019;234(6):7903–14. https://doi.org/10.1002/jcp.27922.

41. Harn HI, Ogawa R, Hsu CK, Hughes MW, Tang MJ, Chuong CM. The tension biology of wound healing. Exp Dermatol. 2019;28(4):464–71. https://doi.org/10.1111/exd.13460.

42. Veith AP, Henderson K, Spencer A, Sligar AD, Baker AB. Therapeutic strategies for enhancing angiogenesis in wound healing. Adv Drug Deliv Rev. 2019;146:97–125. https://doi.org/10.1016/j.addr.2018.09.010.

43. Das S, Majid M, Baker AB. Syndecan-4 enhances PDGF-BB activity in diabetic wound healing. Acta Biomater. 2016;15(42):56–65. https://doi.org/10.1016/j.actbio.2016.07.001.

44. Marotz J, Kulcke A, Siemers F, Cruz D, Aljowder A, Promny D, Daeschlein G, Wild T. Extended perfusion parameter estimation from hyperspectral imaging data for bedside diagnostic in medicine. Molecules. 2019;24(22):4164.

45. Marotz J, Schulz T, Seider S, Cruz D, Aljowder A, Promny D, Daeschlein G, Wild T, Siemers F. 3D-perfusion analysis of burn wounds using hyperspectral imaging. Burns. 2021;47(1):157–70. https://doi.org/10.1016/j.burns.2020.06.001.

46. Saiko G, Lombardi P, Au Y, Queen D, Armstrong D, Harding K. Hyperspectral imaging in wound care: a systematic review. Int Wound J. 2020;17(6):1840–56. https://doi.org/10.1111/iwj.13474. Epb 2020 Aug 23

47. Yudovsky D, Nouvong A, Pilon L. Hyperspectral imaging in diabetic foot wound care. J Diabetes Sci Technol. 2010;4(5):1099–113. https://doi.org/10.1177/193229681000400508.

48. Wahabzada M, Besser M, Khosravani M, Kuska MT, Kersting K, Mahlein AK, Stürmer E. Monitoring wound healing in a 3D wound model by hyperspectral imaging and efficient clustering. PLoS One. 2017;12(12):e0186425. https://doi.org/10.1371/journal.pone.0186425.

49. Chan KS, Lo ZJ. Wound assessment, imaging and monitoring systems in diabetic foot ulcers: a systematic review. Int Wound J. 2020;17(6):1909–23. https://doi.org/10.1111/iwj.13481.

50. Holmer A, Marotz J, Wahl P, Dau M, Kämmerer PW. Hyperspectral imaging in perfusion and wound diagnostics—methods and algorithms for the determination of tissue parameters. Biomed Tech (Berl). 2018;63(5):547–56. https://doi.org/10.1515/bmt-2017-0155.

Pathophysiology of Burn Wounds

Sebastian P. Nischwitz, Hanna Luze, and Lars-Peter Kamolz

Introduction

Burn trauma remains one of the main causes of posttraumatic fatalities and long-term morbidity. Even though advances to reduce mortality after burns were achieved in recent decades, especially middle- and low-income countries still struggle with the often-devastating sequelae of burns [1]. Fortunately, not every burn has serious consequences and most burns—especially in developed countries—are non-fatal, heal spontaneously, and do not require highly specialized treatment [2, 3]. Even though these developments, which might be attributed to effective prevention strategies, can be considered pleasant, there are still a number of severe burns that should only be treated in highly specialized centers to achieve the best possible outcome [4, 5]. Advances in burn care have enabled the survival of burns of up to 100% total body surface area (TBSA), yet deep burns always leave a mark. The pathognomonic burn scar after a deep dermal injury often mirrors and publicly displays the suffering a patient had to live through and is the reason for long-term psychosocial and physical morbidity [6]. While a normal scar is usually flat, pliable, slightly dyspigmented, and painless, burns entail a particularly high prevalence of hypertrophic scars that are heterogeneously bulky, non-pliable, stiff and contracting, reddish, and often painful or itchy. Depending on the available literature, hypertrophic scars following burns develop in 70–90%, whereas surgery or non-burn trauma shows a decisively lower prevalence of about 30% [6, 7]. This chapter discusses the pathophysiology of burns and the differences to regular wound healing with a focus on local and systemic inflammatory changes.

S. P. Nischwitz (✉) · H. Luze
Division of Plastic, Aesthetic and Reconstructive Surgery, Department of Surgery, Medical University of Graz, Graz, Austria
e-mail: sebastian.nischwitz@medunigraz.at; hanna.luze@medunigraz.at

L.-P. Kamolz
Division of Plastic, Aesthetic and Reconstructive Surgery, Department of Surgery, Medical University of Graz, Graz, Austria

COREMED-Cooperative Centre for Regenerative Medicine, JOANNEUM RESEARCH Forschungsgesellschaft mbH, Graz, Austria
e-mail: Lars.kamolz@medunigraz.at

Burn Trauma

Burns are defined as thermal injuries that are the reaction to increased (or reduced) temperatures the human skin is not able to tolerate unscathed. They result in coagulative necrosis of epidermis, dermis, and deeper tissues. The dimension of the damage is dependent on the temperature, the duration of exposure, as well as the respective resistance of the skin resulting from its thickness. Burns are usually categorized into five subtypes, each with respective causes that show slight differences in the resulting pathologies: flame, scald, contact, chemical, or electrical. While the local damage in flame burns, contact burns, and scalds is delivered by heat energy that is transferred to the cells and causes their imminent destruction, chemical and electrical burns additionally damage the cell membranes by chemical reactions or electric energy. While small burns are usually confined, larger TBSA burns can result in extended damage by local and systemic inflammatory responses that can harm the whole organism. Despite the therapy of choice for every type of burn is the immediate termination by removal of the agent causing the burn, the already transmitted energy or initiated immune reaction may continue to damage further areas.

The Zones of a Burn

The local burn itself can be differentiated into three zones of intensity [8]: the central area (usually the area of direct contact) is defined as the *coagulation zone*. Within this zone, cells are irreversibly destroyed. The adjoining area is the *zone of stasis*, wherein cell metabolism is diminished or has ceased completely, yet the cells are still alive. In the periphery is the *zone of hyperemia* where the perfusion and metabolism are intact and even increased as is in first-degree burns (see below). A few days later, the initially alive cells in the *zone of stasis* may have given in to the damaging effect of the burn, resulting in necrotic tissue as well. This process is also known as burn wound progression resulting in only two zones (necrotic and alive). The peripheral *zone of hyperemia* usually heals, and the cells will have restored their physiological function.

Burn Depth

A significant factor for the evaluation of burn severity, prognosis, and therapy planning is the burn depth. Burn depth can vary within a burn wound whereby the area that experienced the most intense energy transfer typically shows the "deepest" burn.

By definition, **superficial (first-degree) burns** are confined to the epidermis. Dermal structures are intact, and so are the subpapillary and capillary plexus. The burns have a red appearance, are painful, and show blanching when pressure is applied with an accelerated return of the red color upon release, indicating the higher perfusion and hyperemia. Treatment focuses on topical soothing substances and pain medication while surgical interventions are not necessary and scars do not occur.

If the burn also affects dermal structures, the burn is at least a **partial-thickness burn (second degree)**. Second-degree burns are further differentiated in superficial and deep burns. While second-degree burns form blisters as a primary characteristic, superficial second-degree burns only affect the upper layers of the dermis, are erythematous, painful, and blanch to the touch. Their deeper counterparts also form blisters but are less erythematous if at all, do not blanch to touch, and cause reduced but present pain. The difference is found in the affection of reticular dermis with additional damage to hair follicles and nerves. Since dermal structures are damaged, superficial second-degree burns can show a discoloration after spontaneous healing but reepithelize from rete ridges, sweat glands, and hair follicles within 2 weeks. Deep second-degree burns can also heal spontaneously by reepithelization from the remaining hair follicles; however, the process takes usually longer than 3 weeks and shows severe scarring due to the loss of almost complete dermis.

Full-thickness (third-degree) burns involve the whole skin thickness and present themselves without blisters and pain but with a leathery eschar of black, gray, white, or deep red color. Since no skin appendages are retained, these wounds need to heal from the remaining wound edges. Deep second- and third-degree burns typically require a surgical necrectomy and skin grafting.

Sometimes, a **fourth-degree** burn is also added to this list being defined as a burn not only of the entire skin thickness but also of deeper structures like subcutaneous fatty tissue, muscles, fascia, or bones.

Table 1 and Fig. 1 provide a summary and depiction of burn depths, respectively.

The current gold standard is the evaluation of burn depth by experienced specialists. Since the differentiation between superficial and deep partial-thickness burns can be hard to tell, especially given their need for surgical intervention, the term "burn of undefined depth" is sometimes used and repeated evaluations are performed. Moreover, new technologies like Laser Doppler present a possibility of objectively evaluating a burn wound, possibly allowing an earlier definitive decision of treatment. While some studies show superior accuracy of the Laser Doppler as compared to a clinical evaluation, its use in clinical routine could not replace the clinical assessment (to date) [9, 10].

Burn Area

In order to properly assess prognosis and therapy, another important aspect of a burn is the involved TBSA. The TBSA is indicated in percentage, whereas first-degree burns are not considered. The TBSA does not concern the outcome concerning resulting scars and is therefore described here for the sake of completeness. In clinical

Table 1 Summary of the different burn degrees and their characteristics

Burn degree	Clinical characteristics	Involved tissues	Outcome
Superficial (I°)	Erythema, edema, pain	Epidermis	Healing within a few days without scar
Superficial partial thickness (IIa°)	Blisters, erythema, blanching to touch, pain	Superficial dermis (stratum papillare)	Healing in 1–3 weeks with low-profile scar
Deep partial thickness (IIb°)	Blisters, no erythema or blanching to touch, reduced sensitivity/pain, loose hair	Deep dermis (stratum reticulare)	Spontaneous healing possible after more than 3 weeks—frequent pathologic scarring
Full thickness (III°)	Dry, leathery eschar, no pain, no hair	Full-thickness skin	Usually requires surgical intervention—more frequent pathologic scarring
IV°	Charred tissue	Deeper tissues (fat, fascia, muscle,…)	Surgical intervention mandatory

° degree

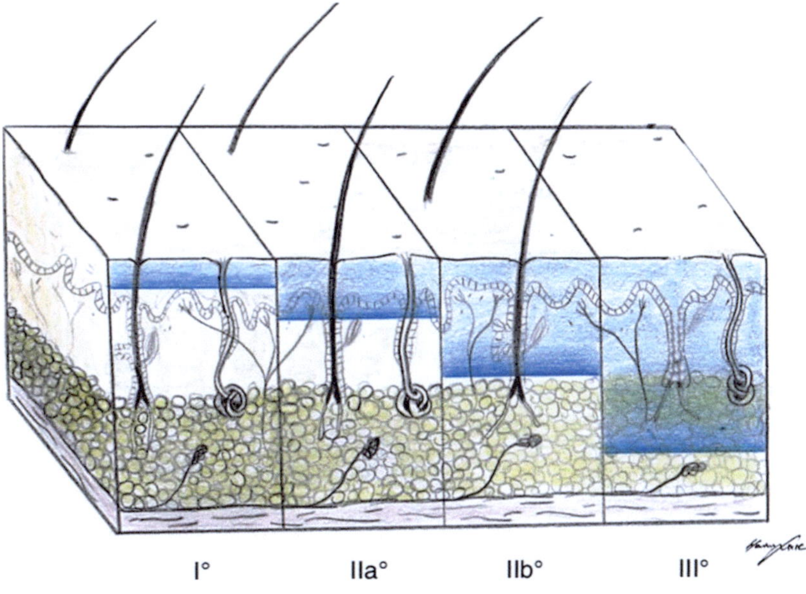

Fig. 1 Schematic depiction of burn depths (© Hanna Luze)

practice, the rule of 9s has proven useful [11]. Specific body regions in an adult are allocated 9% (head, left arm, right arm) or 18% (anterior trunk, posterior trunk, left leg, right leg), and the genitalia counts for 1%, which allows a quick estimation of a burn size. Another useful technique is to consider the palm (including the fingers) of the patient to be 1% TBSA, allowing a feasible estimation of mixed depth or smaller-size burns. In newborns and children, these estimations have to take into account the relatively higher surface area of the head compared to the body, having resulted in adaptations such as the Berkow formula.

Pathophysiology of Burn Wound Healing

Burn wounds show some particularities that distinguish them from incisional wounds: burn wounds are usually much larger and show a horizontal direction in contrast to the vertical direction of incisional wounds. If specific TBSA are involved, a burn can result in the systemic burn disease, which will not be covered in this chapter. Moreover, blood loss is typically much lower than in other acute wounds, given the coagulational effect of the heat, which also leads to an initial sterility of the wound [12]. Consequently, the resulting necrosis and destruction of widespread skin barrier make them prone to infections; that risk is furthermore increased by the generally altered immune status of burn patients. Since the general wound healing cascade is comparable to the one in non-burn wounds, we would like to refer the reader to the respective chapter in this book for details. However, to allow a proper understanding of burn wound healing and show up the relevant aspects thereof, a short summary is given at the risk of repetition.

Phases of Wound Healing

While a human fetus shows scarless wound healing [13], once a human is born, wound healing occurs in three phases that ultimately yield a scar: the inflammation, proliferation, and remodeling phases. A disturbance of the physiological course of wound healing at any place typically results in a pathological or excessive scar.

Immediately after the injury, blood platelets aggregate and release cytokines like transforming growth factor beta (TGF-b), platelet-derived growth factor (PDGF), and insulin-like growth factor (IGF) that (among others) attract inflammatory cells like mast cells, macrophages, or neutrophil granulocytes. These cells are required to prevent infection and clear the wound of necrotic tissue and debris. The resulting inflammation is a paramount part in wound healing, yet the extent of the burn can lead to a significantly prolonged and elevated inflammation.

The platelets are supported by fibrin that clots and creates a scaffold for the following proliferation phase.

The core aspect of the proliferation phase is the accumulation of fibroblasts that replace the fibrin scaffold with extracellular matrix. Fibroblasts are stimulated already in the inflammation phase by TGF-b and PDGF but do not migrate to the scaffold until a competent immune defense is established and the wound is cleared of debris. Inflammation and proliferation phases however overlap and are not strictly separated. Fibroblasts then produce procollagen III as well as other elements of the extracellular matrix like fibronectin or proteoglycans. On a macroscopic level, granulation tissue forms in the proliferation phase. Once a first layer of granulation tissue is formed, fibroblasts transform into myofibroblasts that lead to the constriction of the wound. Additionally, keratinocytes can migrate from the wound edges to cover the wound with epithelium.

Once the wound is closed, the remodeling phase begins. Characteristics of the remodeling phase are the degradation of unorganized collagen III and the replacement thereof with collagen I. Main actors in this phase are matrix-metalloproteinases that are produced by neutrophil granulocytes, fibroblasts, and macrophages and degrade the preliminary collagen. The number of fibroblasts and macrophages is reduced over time, and the collagen scaffold is reinforced and reorganized to produce the final scar.

Particularities in Burns

The primary damaging mechanism in burns is the protein denaturation. This damaging process is quickly accompanied by an activation of inflammatory mediators. Peptidases and oxidants further damage the already frail endothelial cells and support the tissue necrosis. Another effect thereof is the onset of edema. The more severe the burn (depth, area, and inflammatory response), the more expressed the edema becomes, possibly resulting in a hypovolemic situation, even with adequate fluid resuscitation. This process stimulates the activation of neutrophils and xanthinoxidase, which in turn leads to an increase of toxic by-products like radicals. These, along with an elevated accumulation of histamine, further intensify endothelial permeability. On a systemic level, these pathways may lead to a subsequent burn disease with systemic sequelae up to multiorgan failure and death. For further information on the systemic level, please refer to the literature in Recommended Reading below.

The above-mentioned processes are the reason why the inflammatory phase in burns can be considered abnormal as compared to the wound healing process in incisional wounds. While wounds may heal, a prolonged presence of inflammatory cells in burn wounds and increased proinflammatory cytokines years after trauma prove the persistence of the inflammatory phase long after completed wound healing. With burn wounds being exposed to an increased and sustained influence of the inflammatory phase, the respective cells exert their activity for a prolonged period of time as well. TGF-b or matrix-metalloproteinases are only two of the key mediators that heavily regulate pro- and antifibrotic effects. While the exact pathomechanism of hypertrophic scar formation is not yet elucidated, several treatment strategies focus on the reduction of the inflammatory response in scars. With

prolonged healing time and bacterial colonization, two of the most commonly known risk factors for pathologic scarring are inherently present in burn wounds, with others such as young age being patient-dependent and skin stretch being technique-dependent [14, 15]. Thereby, the increased risk for pathologic scars can at least partially be explained.

Conclusion

In this chapter, the fundamentals of burn wounds and burn wound healing have been discussed. The mechanism of cell destruction by thermal energy leads to three different zones that show distinctive responses in terms of wound healing. Overall, burn wounds show an increased and prolonged course of the inflammatory phase. With burns yielding an enormously higher prevalence of hypertrophic scars, therapeutic approaches understandably focus on inflammatory control. Future research needs to comprehensively elucidate pathologic scar pathophysiology and the exact local alterations that follow a burn injury.

References

1. Mock C, Peck M, Peden M, Krug E. A WHO plan for burn prevention and care. 2008. https://apps.who.int/iris/bitstream/handle/10665/97852/9789241596299_eng.pdf?sequence=1&isAllowed=y. Accessed 6 Feb 2022.
2. Rennekampff HO, Mirastschijski U, Aumann E, et al. Improvement in burn wound care: summary of the AWMF guideline for the treatment of thermal injuries in adults. Handchirurgie Mikrochirurgie Plastische Chirurgie. 2020;52(6):497–504. https://doi.org/10.1055/a-1230-3866.
3. Brigham PA, McLoughlin E. Burn incidence and medical care use in the United States: estimates, trends, and data sources. J Burn Care Rehabil. 1996;17(2):95–107. https://doi.org/10.1097/00004630-199603000-00003.
4. Depamphilis MA, Cauley RP, Sadeq F, et al. Surgical management and epidemiological trends of pediatric electrical burns. Burns. 2020;2020:005. https://doi.org/10.1016/j.burns.2020.03.005.
5. Atiyeh BS, Costagliola M, Hayek SN. Burn prevention mechanisms and outcomes: pitfalls, failures and successes. Burns. 2009;35(2):181–93. https://doi.org/10.1016/J.BURNS.2008.06.002.

6. Finnerty CC, Jeschke MG, Branski LK, Barret JP, Dziewulski P, Herndon DN. Hypertrophic scarring: the greatest unmet challenge following burn injury. Lancet. 2016;388(10052):1427. https://doi.org/10.1016/S0140-6736(16)31406-4.

7. Arno AI, Gauglitz GG, Barret JP, Jeschke MG. Up-to-date approach to manage keloids and hypertrophic scars: a useful guide. Burns. 2014;40(7):1255–66. https://doi.org/10.1016/J.BURNS.2014.02.011.

8. Jackson DM. The diagnosis of the depth of burning. Br J Surg. 2005;40(164):588–96. https://doi.org/10.1002/bjs.18004016413.

9. Hop MJ, Stekelenburg C, Hiddingh J, et al. Cost-effectiveness of laser Doppler imaging in burn care in The Netherlands; a randomised controlled trial. Value Health. 2014;17(7):A608. https://doi.org/10.1016/J.JVAL.2014.08.2125.

10. Holland AJA, Martin HCO, Cass DT. Laser Doppler imaging prediction of burn wound outcome in children. Burns. 2002;28(1):11–7. https://doi.org/10.1016/S0305-4179(01)00064-X.

11. Wallace AB. The exposure treatment of burns. Lancet. 1951;257(6653):501–4. https://doi.org/10.1016/S0140-6736(51)91975-7.

12. Strudwick XL, Cowin AJ. The role of the inflammatory response in burn injury. Hot Top Burn Inj. 2017;2017:71330. https://doi.org/10.5772/INTECHOPEN.71330.

13. Longaker MT, Whitby DJ, Adzick NS, et al. Studies in fetal wound healing, VI. Second and early third trimester fetal wounds demonstrate rapid collagen deposition without scar formation. J Pediatr Surg. 1990;25(1):63–9. https://doi.org/10.1016/S0022-3468(05)80165-4.

14. Lonie S, Baker P, Teixeira RP. Healing time and incidence of hypertrophic scarring in paediatric scalds. Burns. 2017;43(3):509–13. https://doi.org/10.1016/J.BURNS.2016.09.011.

15. Butzelaar L, Ulrich MMW, Mink Van Der Molen AB, Niessen FB, Beelen RHJ. Currently known risk factors for hypertrophic skin scarring: a review. J Plast Reconstr Aesthet Surg. 2016;69(2):163–9. https://doi.org/10.1016/J.BJPS.2015.11.015.

Recommended Reading

Marc G. Jeschke, Lars-Peter Kamolz, Folke Sjöberg, Steven E. Wolf. Handbook of Burns Volume 1 - Acute Burn Care. Springer Nature.

Lars-Peter Kamolz, Marc G. Jeschke, Raymund E. Horch, Markus Küntscher, Pavel Brychta. Handbook of Burns Volume 2 - Reconstruction and Rehabilitation. Springer Nature.

Mechanobiology and Mechanotherapy of Cutaneous Scarring

Rei Ogawa

Core Messages

- Mechanical force can be an important cause of pathological scar development and progression.
- The pathogenic mechanical forces on scars/wounds include stretching tension, shear force, scratching, compression, hydrostatic pressure, and osmotic pressure.
- The importance of mechanical forces in pathological scar formation and progression is demonstrated by the fact that keloids grow horizontally in the predominant direction(s) of tension on the wound/scar.
- Another line of evidence is the hypertrophic scar mouse model, which develops heavy scars when the edges of a cutaneous incision are repetitively stretched.
- Tension reduction surgery, which is a form of mechanotherapy, is an effective treatment for pathological scars.

Introduction

Cutaneous wound healing involves several overlapping phases, the first of which is an inflammatory phase whose purpose is to clean and close the wound. The local inflammation is derived from the blood vessels in the wound, which become permeable after wounding. This allows inflammatory soluble factors and many types of immune cells in the circulation to enter the wound bed. Thus, during this early phase of wound healing, circulating cells accumulate in the damaged area. These changes drive the activation and proliferation of resident cells, including collagen-secreting fibroblasts whose products fill the defect. The last phase of wound healing is the remodeling phase. Over several months, this phase produces first the immature and then the mature scar, which has regained much of the original strength of the tissue. These scars mainly consist of dermal-like collagens (particularly type I collagen) that are covered by epidermis.

However, in some cases, wound healing does not start or progress normally, thereby producing scars with contour defects. Figure 1 shows the three main types of abnormal scars. The first type is characterized by skin hollows and is called an atrophic scar. This scar is caused by local inflammation such as chickenpox and acne that differs from the inflammation that is produced after normal wounding. This inflammatory profile induces more collagen degradation than normal, thus generating a depressed scar. In other words, atrophic scars occur when the breakdown of collagen fibers exceeds their production. The two other abnormal scars are characterized by abnormal elevation. They are called hypertrophic scars and keloids and arise due to local, systemic, and genetic factors; the inflammatory phase does not

R. Ogawa (✉)
Department of Plastic, Reconstructive and Aesthetic Surgery, Nippon Medical School, Tokyo, Japan
e-mail: r.ogawa@nms.ac.jp

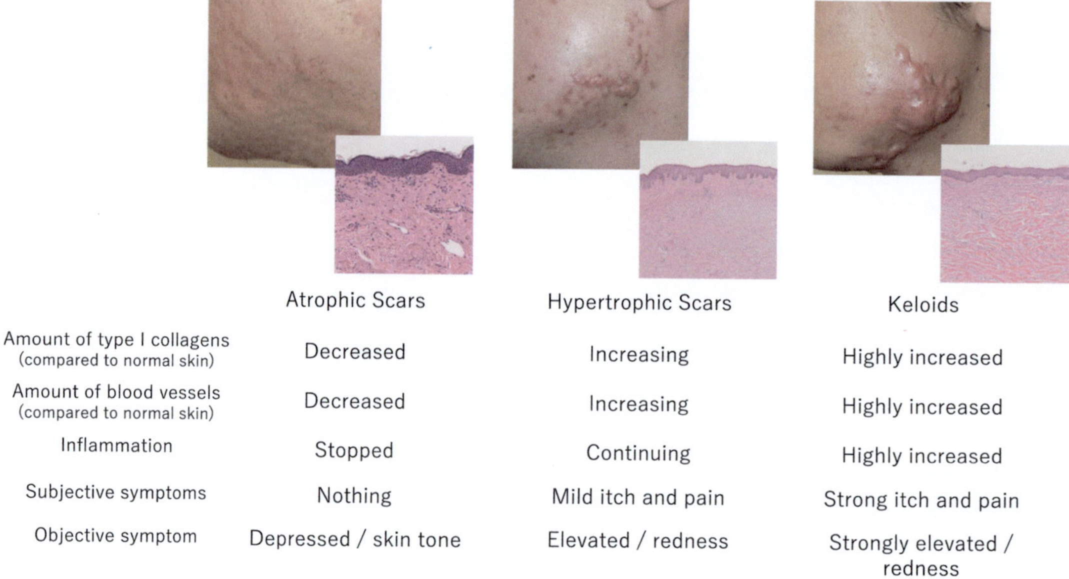

	Atrophic Scars	Hypertrophic Scars	Keloids
Amount of type I collagens (compared to normal skin)	Decreased	Increasing	Highly increased
Amount of blood vessels (compared to normal skin)	Decreased	Increasing	Highly increased
Inflammation	Stopped	Continuing	Highly increased
Subjective symptoms	Nothing	Mild itch and pain	Strong itch and pain
Objective symptom	Depressed / skin tone	Elevated / redness	Strongly elevated / redness

Fig. 1 The three main scar types that are characterized by contour defects

Fig. 2 Appearance of typical hypertrophic scars and keloids. (**a**) A typical hypertrophic scar. (**b**) Typical keloids. In typical hypertrophic scars, the inflammation is not strong and often resolves spontaneously over time. Consequently, the scar stiffness, elevation, and redness are generally limited to the initial wound area. By contrast, typical keloids associate with strong and prolonged inflammation and their stiffness, elevation, and redness invade the normal skin around the initial wound

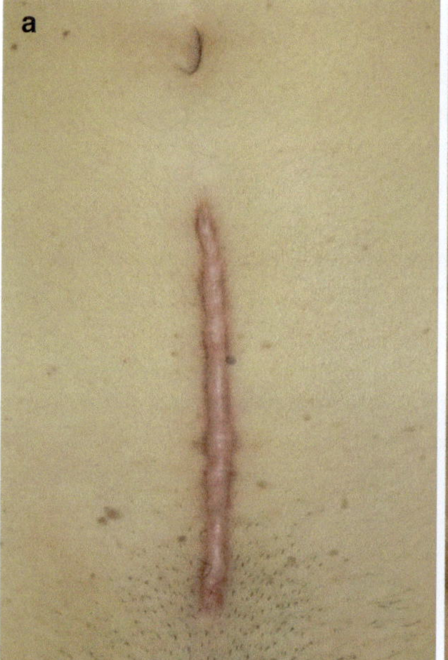
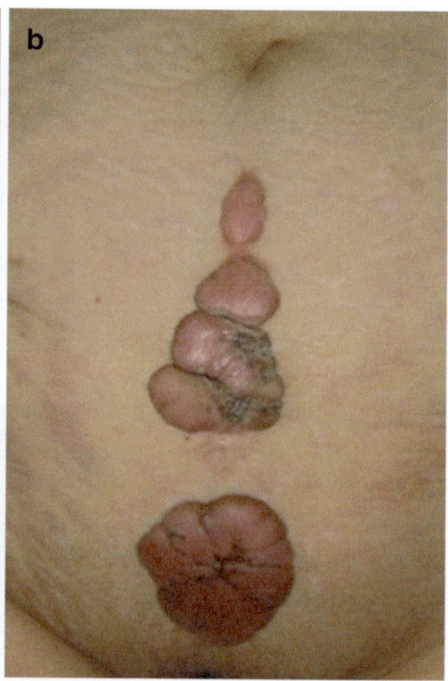

subside. Instead, it provokes the unrelenting accumulation of collagen fibers, blood vessels, and nerve fibers and prevents the remodeling phase from engaging properly. This produces a pathologically immature scar that is red, elevated, hard, and painful [1] (Fig. 2).

Role of Mechanobiology in Cutaneous Scarring

Of the multiple factors that have been implicated in prolonging the inflammatory stage in wound healing in recent years [2, 3], a particularly

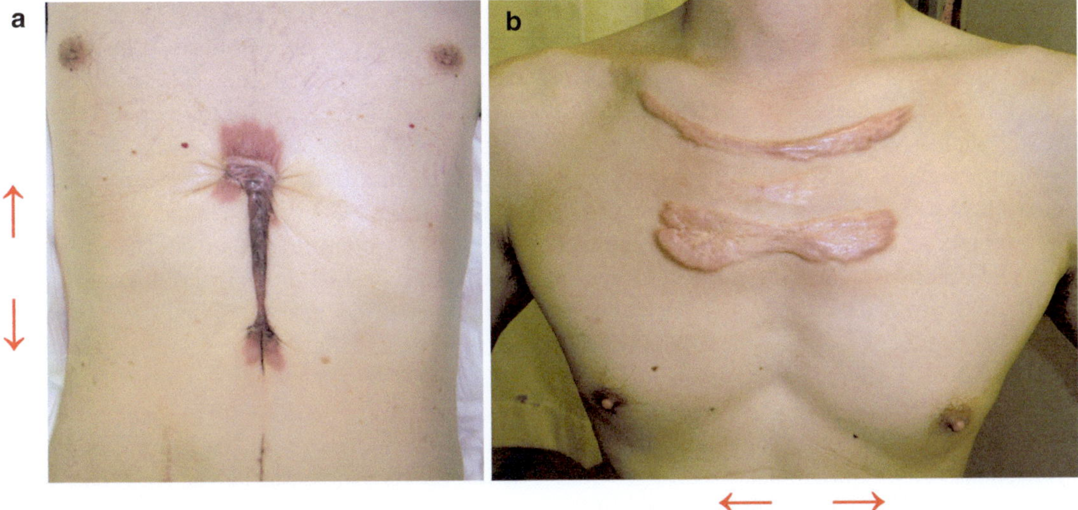

Fig. 3 Keloids often spread in the prevailing direction(s) of skin tension. (a) A typical keloid after abdominal surgery. (b) Typical keloids caused by folliculitis on the chest. The skin tension on the abdomen runs along the long axis of the body and is produced by sitting and standing. This causes strong stretching and growth of abdominal surgical scars in the cranial and caudal directions. By contrast, the chest wall is subjected to strong skin tension in the horizontal direction that is caused by upper limb movements. As a result, chest keloids tend to spread horizontally

important one may be mechanical force: as will be discussed in more detail further below, this is shown by the fact that mechanical force can strongly shape the horizontal growth directions of keloids [4–7] (Fig. 3). The importance of mechanical forces in pathological scar formation is also supported by the empirically acquired clinical realization that these scars can be prevented from arising after surgery by tension-reducing procedures that stabilize the wound [8]. These procedures include tension reduction suturing, where the first sutures are placed on the deep fasciae, thereby inducing a close approximation of the wound edges; this relieves the intrinsic tension on the dermis, which is where pathological scarring commences. Another tension-reducing surgical procedure is z-plasty, which effectively relieves the tension on the wound edges that is generated by body movements. A postoperative technique, namely, taping fixation, can further limit these extrinsic forces on the wound.

These observations together support the notion that heavy scarring can result when the mechanical forces on and in the wound/scar are strong and/or repetitive. To understand why, it is important to discuss how cells and tissues can sense and respond to mechanical forces. This knowledge will also help us to identify effective mechanotherapeutic strategies that prevent or ameliorate pathological scarring.

Cellular and Tissue Responses to Mechanical Forces

The mechanical forces on scars/wounds include stretching tension, shear force, scratching, compression, hydrostatic pressure, and osmotic pressure [5]. In the case of cutaneous scars on the body surface, stretching tension is the main mechanical force that shapes pathological scar development. These forces are all perceived by mechanosensors on and in the cells that reside in the extracellular matrix of the wound/scar. Mechanoreceptors on nerve fibers also recognize these forces and shape the responses of the tissue [9].

In relation to cellular responses, several mechanosensors have been identified in wound/scar cells. Some are mechanosensitive molecules on the cell membrane that receive mechanical stress-induced signals from other cells: examples are ATP hemichannels and Ca^{2+} ion channels. Others are molecules that sense mechanical changes in the surrounding extracellular matrix; examples are cell adhesion molecules such as integrin (Fig. 4) and cytoskeletal components such as actin filaments, which respond with polymerization and depolymerization. These molecules act together when the extracellular matrix is contorted by mechanical forces such as skin tension: in wounds/scars, these matrix changes are detected by the mechanosensors on fibroblasts and endothelial cells. These sensors in turn initiate mechanosignaling pathways in these cells that promote molecular changes such as gene transcription, fibroblast proliferation, local angiogenesis, and changes in epithelial cell behavior that induce epithelialization. The main cellular mechanosignaling pathways in wounds/scars are the integrin, MAPK/G protein, TNF-α/NF-κB, Wnt/β-catenin, interleukin, calcium ion, TGFβ/Smad, and FAK signaling pathways [9] (Fig. 5).

Sensory nerve fibers in the skin also play important roles in the responses of wound/scar tissue to mechanical forces. These fibers bear mechanosensitive nociceptors that produce the somatic sensation of mechanical force [10] (Fig. 6). When these mechanosensitive nociceptors are triggered by mechanical stimuli on or around the wound, they emit electrical signals that are received by the dorsal root ganglia. The cell bodies of the afferent spinal neurons in the dorsal root ganglia then transmit the electrical signals to their peripheral terminals, which innervate the skin and are often in physical contact with cells in the skin. The terminals release neuropeptides, including substance P, calcitonin gene-based peptide (CGRP), neurokinin A, vasoactive intestinal peptide, and somatostatin, which then directly shape the behavior of the surrounding skin cells, including keratinocytes, fibroblasts, Langerhans cells, mast cells, endothelial cells, and infiltrating immune cells. This induces cellular proliferation, cytokine production, altered antigen presentation, mast cell degradation, and sensory neurotransmission. In particular, neuropeptides increase vascular permeability in both normal and pathophysiologi-

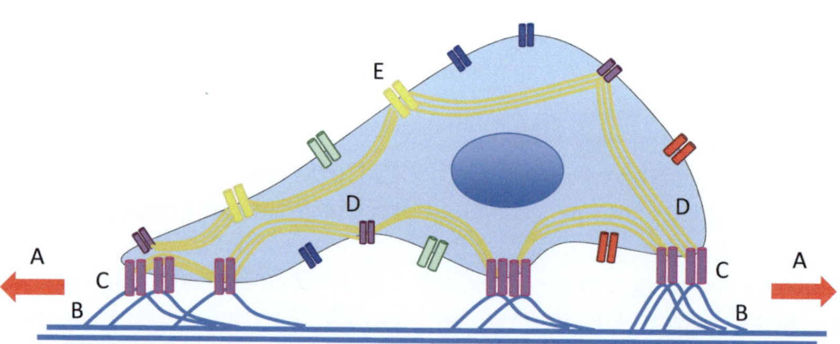

Fig. 4 Schematic depiction of the mechanosensors on skin cells that sense extrinsic mechanical forces. Skin tension (**a**) distorts/stretches the local extracellular matrix (**b**). This architectural change is detected by mechanosensors on cells within the matrix; examples are cell adhesion molecules (**c**). Cellular actin filaments also register this matrix change (**d**). In addition, the cells are alerted by molecular signals from other mechanically triggered cells, which bind to other mechanosensors on the cell surface; these sensors include ATP hemichannels and Ca^{2+} ion channels (**e**). These mechanosensors initiate mechanosignaling pathways that lead to a large variety of gene expression changes

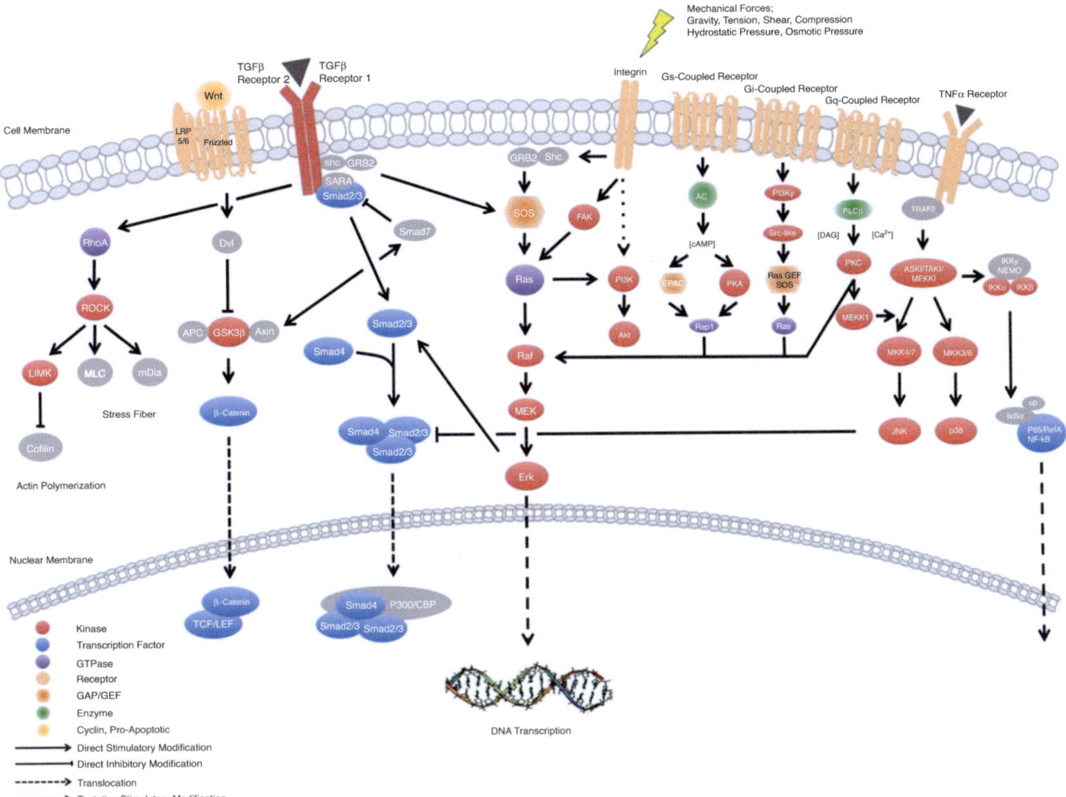

Fig. 5 Mechanosignaling pathways in cells subjected to mechanical forces. When the mechanosensors in or on skin cells are triggered, they activate various mechanosignaling pathways that then regulate cell proliferation, angiogenesis, and epithelialization. (This figure is from reference [9] with copyright permission from the publisher)

cal conditions [10]. All of these effects result in neurogenic inflammation.

Thus, mechanical forces can induce local cellular responses and neurogenic inflammation/neuropeptide activity that together promote local inflammation [9]. As will be described below, when these mechanical forces are persistent and/or strong, they can both augment and prolong local immune responses that hamper the normal wound-healing process.

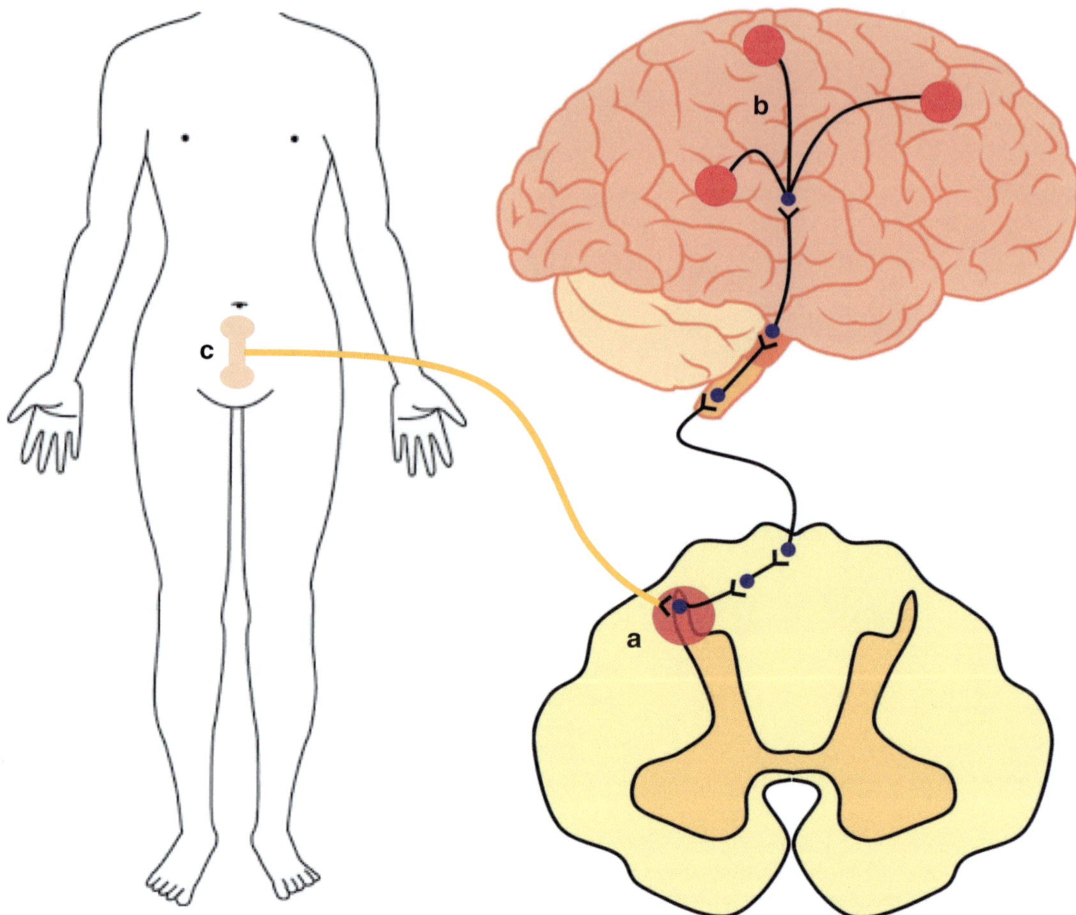

Fig. 6 Mechanosensitive nociceptors shape somatic sensations and tissue responses to mechanical forces. Mechanosensitive nociceptors in tissues like skin respond to external mechanical forces such as tension by converting the mechanical stimuli into electrical signals that travel to the spinal cord dorsal root ganglia, which contain their cell bodies (**a**). Thus, when a scar (**c**) is subjected to mechanical force, the mechanosensitive nociceptors in/around the scar send a signal to the spinal cord, which transmits it to the brain (**b**). This produces the somatic sensations (e.g., pain and/or itch) that associate with the mechanical force. Simultaneously, electrical signals return from the dorsal root ganglia (**a**) to the mechanosensitive nociceptors in/around the scar (**c**). They release neuropeptides from their peripheral terminals, which are often in physical contact with cells in the scar, including epidermal and dermal cells. Consequently, the neuropeptides can induce neurogenic inflammation that promotes pathological scar formation and progression

Role of Mechanobiology in the Development of Pathological Scars

The traditional view of hypertrophic scars and keloids is that they are distinct entities. Thus, the so-called typical keloids grow beyond the confines of their original wounds and demonstrate the accumulation of dermal thick eosinophilic collagen bundles and dermal nodules. By contrast, the classical hypertrophic scars grow within the wound boundaries and are characterized histologically by dermal nodules alone (Fig. 2). However, both hypertrophic scars and keloids are characterized by prolonged inflammation and aberrant extracellular matrix accumulation.

Moreover, there are many so-called atypical cases that bear the clinical and histological characteristics of both scar types; these cases can pose significant diagnostic difficulties for even senior clinicians. It is possible that hypertrophic scars and keloids are often believed to be distinct entities because keloids are relatively uncommon in Caucasian populations and thus the atypical cases are rarely seen. However, in Asian countries, keloids are very common and atypical cases are encountered frequently. We currently believe that hypertrophic scars, atypical intermediate-type scars, and keloids are successive stages or alternative forms of the same underlying fibroproliferative pathology. We also believe that a variety of proinflammatory risk factors dictate whether a scar progresses into a more severe form or develops into one or the other classical form [11].

As mentioned above, one of these risk factors is mechanical force. Several lines of evidence support the importance of this factor in pathological scarring. First, as described in more detail further below, when incisions on experimental animal models are subjected to mechanical force, they develop hypertrophic scars [12]. Second, an analysis of Asian patients showed that keloids tend to occur at specific sites (the anterior chest, shoulder, scapular, and lower abdomen-suprapubic regions) that are characterized by constant or frequent mechanical forces, including skin stretching due to daily body movements [5]. These movements include the upper limb movements that horizontally stretch the skin on the anterior chest, shoulder, and scapula. Similarly, the sitting and standing motions stretch the skin on the lower abdomen and suprapubic regions hundreds of times a day. By contrast, the scalp and anterior lower leg, which have little skin tension because of the underlying bone, rarely develop keloids, even when the patients have extensive keloids or hypertrophic scars [13]. This is also true for the upper eyelid, which experiences little tension during the opening and closing of the eyes. Third, keloids on specific locations develop characteristic keloid shapes because they grow horizontally along the direction(s) of the predominant forces on the wound/scar (Fig. 3). Thus, anterior chest keloids develop into a "crab's claw" or "butterfly" shape while keloids on the upper arm keloids form a "dumbbell"-like shape that runs along the long axis of the arm.

Classical keloids exhibit stronger and more prolonged inflammation than classical hypertrophic scars. This together with the strong link between inflammation and mechanical force suggests that keloid and hypertrophic scars differ in terms of how much skin tension is placed on the wound/scar and how strong the resulting inflammation is. In other words, keloids may result when the tension on the wound/scar is strong and/or highly repetitive and induces profound inflammation. By contrast, hypertrophic scars may be due to different and/or weaker mechanical forces that lead to a more muted or qualitatively different inflammation. This is supported by our finite element analysis of the mechanical force distribution around keloids: this showed that the keloid region with the highest skin tension (i.e., the leading edge) also exhibited the greatest inflammation [14] (Fig. 7). This explains the tendency of keloids to invade the normal skin in the predominant direction of skin tension and therefore adopt body region-specific shapes [13].

It should be emphasized that other factors may also contribute to the ultimate inflammatory status of a wound/scar; these factors include genetics and systemic factors such as hypertension [2]. These factors may promote/aggravate or conversely downregulate the inflammation induced by mechanical tension.

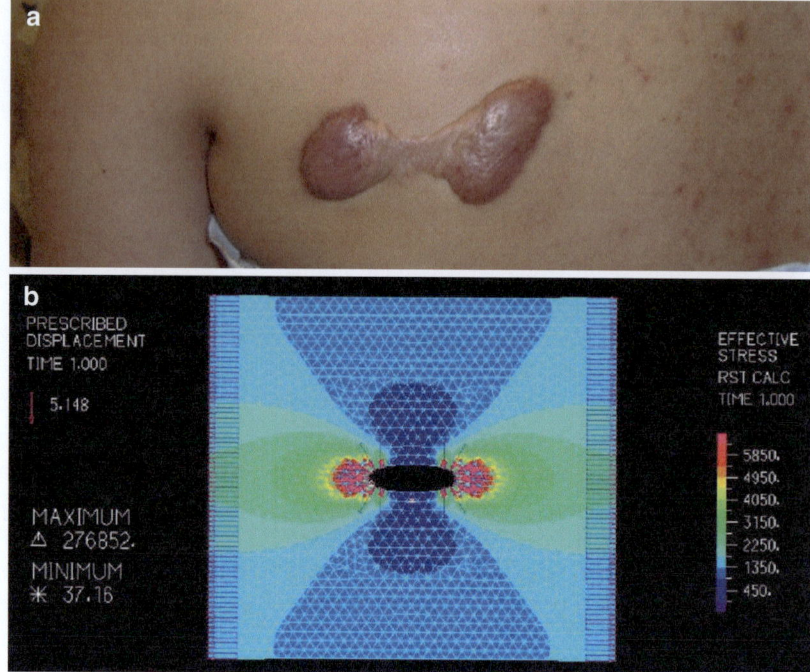

Fig. 7 Close overlap of the distributions of keloid inflammation and the surrounding mechanical forces. (**a**) A mechanosensory scapular keloid. (**b**) Finite element analysis of the mechanical force on the scapular keloid. The inflamed, elevated parts of the keloid (**a**) overlap with the regions of high tension in the keloid (red color in **b**). Thus, high skin tension may prolong and amplify the inflammation in the keloid periphery. (The figure is from reference [14] with copyright permission from the publisher.)

A Pathological Scar Animal Model That Is Based on Mechanotransduction

Many attempts have been made to generate murine, rat, or rabbit models of pathological scars. However, since these scars are generally characterized by acute inflammation rather than chronic inflammation, they are often immature and fail to develop the clinical and pathological features of human pathological scars. An exception is the hypertrophic scar mouse model. In this model, pathological scars are generated from a cutaneous incision by subjecting its edges to repetitive daily stretching for several weeks. These scars resemble human hypertrophic scars pathologically and clinically. A study with this model showed that the tension associates with less apoptosis; it also observed that inflammatory cells play an important role in this mechanical force-induced skin fibrosis [12]. Moreover, other studies with this model demonstrate that pathological scar development involves active interactions between cellular mechanosignaling pathways and the extracellular matrix, and that there is considerable crosstalk between these mechanosignaling pathways and the hypoxia, inflammation, and angiogenesis pathways [9].

Mechanotherapy for Scar Prevention and Treatment

The finding that stretching tension on wounds/scars can provoke and augment pathological scarring has significantly shaped our surgical and postoperative approaches, both in normal and scar-revision surgeries, as follows.

Stabilization Materials

To limit skin stretching and exposure to external mechanical stimuli during wound healing/scarring, wounds and immature scars should be covered by fixable materials such as tape, bandages, garments, or silicone gel sheets. Several randomized controlled trials have shown that such wound stabilization reduces the incidence of hypertrophic scars and keloids. Our finite element analy-

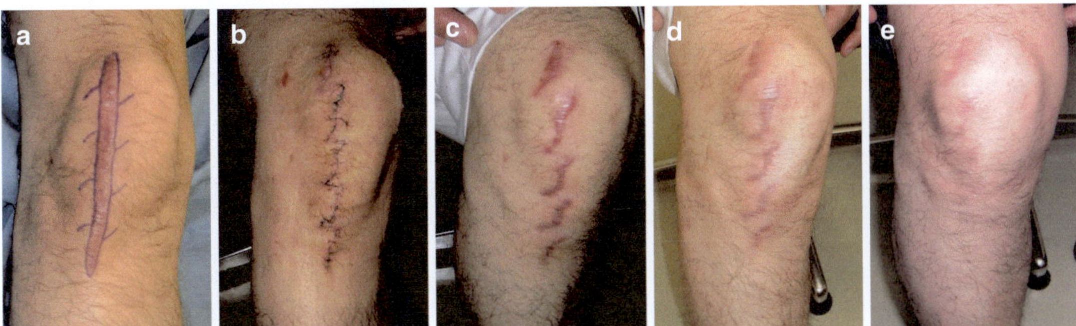

Fig. 8 Z-plasties effectively reduce tension on knee hypertrophic scars. (**a**) Design of the incisions needed to remove the scar and apply z-plasties. (**b**) Two weeks after surgery. (**c**) Three months after surgery. (**d**) Six months after surgery. (**e**) Twelve months after surgery. A Z-plasty breaks up a linear scar, thus reducing the tension along the long axis of the scar. This reduces inflammation and promotes the healing of the hypertrophic scar

sis of the mechanical forces around scars also showed that silicone gel sheeting reduces the tension at the scar edges [15].

Sutures

Keloids and hypertrophic scars arise from the reticular dermis. Since mechanical tension may be an etiological factor for these abnormal scars, we routinely close surgical wounds with subcutaneous/fascial tensile reduction sutures that place tension on the deep and superficial fascial layers rather than the dermis. Subsequently, few, if any dermal sutures are needed, especially if the deep sutures draw the wound edges together. This approach is especially mandatory in patients with other keloid risk factors such as a genetic predisposition.

Z-Plasty, Skin Grafting, and Local Flaps for Scar Revision Surgery

Keloids are highly prone to recurrence after scar revision surgery due to ongoing skin tension on the scars left by the revision surgery. Therefore, our current approach is to use surgical procedures that effectively reduce the tension on the scar, followed by postoperative radiotherapy that dampens the surgery-induced inflammation [3,

16, 17]. A good choice is the Z-plasty, which disrupts the line of tension on linear scars (Fig. 8). Skin grafts are also a good choice. Full-thickness skin grafts have better outcomes than split-thickness skin grafts, which have a higher risk of secondary contracture. However, if there is normal skin nearby, local flaps should be chosen rather than full-thickness skin grafts: they result in contracture much less often and the aesthetic outcomes are better. If a local flap is selected, one can choose between an island flap and a skin-pedicled flap. The geometry of the scar and other patient-specific characteristics shape this decision to some extent. However, skin-pedicled flaps are often the best choice because they expand better than island flaps due to their connection with normal skin, which is much more elastic than the scar tissue surrounding the perimeter of island flaps. Thus, skin-pedicled flaps more effectively release the tension of the scar.

Conclusion

It is increasingly clear that mechanical forces on the skin promote scarring, and that this is due to mechanosensitive cellular behavior that promotes local inflammation and prevents the normal transition to wound remodeling. These observations have led us to focus on reducing skin tension in both normal surgery and keloid/hypertrophic scar revision surgery by using subcutaneous/fascial tensile reduction sutures. In addition, z-plasties and skin flaps effectively release the tension on the scar and can be used to successfully treat big scars.

References

1. Huang C, Murphy GF, Akaishi S, Ogawa R. Keloids and hypertrophic scars: update and future directions. Plast Reconstr Surg Glob Open. 2013;1(4):e25.
2. Huang C, Ogawa R. Systemic factors that shape cutaneous pathological scarring. FASEB J. 2020;34(10):13171–84.
3. Ogawa R, Dohi T, Tosa M, Aoki M, Akaishi S. The latest strategy for keloid and hypertrophic scar prevention and treatment: the Nippon Medical School (NMS) protocol. J Nippon Med Sch. 2021;88(1):2–9.
4. Ogawa R. Keloid and hypertrophic scarring may result from a mechanoreceptor or mechanosensitive nociceptor disorder. Med Hypotheses. 2008;71(4):493–500.
5. Ogawa R. Mechanobiology of scarring. Wound Repair Regen. 2011;19(Suppl 1):s2–9.
6. Wong VW, Rustad KC, Akaishi S, Sorkin M, Glotzbach JP, Januszyk M, Nelson ER, Levi K, Paterno J, Vial IN, Kuang AA, Longaker MT, Gurtner GC. Focal adhesion kinase links mechanical force to skin fibrosis via inflammatory signaling. Nat Med. 2011;18(1):148–52.
7. Harn HI, Ogawa R, Hsu CK, Hughes MW, Tang MJ, Chuong CM. The tension biology of wound healing. Exp Dermatol. 2019;28(4):464–71.
8. Ogawa R, Akaishi S, Huang C, Dohi T, Aoki M, Omori Y, Koike S, Kobe K, Akimoto M, Hyakusoku H. Clinical applications of basic research that shows reducing skin tension could prevent and treat abnormal scarring: the importance of fascial/subcutaneous tensile reduction sutures and flap surgery for keloid and hypertrophic scar reconstruction. J Nippon Med Sch. 2011;78(2):68–76.
9. Huang C, Akaishi S, Ogawa R. Mechanosignaling pathways in cutaneous scarring. Arch Dermatol Res. 2012;304(8):589–97.
10. Akaishi S, Ogawa R, Hyakusoku H. Keloid and hypertrophic scar: neurogenic inflammation hypotheses. Med Hypotheses. 2008;71(1):32–8.
11. Huang C, Akaishi S, Hyakusoku H, Ogawa R. Are keloid and hypertrophic scar different forms of the same disorder? A fibroproliferative skin disorder hypothesis based on keloid findings. Int Wound J. 2014;11(5):517–22.
12. Aarabi S, Bhatt KA, Shi Y, Paterno J, Chang EI, Loh SA, Holmes JW, Longaker MT, Yee H, Gurtner GC. Mechanical load initiates hypertrophic scar formation through decreased cellular apoptosis. FASEB J. 2007;21(12):3250–61.
13. Ogawa R, Okai K, Tokumura F, Mori K, Ohmori Y, Huang C, Hyakusoku H, Akaishi S. The relationship between skin stretching/contraction and pathologic scarring: the important role of mechanical forces in keloid generation. Wound Repair Regen. 2012;20(2):149–57.
14. Akaishi S, Akimoto M, Ogawa R, Hyakusoku H. The relationship between keloid growth pattern and stretching tension: visual analysis using the finite element method. Ann Plast Surg. 2008;60(4):445–51.
15. Akaishi S, Akimoto M, Hyakusoku H, Ogawa R. The tensile reduction effects of silicone gel sheeting. Plast Reconstr Surg. 2010;126(2):109e–11e.
16. Ogawa R, Akaishi S, Kuribayashi S, Miyashita T. Keloids and hypertrophic scars can now be cured completely: recent progress in our understanding of the pathogenesis of keloids and hypertrophic scars and the most promising current therapeutic strategy. J Nippon Med Sch. 2016;83(2):46–53.
17. Ogawa R. Surgery for scar revision and reduction: from primary closure to flap surgery. Burns Trauma. 2019;7:7.

Further Reading

Huang C, Akaishi S, Ogawa R. Mechanosignaling pathways in cutaneous scarring. Arch Dermatol Res. 2012;304(8):589–97.
Huang C, Holfeld J, Schaden W, Orgill D, Ogawa R. Mechanotherapy: revisiting physical therapy and recruiting mechanobiology for a new era in medicine. Trends Mol Med. 2013;19(9):555–64.
Ogawa R. Keloid and hypertrophic scars are the result of chronic inflammation in the reticular dermis. Int J Mol Sci. 2017;18(3):606.
Ogawa R, Akaishi S, Kuribayashi S, Miyashita T. Keloids and hypertrophic scars can now be cured completely: recent progress in our understanding of the pathogenesis of keloids and hypertrophic scars and the most promising current therapeutic strategy. J Nippon Med Sch. 2016;83(2):46–53.
Ogawa R, Akita S, Akaishi S, Aramaki-Hattori N, Dohi T, Hayashi T, Kishi K, Kono T, Matsumura H, Muneuchi G, Murao N, Nagao M, Okabe K, Shimizu F, Tosa M, Tosa Y, Yamawaki S, Ansai S, Inazu N, Kamo T, Kazki R, Kuribayashi S. Diagnosis and treatment of keloids and hypertrophic scars-Japan scar workshop consensus document 2018. Burns Trauma. 2019;7:39.

The History of Scar Treatment

Frank Sander, Herbert L. Haller,
Sebastian P. Nischwitz, and Bernd Hartmann

Core Messages

- Scars were considered God-given and meaningful marks in ancient history.
- Early treatments focused on the surgical premise "excise and replace."
- Time helps for many scars.
- Tight is never right.
- Scar therapy is still developing.

Introduction

Due to the large field with numerous steps and inventions related to contemporary scar treatment, the authors outline only some essential parts of their development. This is not a complete report by any means.

Fire and war are a part of the history of human civilization's origin and are often linked to divinity. The taming of fire initiated the start of human society, and the preservation of fire was attributed to the Greek goddess Hestia [1]; later, in the Roman mythology, it was attributed to Vesta. In the bible, god talks to Moses through a burning thorn bush as a sign of divinity and commands him to spread his commandments. Hephaistos, the Greek son of Zeus and Hera, was the God of blacksmiths and fire and was a disappointment to his mother due to his notorious ugliness. Zeus threw him out of the Olympus, and he was severely hurt and disabled since. Prometheus stole the fire from Zeus, who wanted to punish humanity by withholding fire due to an insufficient sacrifice. As revenge, Zeus sent Pandora's box to the earth, bringing plagues and evil over humankind.

The ambivalence of fire is reflected by the fact that the ugliest God (Hephaistos—god of fire) married or had to marry Aphrodite, the most beautiful goddess in Olympus.

Nearly every culture adores its fire gods, and the fire was the beginning of civilization. Fire has always been used in both peace and martial techniques. It has to be assumed that at least some people in history have survived their injuries and had to deal with the consequences of scars and contractures with consecutive disabilities. Interestingly, as non-historians, the authors could not find reports on surgical scar treatment in the antique literature. Treatment of wounds and scars in the antique literature may have been mainly based on plants and herbs [2, 3] that are well known for the treatment of wounds.

F. Sander (✉) · B. Hartmann
Burn Center and Plastic Surgery, BG Klinikum
Unfallkrankenhaus Berlin, Berlin, Germany
e-mail: frank.sander@ukb.de; bernd.hartmann@ukb.de

H. L. Haller
HLMedConsult, Leonding, Austria
e-mail: herbert.haller@liwest.at

S. P. Nischwitz
Division of Plastic, Aesthetic and Reconstructive
Surgery, Department of Surgery, Medical University
Graz, Graz, Austria
e-mail: sebastian.nischwitz@medunigraz.at

S. P. Nischwitz et al. (eds.), *Scars*, https://doi.org/10.1007/978-3-031-24137-6_5

Some religions declared the consequences of trauma as supernatural or god-given, so treatment was frequently combined with spells and magical practices [4]. Priests acted as spiritual healers and received sacrificial offers from the suffering victims. Surgery was limited to a few indications, and the ones performing it were not doctors, but wound surgeons "chirurgos" or later "baders" who were trained craftsmen, while surgery was forbidden for the studied medics, mostly by clerical ranks. This was confirmed at the Council of Tours in 1163 [5]. Trying to treat physical blemishes as a consequence of a god-given punishment might even have been dangerous for those trying to do so.

Going away from myth, it is impressive that even the oldest historical sources of medical history, the Codex Hammurabi (Babylonia, eighteenth century BC), deals with surgery, although not on scars, but also social and honorary aspects, as well as punishment for maltreatment [6].

Scars were not always considered disturbing in several different cultures. Ornamental scars are often part of certain forms of body modifications. In Central and East Africa and Papua New Guinea, scars have traditional social and clan affiliations or ritual initiation ceremonies. In Western societies, modern forms of scarification, such as cutting or branding, are common procedures in youth groups and subcultural scenes.

While these ornamental scars are usually the results of intentional trauma, non-intentional trauma, such as large burns, do not account for that. Indeed, the survival of burns has been the leading problem in previous times. Higher survival rates have been achieved only in the last century with advances in burn treatment such as antibiotics, fluid management, and skin transplant techniques. Since then, burn scar treatment has become essential for the quality of life. To date, the holy grail of scar-less wound healing has not been found.

Preconditions

Preconditions essential for treating burn scars were always the underlying medical theories, the beliefs, and the contemporary societies' medical abilities. *Veda medicine* from India is an excellent example of an existing way of dealing with diseases. The body as a microcosm contained three substances as reflections of the macrocosm—air, phlegm, and bile—that had to be balanced for good health and produced the body's seven primary components [7]. Treatment was based on diverting the evil by emetics, purgatives, sneezing powders, water, and oil enemas. According to the later Greek teaching of "dyscrasia," bleeding, leeching, and cupping were used. Interestingly, the modified methods are still in successful use for minor burn scars therapy such as vacuum massage or micro-needling.

Anatomy

As one of the basic sciences for surgeons, human anatomy is often hampered by religious and social commandments that do not allow autopsy, as it was in India. The first known sections of humans were performed about 300 BC in Egypt. Herophilos from Chalkedon (325–255 BC) and Erasistratos from Keos (305–250 BC) [8], anatomists at the medical school in Alexandria, performed sections of dead bodies, and some suspect that they also did vivisections [9]. Their intentions did not result in scientific anatomy, and neither did the Egyptian mummifications, where the body's surface was kept intact, and the guts and brain were removed through keyhole incisions. Nevertheless, this could be done only for some decennia and was stopped due to resistance from other scientific branches.

Later, in the Hellenistic and Roman periods, around 160 AD, Galenus of Pergamon (ca. 129–210) is an example of such restrictions. His results remained the foundation of medical science for a long time. Celsus (25 BC–50 AD) and Galenus used grafts to repair skin defects after infections or replace the foreskin in Jewish people, who wanted to be accepted by Romans [10]. He derived his anatomy from apes, and his anatomical work was not disputed for centuries [11]. Even in the seventeenth century, his anatomical work was used to teach students at universities. Andreas Vesalius (1514–1564), a Flemish anatomist of the Renaissance, was the first to realize and demonstrate that Galenus had never done a section of the human body. The anatomy Galenus taught was hence not solid. Leonardo da Vinci (1452–1519) also performed secret sections, created very detailed paintings, and started advanced anatomical documentation [12].

As previously described, the development of surgery interfered with the dogma of human integrity as God's work. Tagliacozzi (1546–1599) described the repair of mutilated noses using a flap taken from the inner arm. This method was later known as the "Italian method for complete nose repair." He was exhumed and transferred from the church's burial site of St. Giovanni Battista to avoid desecrating the holy ground after performing these blasphemous deeds.

Anesthesia

The development of reconstructive surgery and scar reconstruction is closely linked to sufficient anesthesia and analgesic techniques—methods of regional and local anesthesia supplemented the current methods of general anesthesia. Essential analgesic medication such as alcohol, poppy seed extractions, and mandragora was used for minor surgical interventions before the first operation under the use of ether fumes in 1842, which was performed by the American surgeon Crawford William Long (1815–1878) [14].

In 1848, John Snow (1813–1858) provided analgesia during childbirth to Queen Victoria using chloroform in an open drop method, which gave credibility to the new method [13]. Other forms of inhalation anesthetics and modifications of the techniques followed, and the surveillance methods for anesthesia, such as pulse control, were developed. Ethen, cyclopropane, and halothane are frequently used. Sir Frederick Hewitt (1857–1916) published the first "Textbook on Anesthesia" [14] in 1893 and developed an oral device, the "airway restorer," to keep the airways open while under anesthesia. He recognized that nitric oxide and air mixture developed a hypoxic condition, so he designed an apparatus to deliver oxygen and nitric oxide in various proportions [13]. During this time, ether was popular due to its intoxicating effects and was used as recreational drug. Nitric oxide was demonstrated to allow painless operations in 1844 [15].

Intravenous anesthesia was first performed by the French surgeon and physiologist Pierre–Cyprien Ore (1828–1889) in 1874, who successfully used chloral hydrate [16]. With the development of barbiturates for intravenous application, intravenous anesthesia was invented, and Johann Nepomuk Ritter von Nussbaum (1829–1890), an Ordinarius of surgery in Munich, first used opioids in 1878 to prolong and increase the effect of inhalation anesthesia. He was the inventor of the so-called balanced anesthesia [17].

August Bier (1861–1949), a holder of surgical professorship in Greifswald and Bonn, developed local forms of anesthesia in 1908 as a regional form of intravenous anesthesia, called Bier's block [18]. He used tourniquets to separate intravenously applied lidocaine from the general circulation. Peripheral local forms of nerve blocks and epidural and spinal anesthesia were developed and facilitated surgical procedures, as they did not afford a high-tech outfit, which is necessary to provide general anesthesia.

Circulation

Physiological knowledge, on which our current surgery is based, has been missing for centuries. Since Galenus, people knew that blood flows through the arteries and veins and not pneuma or air. The apparent idea of circulating blood was stated nearly 1500 years later by William Harvey (1578–1657) [19]. Until this, the pulse was thought to be an active expansion of the arteries caused by pneuma.

Vascular surgery was a development of the last century, although the first steps were described in 1877 in Leningrad by Nicolai V. Eck (1849–1908) [20], who performed the first documented anastomosis of two blood vessels in a dog [21]. In 1896, the first successful arterial repair was operated by John Benjamin Murphy (1857–1916) in Chicago using an invagination technique after a gunshot wound. Different methods were developed mostly leaving coats of the vessels untouched, until Dörfler propagated the inclusion of the intima, as he could show no interference with the patency of the lumen; successful sutures of arteries and veins have been performed since 1905 [21]. In 1912 Alexis Carrel (1873–1944) was honored with the Nobel Prize in Medicine for his work about suturing of vessels and organ transplantation.

Skin Transplantation

Skin transplants were first described around 1500 BC in the Papyrus Ebers [6], but stories on their practical uses began with nose replants. Full-thickness transplantations were sporadically described, but the general opinion, as commented by Guy de Chauliac (1298–1368), was that a nose, totally cut off, could not be replanted successfully [22]. Single cases of success were described but assumed falsehoods (Lefranchi, approximately 1400). Robert Hooke (1635–1702), in 1683, performed the first animal study [10] with the successful transplantation of a cock's spur onto its head; unfortunately, his study in a dog failed. The Milanese physician Giuseppe Baronio (1759–1811) published the first successful experiments with sheepskin in 1804. Sir Astley Paston Cooper (1768–1841), the personal physician of King George IV and later Queen Victoria, described the first successful skin grafts in humans in 1817, as did Christian Heinrich Buenger (1782–1842), a surgeon and professor of Anatomy in Marburg, Germany, in 1821 [23]. Although they were mentioned in the paper by Jacques-Louis Reverdin (1842–1929), they did not receive the acceptance of the surgical society, and the merits were attributed to Reverdin, resulting in the *Reverdin grafts* [10, 24]. Reverdin implanted "pinch grafts" which he described as epidermal grafts, but were later seen to be full-thickness grafts in 1869. He realized that each graft had limited epithelialization power, and described epithelialization from the surrounding wound edges. He used it in granulation tissues and fresh wounds. Grafts can be taken from other body areas, from amputated limbs as autografts, or from other humans as allografts. The method is still used in some indi-

cations (e.g., chronic ulcers), yet resulting contractures were no different than in non-grafted wounds, and the scars did not show the desired stability and cosmetic outcome [25]. The pinch grafts were followed by *Ollier's graft* (Louis Léopold Ollier, 1830–1900) [26], a "dermo-epidermal" split-thickness skin graft in the form of 4- to 8-cm^2 stripes, which were used to close wounds. According to Albert Ehrenfried (1880–1951) [27, 28], this resulted in faster epithelialization, less scar formation, and less contraction. The *Ollier graft* was further modified by Carl Thiersch (1822–1895): He used split-thickness skin graft of 0.2–0.25 mm by tangential excision, and thereby also reduced the granulation tissue, anticipating the granulation tissue's role in the subsequent contraction. The *"Thiersch Graft"* was the standard procedure for skin grafting for nearly 100 years [25], which reduced donor site complications as well. George Lawson (1831–1903) was the first to describe full-thickness graft use to repair the eyelid's skin defects in 1871. John Reissberg Wolfe (1823–1904) from Glasgow published this method in 1875; Friedrich von Esmarch (1823–1908) [29] described its usage in other plastic surgical operations on the face simultaneously, and Fjedor Krause (1857–1937), founder of modern neurosurgery, established full-thickness grafts for any reconstructive purposes in 1893 [30].

Methods such as micro-dermagrafting proposed by Cicero Parker Meek (1914–1979, Meek-Grafting) [39] in 1958 did not gain relevance as an isolated method in scar reconstruction due to the limited cosmesis of the results [40]. However, it is still used in larger burns or complicated ulcers considering that the graftable area is maximized while the donor site defects remain relatively small.

The most commonly used graft type nowadays is an unmeshed sheet graft with different thicknesses. The reduced availability of healthy skin forced the development of alternatives, resulting in dermal transplants, which were secondarily grafted with split-thickness skin, as it was realized that the minor quality of the transplanted epidermis was based on the lack of soft and pliable dermis. This was later expressed by the words: "Epidermis is life and dermis is quality of life," attributed to Michel Rives.

Technical Development

Technical advancements were crucial for the proper harvest of split skin. In 1920, Finociette developed a knife to facilitate the harvesting of homogenous split skin [31]. In 1934, Humby's knife followed, combined with a frame to produce a flat donor site [32]. Subsequently, different knives were developed, and after Reese [33] and Padgett's drum dermatome [32], which used glue to harvest and transport skin, H. M. Brown developed a power-driven dermatome during World War II during his Japanese imprisonment [34], which allowed surgeons to remove larger pieces of skin faster [32].

The Swiss professor Otto Lanz (1865–1935) first described meshed skin grafts in 1907 and developed a device which he called "Hautschlitzapparat," reminiscent of the scarificator used with cupping to extract blood from inflammation [35]. Beverly Douglas (1891–1975) reported the use of a sieve graft in extended skin loss cases in 1930 [36], and his publication started the graft's success [37]. These were followed by Stryker and Padget's dermatomes, which were electrically driven. The development of dermatomes is still ongoing, with circular ones for accelerated excisions developed in recent years [38].

History of the Understanding of Skin Tension and Scar Prophylaxis

The avoidance of scars by preserving healthy tissue and reducing donor sites is an essential step in the prophylaxis of scar development. Nowadays, knives are replaced by enzyme-based debridement in some indications [41, 42]. This avoids the resection of healthy tissue for the complete removal of necrosis and escharotomies in many cases [43], but this method is rarely used in reconstructive surgery.

Based on the observations by Guillaume Dupuytren (1777–1835) [44] and Joseph-François Malgaigne (1806–1865), who noted that a rounded body awl produced not round but rather linear clefts, the Austrian anatomist Karl Langer von Edenberg (1819–1887) published his observations in 1961 on the anatomy and physiology of the skin with a detailed description of the tension lines of the skin [45]. He recognized that the form of skin defects was dependent on the direction of the dermal fibers under the papillary layer of the skin. The dermal fibers were arranged in a longitudinal or rhomboidal form dominant in high-mobility areas of the skin. In 1895, Theodor Kocher (1841–1917) promoted Langer's lines as a direction for skin incisions and excisions [46] predominantly at the trunk, but not at the extremities. In 1927, the dermatologist Felix Pinkus (1868–1947) described the main folding lines of the skin and the wrinkle lines produced by pinching the skin. These lines were related by Kraissl in 1949 to the underlying muscle fascia, as the connective tissue was fixed to the fascia. Kraissl [47] recommended surgical incision lines perpendicular to the underlying muscle fiber direction. Borges described the "relaxed skin tension lines" based on the aforementioned findings in 1962. These lines follow the skin folding lines in the face and at the trunk [48, 49]. On these grounds, incision lines and techniques for the avoidance of increased skin tension and resulting hypertrophic scars have been developed and are still a field of discussion.

Identification of the Myofibroblast

Avoidance of scars refers to the avoidance of mechanical forces in a scar, based on the research work of Alexis Carrel [50, 51]. During World War I, in 1915, due to insufficient knowledge about the treatment of infected wounds, and with money from the Rockefeller Foundation and cooperation with the French military, Carrel established an experimental hospital in Compiegne, just 12 miles from the front lines [51]. Together with the British chemist, Henry

Drysdale Dakin (1880–1952), they developed the Carrel–Dakin method to treat easily infected wounds to not result in gangrene. When the Americans entered the war, they established a demonstration hospital in Manhattan where they taught their very successful treatment method. The increased number of survivors with scars of any type heightened interest in the pathophysiology of scars. In 1908, Carrel et al. studied wound sizes and the resulting cicatrization [50]. They recognized the correlation between the size of the wound and the velocity of repair, as well as the importance of contraction and epithelialization. In standardized wounds, the initial wound size was measured and compared to the scar size. Thus, they realized that wound contracture is a part of the routine wound healing.

Myofibroblasts' pathophysiological foundation of shrinking wounds, how scars react to tension [82], and the role of ongoing inflammation were initially unknown. Wound contracture can occur even without myofibroblasts [52]; the mechanism of myofibroblast generation and inhibition is an ongoing research topic [53].

In 1971, modified fibroblasts with smooth muscle-like structures in the granulation tissues of healing wounds were described by Gabbiani [54, 55], which he denoted as "myofibroblast." He stated that "the contractile activity of myofibroblasts is a crucial factor for connective tissue remodeling during wound healing and creates a stressed matrix, which in turn promotes myofibroblast differentiation in a mechanical feedback mechanism."

Myofibroblasts can originate from different sources, such as epithelial and endothelial cells, fibroblasts, smooth muscle cells, perivascular adventitia cells, and pericytes [54]. Further research has elucidated the type of myofibroblasts with different contractility. Smooth muscle actin (SMA) can be expressed in stress fibers and contributes to twice the contractility of SMA-negative fibroblasts [56].

Three conditions contribute to the generation of SMA-positive fibroblasts: TGF-β1 in an active form, extra cellular matrix (ECM) proteins such as the ED-A splice variant of fibronectin, and high extracellular mechanical stress during cell remodeling activity from the ECM [56]. Cell matrix junctions called "fibronexus" in vivo and in vitro and "supermature focal adhesions (FAs)" transfer the mechanoreception and small adherin-type cell adhesions form larger cell adherin-type junctions. The incorporation of α-SMA in pre-existing actin stress fibers occurs only when the substrate stiffness of ECM allows for the generation of supermature FAs [56]. Further research on this topic is ongoing.

Consequences of Surgery

Transferred into surgery, the most crucial prophylaxis methods are tension-free wound closure and a reduction of inflammation via reductions in mechanical stress [57].

Surgical methods to avoid tension and noninvasive treatment methods with dressings, which reduce oxidative stress and ongoing inflammation [58–61], are still being developed.

Surgical Toolbox

The Excision and Grafting of Scars

The observation that some scars are prone to contraction and shortened tissues may have influenced the initiation of scar surgery. The first intention might have been to remove the shortened and stiffer tissue by replacing it with "normal," possibly elastic, and new scar tissue.

The Interposition of Tissue

The surgical approach of interrupting scars to resolve contractures is to interpone healthy tissue. To date, this fundamental principle of scar treatment is used in different ways, either in the interposition of pediculated multi-layer flaps or by bringing in tissue using different modalities such as laser punction, or micro-needling, creating holes filled with regenerative tissue that does not have the contractile properties of the original scars.

Flap Surgery

Transposition Flaps and Z-Plasty

After precursors with single transposition flaps by Johann Karl Georg Fricke (1970–1841) in 1829 and William Edmonds Horner (1793–1853) in 1837 [62], Charles-Pierre Denonvilliers (1808–1872) first described the Z-Plasty in 1856, originally using it for eyelid corrections; it evolved to be a "working horse" in plastic surgery. Surgery using different kinds of flaps to resolve scars demonstrates the close link between scar correction procedures and the history of plastic surgery. Historically, the development of different flaps did not correct scar issues; but rather, the flaps simply corrected the patient's outer appearance and covered more significant defects [63].

Distant Flaps

The first corrections of nose and earlobe defects can be traced to Sushruta and the old-Indian healing art [64, 65], in approximately 600 BC. After pediculated random-pattern flaps were developed as advancement flaps, cross-leg, first performed by Frank Hastings Hamilton (1813–1886) in 1854, cross-arm, or even wandering flaps with a limited length-to-width ratio [19] followed. The consecutive steps were axially vascularized flaps: used as pre-expanded or later as free or perforator-based flaps [66–68]. The introduction of the operative microscope in the early 1960s enabled microvascular surgical procedures [21].

Milestones in Flap Development

Pedicled and free flaps were performed with increasing expertise in microvascular anatomy and microsurgery, and free flaps became the problem-solvers in scar treatment, often combined with extensive scar excision.

Igino Tansini (1855–1943) first described myocutaneous breast reconstruction by including the latissimus dorsi muscle in 1896, respectively, in 1906 [69]. His primary intention was to cover skin defects after breast surgery. After problems with the initial flap design, he studied the vascular situation of the trunk and identified the Arteria circumflexa scapulae as the feeding artery of his planned flap. As the artery also perfuses parts of the M. latissimus dorsi, this myocutaneous flap provided good skin defect repair after total mastectomy with parts of the pectoral muscle removed [69].

Unaware of Tansini's technique, Olivari introduced the term "Latissimus flap" in 1976 [70]. This pedicled island flap was increasingly used to reconstruct the breast and thoracic defects, and multiple other indications in reconstructive surgery were treated with the free latissimus dorsi flap procedure. The fasciocutaneous pedicled and the later-developed free axillary flaps, such as the scapular and parascapular flaps derived from the subscapular axis, are commonly used in plastic surgery. However, the enthusiasm for different free flaps for the correction of scars was soon diminished due to high donor site morbidity and limited cosmetic results with often thick flaps.

Fascial flaps such as the free temporal fascial flap (Smith 1980, Brent 1984) and the Serratus fascial flap (Wintsch 1986) have a thinner character, yet they require additional autologous split-thickness skin coverage. These flaps enable scar reconstruction on the dorsum of the hands and feet, with improved functionality and fewer cosmetic disadvantages. Different flaps were recommended in cervicothoracic and axillary contractures with the elasticity and thickness of the skin to be replaced being considered.

Perforator Flaps

Based on studies by Manchot [71] and Salmon [72], the era of perforator flaps began in the mid of the 1980s. Taylor and Palmer [73] defined static vascular territories, calling them angiosomes, which offered and explained a new approach to flap designs [74–77]. In 1984, Song introduced a free thigh flap based on a septocutaneous artery. This flap was later called the anterolateral thigh (ALT) flap and proved to be a stable and versatile flap that is still frequently used [78]. Koshima and Soeda described an inferior epigastric artery pediculated flap in 1989 [74], which was later called the deep inferior epigastric perforator (DIEP) flap [75]. The thoracodorsal artery perforator (TDAP) flap is a perforator-based advancement of the Latissimus dorsi flap without the muscle portion, as described in 1995 [79].

In 2009, Saint-Cyr defined multiple perforasomes as the vascular territories of the perforators [80]. The propeller flap method was generated based on perforator vessels [81]. The propeller perforator flaps follow the definition of a skin island with two paddles where the demarcation limit between them is the perforator. The main advantages of the perforator flaps were the "sparing of the source artery and underlying muscle and fascia, the combining of the excellent blood supply of a musculocutaneous flap with the reduced donor-site morbidity of a skin flap and the replacing like with like" [82].

Some free flaps often result in clumsy and bumpy areas in which the thickness must be reduced. They must also be adapted and combined with other methods such as Z-plasties in order to provide acceptable results in further procedures and to not create problems with the methods chosen to solve others. In 2011 at the ECPB (European Club of Pediatric Burns) meeting in Zürich, Donalan generated the idiom of "SAD faces" (Surgically Acquired Deformity) and established the principles of facial burns reconstruction (see Table 1).

Skin Substitutes

Dermal Templates

The restoration of the dermal layers has become a clear focus of burn scar reconstruction [83]. In the 1970s, biosynthetic or fully synthetic dermal templates were developed. Integra® [84] as a dual-step procedure and Matriderm® [85] as a single-step procedure, and the recently developed

Table 1 Some important rules for scars treatment

Stay calm; things will get better
Scar excision is an oxymoron
Scars are your friends
Relaxed scars are happy scars
Tight is never right
Sins of commission are the worst
A normal-looking face with scars is better than a grotesque face with fewer scars

(Courtesy of Mattias Donelan, ECPB 2014 Boston)

Biological Technical Matrix (BTM) [86] added additional tools to the armamentarium of burn scar improvement methods and partly provided long-term results of more than 10 years [87]. Multiple dermal substitutes were tested, reached product status, and were competing as sufficient dermal substitutes [88–90]. Different prototypes for developing a skin substitute with an increased antiscar and antimicrobial capabilities were compared in terms of their physical properties, impact on healing, inflammation, fibroblast, and myofibroblast differentiation, and mesenchymal stem cell growth, all without long-term results or a definitive advantage established [91–94]. However, the limiting components remained infection and contracture.

Seeding on Dermal Templates

Research on seeding noncultivated keratinocyte suspensions on different templates is ongoing [95–99]. Larson created a suspension with BTM® [100], a foam from polyurethane, and RECELL® [101] in 2020. The method used by Stratagraft® involving the use of NIKS cells, which are pathogen-free, long-lived, and consistent human keratinocyte progenitors [102–104], is solving the challenge of acute nonavailable epidermal cells. Another method is to use fully tissue-engineered skin substitutes. As scar reconstruction is usually a planned procedure, there is time to prepare the substitute, which may take several weeks. Modern tissue engineering has resulted in extracorporeally created skin with epidermal, dermal, and subcutaneous layers [105]. Development is still ongoing, and a single-step procedure without a long waiting period available in the OR is currently under investigation for burns (SkinTE®) [106].

Full Skin Substitutes

Skin substitutes cannot only be used to extend treatment windows to avoid the development of bad scars, but they can also be used as fillers of defects following scar excision. As scar reconstruction can be planned as a dual-step procedure, bioengineered skin can be developed for definitive operations.

Developed by the Zurich Tissue Biology Research Unit International Cooperation at the University Children's Hospital, denovoSkin® is a promising bio-engineered personalized dermo-epidermal skin graft. Auspicious results from case reports are currently in the publishing process, and phase I and II studies are ongoing in the Netherlands and Switzerland [107].

SkinTE® is a fully autologous skin product. After taking a full-thickness sample from the patient's skin, it will be sent back within 48–72 h with a syringe, and the final cream-like product can then be applied to the wound. After 12 weeks, the regenerated skin was of good quality, which was "grossly equivalent to healthy skin with skin appendages and sensation and pigmentation" [108, 109]. Trials are registered and recruiting venous leg ulcers and diabetic foot ulcers for treatment [110]. Recently, the company published the first results of a burn study [106] with promising results.

An engineered skin substitute (ESS) is an autologous skin substitute from fibroblasts and keratinocytes attached to a collagen-based scaffold. In 2017, Boyce reported on 15 subjects with full-thickness burns with a mean TBSA of 76.9%. The mean percentage of closed TBSA with ESS was 29.9%. The results indicated a significant reduction in mortality and the requirements for skin harvesting [111]. The results of ongoing studies are expected soon [112].

Stratagraft® is a high-tech product used in skin development that uses different cells for the epidermal layer. A dermal–epidermal graft consists of a dermal equivalent from human dermal fibroblasts and a fully stratified biologically active dermis derived from NIKS cells; Centanni demonstrated its effectiveness in patients with traumatic wounds [103]. It has been successfully used in patients with deep partial-thickness burns [113].

The development of dermal and epidermal substitutes to cover significant defects, even after the excision of inadequate burn scars, raises many currently unresolved issues such as pigmentation, sensibility, heat regulation, and finally, cost-effectiveness.

Allotransplantations

With increasing knowledge about immunology and immune suppression, vascularized composite tissue allotransplantation (VCA) has become an option as a surgical solution for traumatic extremity loss [114] as well as disfiguring and disabling scars after facial injuries. In November 2005, Jean Michelle Dubernard et al. carried out the first partial face transplantation in a patient who suffered severe consequences after a dog bite [115, 116]. The first near-total face transplant was performed in Cleveland by a group led by Maria Siemionow in 2008 [117], followed by full-face transplantations in 2010 in Spain and France and 2011 by Bohdan Pomahac in Boston [118]. The significant limiting aspect of this type of surgery is the life-long immunesuppressive medication [119].

Nonsurgical Toolbox

Laser

The precursor of Lasers (Light Amplification by Stimulated Emission of Radiation) was the Maser (Microwave Amplification by Stimulated Emission of Radiation) in the mid-1950s at the Lomonosov-University Moscow (Russia) and the Columbia University (USA) by Nikolai Gennadijewitsch Bassow and Alexander Michailowitsch Prochorow, and Charles Hard Townes [120]. In 1964, they were honored with the Nobel Prize in Physics for their fundamental research in quantum electronics [121].

The first functioning Laser was developed in 1960 by Theodore Herold Maiman [122]. First medical applications were described in the field of ophthalmology in 1961 [123]. Two years later, the first reports about laser treatment of the skin were published by Goldman et al. [124]. Publications of laser treatments of scars followed about 30 years later.

Non-ablative flashlamp-pumped pulse dye lasers (FPDLs) are used in different scar types, such as hypertrophic and burn scars, which are usually associated with hyperemia [125–127].

Ablative lasers such as the CO_2-laser have also been used for scar resurfacing and for the treatment of atrophic scars [128, 129]; they have become sufficient parts of therapeutic concepts together with cryotherapy, compression, or corticosteroid injection. Non-ablative lasers are also used to treat acne scars by creating an interwoven collagen structure in the scar dermis, which is comparable to normal skin [130]. In the treatment of trauma and burn scars, ablative and non-ablative lasers have positive effects on scar contracture, pigmentation, and pruritus.

Fractional laser application that induces fractional photothermolysis creates numerous thermal injury zones with diameters of less than 500 μm. Epidermal and dermal tissues fill the holes with regenerative cells from the surroundings, showing an elevation of heat shock proteins over several months. The collagens created are type III and fetal collagen, while collagen type I is reduced [131].

Micro-needling

Similar principles as in fractional ablative laser treatment apply in medical needling techniques. Orentreich first described subcision and dermal needling for scars in 1995 [132]. Furthermore, in 2005, Fernandes described the percutaneous collagen induction therapy, and in 2009, Aust treated hypertrophic scars with medical needling. The prick initiates the wound healing cascade, releasing growth factors by macrophages and initiates the proliferation of fibroblasts, keratinocytes, and melanocytes, resulting in an increased epidermal thickness [133, 134] and improved scar pigmentation. The inflammatory process is curbed, and during the maturation and remodeling phase, collagen type III is replaced by type I, while collagen cross-links with increasing tensile strength are formed.

Fat Grafting

Fat grafting is a method of transferring different preparations of fat as a graft to correct volumetric deficits with different therapeutic principles. Fat grafting per se can also be considered a surgical treatment method.

Fat grafting was first mentioned in 1893 by Franz Neuber [135]. Vincenz Cerny (1842–1916) transferred a patient's lipoma for breast reconstruction [136] and Charles Conrad Miller (1926) infiltrated fat tissue through small cannulas [137].

By introducing liposuction in Europe in the early 1980s, plastic surgeons realized the value of the "waste" product that was initially used to fill depressive defects or body contouring issues described by Illouz in 1986 [138]. The cumulative source of mesenchymal stem cells in fat tissues is the background of autologous fat transfer in scar remodeling. Fat transfer results in a reduction of pain and increased elasticity of the scar. Aesthetic and functional improvements [139] were positive side effects of the method.

Other Scar Treatment Modalities

Further conservative supportive measures in scar treatment should be noted, including pressure therapy with compression garments, occlusive or silicone treatments, local injections, radiation, and physiotherapeutic options such as massage. It is difficult to relate these options to the history of scar treatment. These methods are thoroughly discussed in the respective chapters.

Conclusion and Outlook

The treatment of scars was severely limited in the history of humankind. Treatment with balms, creams, or plant extracts followed the current state of science and histopathological knowledge. Although the foundations today seem very different from earlier ones, similar procedures are now explained with a different scientific background. An example of this might be the bloody cupping of a scar, done to "dissipate heat" in ancient times. Nowadays, our pathophysiological understanding explains the ingrowth of new tissue and the release of growth factors for creating new tissue, the interruption of scars, tension release, and reduction of redness and swelling as the mechanism of action of needling or microincisions.

The effects of many methods were evaluated over time, and some were the standards for scar treatment. Compression, massage, treatment with light, physiotherapy and occupational therapy, psychological and social support, and other methods were the primary methods to treat scars out of necessity. Successful surgical methods were developed later, requiring preconditions and tools, as described in the chapters above. The recent advances in pathophysiology, primarily advancements in our understanding of scar pathogenesis and the biomechanical reactivity of cells as well as the avoidance of ongoing inflammation at the cellular level, appear to be crucial for all methods. Modern methods allow nearly every scar to be treated and improved in one way or another.

The search for the holy grail of scar-less wound healing and reverting scars into intact skin without visible changes is ongoing and possibly never successful. It will require much more successful basic and clinical research, as well as modesty in judging the results. Meanwhile, it should be accepted that minimizing the patient's suffering and not the surgeon's ambition should be the driving force of a treatment.

"Primum non nocere, secundum cavere, tertium sanare" is a historical principle of a Hippocratic tradition that is still valid. Time has not changed these fundamental aspects. Even the best methods of scar correction should not distract from the fact that prophylaxis is better than the best treatment.

References

1. Hestia—Wikipedia. https://en.wikipedia.org/wiki/Hestia. Accessed 28 Apr 2021.
2. Brown DA, Gibran NS. History of wound care. In: Handbook of burns, volume 1. Acute burn care. New York: Springer; 2012.
3. Petro JA. An idiosyncratic history of burn scars. Semin Cutan Med Surg. 2015;34:2–6. https://doi.org/10.12788/j.sder.2015.0140.
4. Britannica. History of medicine | History & Facts | Britannica. https://www.britannica.com/science/history-of-medicine#ref35642. Accessed 21 Mar 2021.
5. Wikipedia. Chirurgie. https://de.wikipedia.org/wiki/Chirurgie. Accessed 23 Mar 2021.
6. Dawson WR. The papyrus ebers. J R Asiat Soc Great Britain Ireland. 1936;68:179–84. https://doi.org/10.1017/s0035869x00077108.
7. History of medicine—Traditional medicine and surgery in Asia | Britannica. https://www.britannica.com/science/history-of-medicine/Traditional-medicine-and-surgery-in-Asia#ref35645. Accessed 21 Mar 2021.
8. Herophilos von Chalkedon—Wikipedia. https://de.wikipedia.org/wiki/Herophilos_von_Chalkedon. Accessed 23 Mar 2021.
9. Gehrig R. Die Geschichte der Anatomie. Zürich: Cranioschule KmG; 2005.
10. Ang GC. History of skin transplantation. Clin Dermatol. 2005;23:320–4. https://doi.org/10.1016/j.clindermatol.2004.07.013.
11. On Medicine—World Digital Library. https://www.wdl.org/en/item/11618/. Accessed 28 Apr 2021.
12. Nova A. Die anatomischen Zeichnungen Leonardo da Vincis als Erkenntnismittel und reflektierte Kunstpraxis 1. Zeitsprünge Forschungen Zur Frühen Neuzeit. 2005;9:101–30.
13. Anesthesia and Queen Victoria. https://www.ph.ucla.edu/epi/snow/victoria.html. Accessed 24 Apr 2021.
14. Anaesthetics and their administration: a text book/ by the late Sir Frederic W. Hewitt.—University of Queensland. https://search.library.uq.edu.au/primo-explore/fulldisplay?vid=61UQ&search_scope=61UQ_All&tab=61uq_all&docid=61UQ_ALMA21103452610003131&lang=en_US&context=L. Accessed 28 Apr 2021.
15. Erving HW. The discoverer of anæsthesia: Dr. Horace Wells of Hartford. Yale J Biol Med. 1933;5:421–30.
16. Thoughts on the 150th anniversary of anesthesia. https://pubmed.ncbi.nlm.nih.gov/8992901/. Accessed 20 June 2021.
17. Balanced anesthesia | Definition of balanced anesthesia by Medical dictionary. https://medical-dictionary.thefreedictionary.com/balanced+anesthesia. Accessed 27 Apr 2021.
18. Brown EM, McGriff JT, Malinowski RW. Intravenous regional anaesthesia (Bier block): review of 20 years' experience. Can J Anaesth. 1989;36:307–10. https://doi.org/10.1007/BF03010770.
19. Bolli R. William Harvey and the discovery of the circulation of the blood: part II. Circ Res. 2019;124:1300–2. https://doi.org/10.1161/CIRCRESAHA.119.314977.
20. Konstantinov IE. Eck-Pavlov shunt: the 120th anniversary of the first vascular anastomosis. Surgery. 1997;121:640–5. https://doi.org/10.1016/S0039-6060(97)90052-0.
21. Rickard RF, Hudson DA. A history of vascular and microvascular surgery. Ann Plast Surg. 2014;73:465–72. https://doi.org/10.1097/SAP.0b013e3182710027.

22. Hauben DJ, Baruchin A, Mahler D. On the history of the free skin graft. Ann Plast Surg. 1982;9:242–6. https://doi.org/10.1097/00000637-198209000-00009.

23. Klasen HJ. History of free skin grafting. New York: Springer; 1981. https://doi.org/10.1007/978-3-642-81653-6.

24. Zheng H, Watkins B, Tkachev V, Yu S, Tran D, Furlan S, et al. The Knife's edge of tolerance: inducing stable multilineage mixed chimerism but with a significant risk of CMV reactivation and disease in rhesus macaques HHS public access. Am J Transplant. 2017;17:657–70. https://doi.org/10.1111/ajt.14006.

25. Singh M, Nuutila K, Collins KC, Huang A. Evolution of skin grafting for treatment of burns: Reverdin pinch grafting to Tanner mesh grafting and beyond. Burns. 2017;43:1149–54. https://doi.org/10.1016/j.burns.2017.01.015.

26. Louis Léopold Ollier—Wikipedia. https://en.wikipedia.org/wiki/Louis_Léopold_Ollier. Accessed 27 Apr 2021.

27. Ehrenfried A. https://www.whonamedit.com/doctor.cfm/1954.html. Accessed 4 July 2021.

28. Ehrenfried A. Reverdin and other methods of skin-grafting. Boston Med Surg J. 1909;161:911–7. https://doi.org/10.1056/NEJM190912231612601.

29. von Esmarch F. https://en.wikipedia.org/wiki/Friedrich_von_Esmarch. Accessed 4 July 2021.

30. Kohlhauser M, Luze H, Nischwitz SP, Kamolz LP. Historical evolution of skin grafting—a journey through time. Medicina (Lithuania). 2021;57:1–14. https://doi.org/10.3390/medicina57040348.

31. Zuo KJ, Medina A, Tredget EE. Important developments in burn care. Plast Reconstr Surg. 2017;139:120e–38e. https://doi.org/10.1097/PRS.0000000000002908.

32. Menon S, Li Z, Harvey JG, Holland AJA. The use of the Meek technique in conjunction with cultured epithelial autograft in the management of major paediatric burns. Burns. 2013;39:674–9. https://doi.org/10.1016/j.burns.2012.09.009.

33. Santoni-Rugiu P, Sykes PJ. A history of plastic surgery. Berlin: Springer; 2007. https://doi.org/10.1007/978-3-540-46241-5.

34. Ameer F, Singh A, Kumar S. Evolution of instruments for harvest of the skin grafts. Indian J Plast Surg. 2013;46:28–35. https://doi.org/10.4103/0970-0358.113704.

35. Stark RB. John Davies Reese and the Reese dermatome. Ann Plast Surg. 1979;2:80–3. https://doi.org/10.1097/00000637-197901000-00014.

36. Chick LR. Brief history and biology of skin grafting. Ann Plast Surg. 1988;21(4):358–65.

37. Haeseker B. Forerunners of mesh grafting machines. From cupping glasses and scarificators to modern mesh graft instruments. Br J Plast Surg. 1988;41:209–12. https://doi.org/10.1016/0007-1226(88)90056-2.

38. Vandeput J, Nelissen M, Tanner JC, Boswick J. A review of skin meshers. Burns. 1995;21:364–70. https://doi.org/10.1016/0305-4179(94)00008-5.

39. Douglas B. The sieve graft—a stable transport for covering large skin defects. Surg Gyn Obstet. 1930;50:180.

40. Savetamal A, Wenta S. 660 Decreasing burn excision time by using a circular dermatome. J Burn Care Res. 2021;42(Supplement_1):S185–6.

41. Edmondson SJ, Ali Jumabhoy I, Murray A. Time to start putting down the knife: a systematic review of burns excision tools of randomised and non-randomised trials. Burns. 2018;44:1721–37. https://doi.org/10.1016/j.burns.2018.01.012.

42. Rosenberg L, Krieger Y, Bogdanov-Berezovski A, Silberstein E, Shoham Y, Singer AJ. A novel rapid and selective enzymatic debridement agent for burn wound management: a multi-center RCT. Burns. 2014;40:466–74. https://doi.org/10.1016/j.burns.2013.08.013.

43. Hirche C, Citterio A, Hoeksema H, Koller J, Lehner M, Martinez JR, et al. Eschar removal by bromelain based enzymatic debridement (Nexobrid®) in burns: an European consensus. Burns. 2017;43:1640–53. https://doi.org/10.1016/j.burns.2017.07.025.

44. Cited by Langer 1861; N.A. Über die Verletzungen durch Kriegswaffen.

45. Abyaneh MAY, Griffith R, Falto-Aizpurua L, Nouri K. Famous lines in history: Langer lines. JAMA Dermatol. 2014;150:1087. https://doi.org/10.1001/jamadermatol.2014.659.

46. Kocher TDr. Textbook of operative surgery. London: Adam and Charles Black; 1895.

47. Kraissl CJ. The selection of appropriate lines for elective surgical incisions. Plast Reconstr Surg. 1951;8:1–28. https://doi.org/10.1097/00006534-195107000-00001.

48. Borges AF, Alexander JE. Relaxed skin tension lines, z-plasties on scars, and fusiform excision of lesions. Br J Plast Surg. 1962;15:242–54. https://doi.org/10.1016/S0007-1226(62)80038-1.

49. Borges AF. Relaxed skin tension lines (RSTL) versus other skin lines. Plast Reconstr Surg. 1984;73:144–50. https://doi.org/10.1097/00006534-198401000-00036.

50. Carrel A, Hartmann A. Cicatrization of wounds: I. The relation between the size of a wound and the rate of its cicatrization. J Exp Med. 1916;24:429–50. https://doi.org/10.1084/jem.24.5.429.

51. Selcer P. Standardizing wounds: Alexis Carrel and the scientific management of life in the first world war. Br J Hist Sci. 2008;41:73–107. https://doi.org/10.1017/S0007087407000295.

52. Ibrahim MM, Chen L, Bond JE, Medina MA, Ren L, Kokosis G, et al. Myofibroblasts contribute to but are not necessary for wound contraction. Lab Invest. 2015;95:1429–38. https://doi.org/10.1038/labinvest.2015.116.

53. Kottmann RM, Trawick E, Judge JL, Wahl LA, Epa AP, Owens KM, et al. Pharmacologic inhibition of lactate production prevents myofibroblast differentiation. Am J Phys Lung Cell Mol Phys.

2015;309:L1305–12. https://doi.org/10.1152/ajplung.00058.2015.

54. Ribatti D, Tamma R. Giulio Gabbiani and the discovery of myofibroblasts. Inflamm Res. 2019;68:241–5. https://doi.org/10.1007/s00011-018-01211-x.

55. Gabbiani G, Ryan GB, Majno G. Presence of modified fibroblasts in granulation tissue and their possible role in wound contraction. Experientia. 1971;27:549–50. https://doi.org/10.1007/BF02147594.

56. Hinz B, Phan SH, Thannickal VJ, Galli A, Bochaton-Piallat ML, Gabbiani G. The myofibroblast: one function, multiple origins. Am J Pathol. 2007;170:1807–16. https://doi.org/10.2353/ajpath.2007.070112.

57. Lee HJ, Jang YJ. Recent understandings of biology, prophylaxis and treatment strategies for hypertrophic scars and keloids. Int J Mol Sci. 2018;19:711. https://doi.org/10.3390/ijms19030711.

58. Gürünlüoglu K, Demircan M, Taşçl A, Üremiş MM, Türköz Y, Bag HG, et al. The effects of two different burn dressings on serum oxidative stress indicators in children with partial burn. J Burn Care Res. 2019;40:444–50. https://doi.org/10.1093/jbcr/irz037.

59. Demircan M, Gürünlüoğlu K, Bayrakçı E, Taşçı A. Effects of Suprathel®, Aquacel® Ag or autografting on human telomerase reverse transcriptase expression in the healing skin in children with partial thickness burn. Ann Burns Fire Disasters. 2017;48:49.

60. Demircan M, Gürünlüoğlu K, Gözükara Bağ HG, Koçbıyık A, Gül M, Üremiş N, et al. Pediyatrik yanık hastalarında polilaktik membran veya gümüşlü hidrofiber pansumanların kan ve dokuda interlökin-6, tümör nekrozis faktör-α, transforming büyüme faktörü-b3 düzeylerine etkisi. Ulusal Travma ve Acil Cerrahi Dergisi Turk J Trauma Emerg Surg TJTES. 2020;27:122–31. https://doi.org/10.14744/tjtes.2020.30483.

61. Ogawa R. Keloid and hypertrophic scars are the result of chronic inflammation in the reticular dermis. Int J Mol Sci. 2017;18:606. https://doi.org/10.3390/ijms18030606.

62. Hundeshagen G, Zapata-Sirvent R, Goverman J, Branski LK. Tissue rearrangements: the power of the Z-plasty. Clin Plast Surg. 2017;44:805–12. https://doi.org/10.1016/j.cps.2017.05.011.

63. Bhishagratna K. An English translation of the Sushruta Samhita, based on original Sanskrit text. Toronto: University of Toronto; 1907.

64. Converse JM, Coburn RJ. The twitching scar. Br J Plast Surg. 1971;24:272–6. https://doi.org/10.1016/S0007-1226(71)80068-1.

65. Zeis E. Literatur und Geschichte der plastischen Chirurgie. Leipzig: Wilhelm Engelmann; 2012.

66. Pallua N, Kim BS. Pre-expanded supraclavicular artery perforator flap. Clin Plast Surg. 2017;44:49–63. https://doi.org/10.1016/j.cps.2016.08.005.

67. Pallua N, Wolter TP. Moving forwards: the anterior supraclavicular artery perforator (a-SAP) flap: a new pedicled or free perforator flap based on the anterior supraclavicular vessels. J Plast Reconstr Aesthet Surg. 2013;66:489–96. https://doi.org/10.1016/j.bjps.2012.11.013.

68. Heitland AS, Pallua N. The single and double-folded supraclavicular Island flap as a new therapy option in the treatment of large facial defects in Noma patients. Plast Reconstr Surg. 2005;115:1591–6. https://doi.org/10.1097/01.PRS.0000160694.20881.F4.

69. Maxwell GP. Iginio Tansini and the origin of the latissimus dorsi musculocutaneous flap. Plast Reconstr Surg. 1980;65:686–92. https://doi.org/10.1097/00006534-198005000-00027.

70. Olivari N. The latissimus flap. Br J Plast Surg. 1976;29:126–8. https://doi.org/10.1016/0007-1226(76)90036-9.

71. Manchot C, Daniel RK. The cutaneous arteries of the human body. Plast Reconstr Surg. 1986;77:495. https://doi.org/10.1097/00006534-198603000-00035.

72. Salmon MTG, Tempest M. Arteries of the skin. London: Churchill Livingstone; 1988.

73. Taylor GI, Palmer JH. The vascular territories (angiosomes) of the body: experimental study and clinical applications. Br J Plast Surg. 1987;40:113–41. https://doi.org/10.1016/0007-1226(87)90185-8.

74. Koshima I, Soeda S. Inferior epigastric artery skin flaps without rectus abdominis muscle. Br J Plast Surg. 1989;42:645–8. https://doi.org/10.1016/0007-1226(89)90075-1.

75. Allen RJ, Treece P. Deep inferior epigastric perforator flap for breast reconstruction. Ann Plast Surg. 1994;32:32–8. https://doi.org/10.1097/00000637-199401000-00007.

76. Song YG, Chen GZ, Song YL. The free thigh flap: a new free flap concept based on the septocutaneous artery. Br J Plast Surg. 1984;37:149–59. https://doi.org/10.1016/0007-1226(84)90002-X.

77. Kroll SS, Rosenfield L. Perforator-based flaps for low posterior midline defects. Plast Reconstr Surg. 1988;81:561–6. https://doi.org/10.1097/00006534-198804000-00012.

78. Wei FC, Jain V, Celik N, Chen HC, Chuang DCC, Lin CH. Have we found an ideal soft-tissue flap? An experience with 672 anterolateral thigh flaps. Plast Reconstr Surg. 2002;109:2219–26. https://doi.org/10.1097/00006534-200206000-00007.

79. Angrigiani C, Grilli D, Siebert J. Latissimus dorsi musculocutaneous flap without muscle. Plast Reconstr Surg. 1995;96:1608–14. https://doi.org/10.1097/00006534-199512000-00014.

80. Saint-Cyr M, Wong C, Schaverien M, Mojallal A, Rohrich RJ. The perforasome theory: vascular anatomy and clinical implications. Plast Reconstr Surg. 2009;124:1529–44. https://doi.org/10.1097/PRS.0b013e3181b98a6c.

81. Hyakusoku H, Yamamoto T, Fumiiri M. The propeller flap method. Br J Plast Surg. 1991;44:53–4. https://doi.org/10.1016/0007-1226(91)90179-N.

82. Georgescu AV. Propeller perforator flaps in distal lower leg: evolution and clinical applications. Arch Plast Surg. 2012;39:94–105. https://doi.org/10.5999/aps.2012.39.2.94.

83. van Zuijlen P, Gardien K, Jaspers M, Bos E, Baas D, van Trier A, et al. Tissue engineering in burn scar reconstruction. Burns Trauma. 2015;3:1–11. https://doi.org/10.1186/s41038-015-0017-5.

84. Yannas IV, Burke JF. Design of an artificial skin. I. Basic design principles. J Biomed Mater Res. 1980;14:65–81. https://doi.org/10.1002/jbm.820140108.

85. van Zuijlen PPM, van Trier AJM, Vloemans JFPM, Groenevelt F, Kreis RW, Middelkoop E, et al. Graft survival and effectiveness of dermal substitution in burns and reconstructive surgery in a one-stage grafting model. Plast Reconstr Surg. 2000;106:615–23. https://doi.org/10.1097/00006534-200009030-00014.

86. Wagstaff MJD, Schmitt BJ, Coghlan P, Finkemeyer JP, Caplash Y, Greenwood JE. A biodegradable polyurethane dermal matrix in reconstruction of free flap donor sites: a pilot study. Eplasty. 2015;15:e13.

87. De Angelis B, Orlandi F, D'Autilio FLMM, Scioli MG, Orlandi A, Cervelli V, et al. Long-term follow-up comparison of two different bi-layer dermal substitutes in tissue regeneration: clinical outcomes and histological findings. Int Wound J. 2018;15:695–706. https://doi.org/10.1111/iwj.12912.

88. Moscovici M. Present and future medical applications of microbial exopolysaccharides. Front Microbiol. 2015;6:1–11. https://doi.org/10.3389/fmicb.2015.01012.

89. Martinson M, Martinson N. A comparative analysis of skin substitutes used in the management of diabetic foot ulcers. J Wound Care. 2016;25:S8–17. https://doi.org/10.12968/jowc.2016.25.sup10.s8.

90. Luo X, Kulig KM, Finkelstein EB, Nicholson MF, Liu XH, Goldman SM, et al. In vitro evaluation of decellularized ECM-derived surgical scaffold biomaterials. J Biomed Mater Res Part B Appl Biomater. 2017;105:585–93. https://doi.org/10.1002/jbm.b.33572.

91. Woodroof A, Phipps R, Woeller C, Rodeheaver G, Naughton GK, Piney E, et al. Evolution of a biosynthetic temporary skin substitute: a preliminary study. Eplasty. 2015;15:e30.

92. Woeller CF, Woodroof A, Lacy SH, Cottler PS, Gui JL, Piñeros-Fernandez A, et al. Evaluating a variable porosity wound dressing with anti-scar properties in a porcine model of wound healing. Eplasty. 2018;18:e20.

93. Solanki NS, MacKie IP, Greenwood JE. A randomised prospective study of split skin graft donor site dressings: AWBAT-D™ vs. Duoderm®. Burns. 2012;38:889–98. https://doi.org/10.1016/j.burns.2011.12.022.

94. Wessels Q. Engineered alternative skin for partial and full-thickness burns. Bioengineered. 2014;5:161–4. https://doi.org/10.4161/bioe.28598.

95. Waaijman T, Breetveld M, Ulrich M, Middelkoop E, Scheper RJ, Gibbs S. Use of a collagen-elastin matrix as transport carrier system to transfer proliferating epidermal cells to human dermis in vitro. Cell Transplant. 2010;19:1339–48. https://doi.org/10.3727/096368910X507196.

96. Golinski PA, Zöller N, Kippenberger S, Menke H, Bereiter-Hahn J, Bernd A. Entwicklung eines transplantierbaren Hautäquivalentes auf Basis von Matriderm® mit menschlichen Keratinozyten und Fibroblasten. Handchirurgie Mikrochirurgie Plastische Chirurgie. 2009;41:327–32. https://doi.org/10.1055/s-0029-1234132.

97. Killat J, Reimers K, Choi CY, Jahn S, Vogt PM, Radtke C. Cultivation of keratinocytes and fibroblasts in a three-dimensional bovine collagen-elastin matrix (Matriderm®) and application for full thickness wound coverage in vivo. Int J Mol Sci. 2013;14:14460–74. https://doi.org/10.3390/ijms140714460.

98. ter Horst B, Chouhan G, Moiemen NS, Grover LM. Advances in keratinocyte delivery in burn wound care. Adv Drug Deliv Rev. 2018;123:18–32. https://doi.org/10.1016/j.addr.2017.06.012.

99. Beaudoin Cloutier C, Goyer B, Perron C, Guignard R, Larouche D, Moulin VJ, et al. In vivo evaluation and imaging of a bilayered self-assembled skin substitute using a decellularized dermal matrix grafted on mice. Tissue Eng Part A. 2017;23:313–22. https://doi.org/10.1089/ten.tea.2016.0296.

100. Greenwood JE, Wagstaff MJD. Changing practice in the surgical management of major burns—delayed definitive closure. J Burn Care Res. 2018;39:440.

101. Larson KW, Austin CL, Thompson SJ. Treatment of a full-thickness burn injury with NovoSorb biodegradable temporizing matrix and RECELL autologous skin cell suspension: a case series. J Burn Care Res. 2020;41:215. https://doi.org/10.1093/JBCR/IRZ179.

102. Roy M, King TW. Epidermal growth factor regulates NIKS keratinocyte proliferation through notch signaling. J Surg Res. 2013;185:6–11. https://doi.org/10.1016/j.jss.2013.06.046.

103. Centanni JM, Straseski JA, Wicks A, Hank JA, Rasmussen CA, Lokuta MA, et al. StrataGraft skin substitute is well-tolerated and is not acutely immunogenic in patients with traumatic wounds: results from a prospective, randomized, controlled dose escalation trial. Ann Surg. 2011;253:672–83. https://doi.org/10.1097/SLA.0b013e318210f3bd.

104. Schurr MJ, Foster KN, Centanni JM, Comer AR, Wicks A, Gibson AL, et al. Phase I/II clinical evaluation of StrataGraft: a consistent, pathogen-free human skin substitute. J Trauma. 2009;66:866–73. https://doi.org/10.1097/TA.0b013e31819849d6. Phase.

105. Meuli M, Hartmann-Fritsch F, Hüging M, Marino D, Saglini M, Hynes S, et al. A cultured autologous dermo-epidermal skin substitute for full-thickness skin defects: a phase I, open, prospective clinical trial

in children. Plast Reconstr Surg. 2019;144:188–98. https://doi.org/10.1097/PRS.0000000000005746.

106. Polarity TE. Announces data from head-to-head burn study demonstrating graft take and wound closure with SkinTE treatment | business wire. https://www.businesswire.com/news/home/20200413005104/en/PolarityTE-Announces-Data-from-Head-to-Head-Burn-Study-Demonstrating-Graft-Take-and-Wound-Closure-with-SkinTE-Treatment. Accessed 28 Apr 2021.

107. US National Library of Medicine. Autologous skin substitutes. ClinicalTrialsGov 2020:2020.

108. Granick MS, Baetz NW, Labroo P, Milner S, Li WW, Sopko NA. In vivo expansion and regeneration of full-thickness functional skin with an autologous homologous skin construct: clinical proof of concept for chronic wound healing. Int Wound J. 2019;16:841–6. https://doi.org/10.1111/iwj.13109.

109. Mundinger GS, Patterson CW. Replacement of contracted split-thickness skin graft and keloid scar with a self-propagating autologous skin co-author. PRS Glob Open. 2018;2018:2018.

110. Search of: PolarityTE—List results—ClinicalTrials.gov https://clinicaltrials.gov/ct2/results?cond=&term=PolarityTE&cntry=&state=&city=&dist=. Accessed 13 May 2020.

111. Boyce ST, Simpson PS, Rieman MT, Warner PM, Yakuboff KP, Bailey JK, et al. Randomized, paired-site comparison of autologous engineered skin substitutes and split-thickness skin graft for closure of extensive, full-thickness burns. J Burn Care Res. 2017;38:61–70. https://doi.org/10.1097/BCR.0000000000000401.

112. Safety and efficacy study of autologous engineered skin substitute to treat partial- and full-thickness burn wounds.. ClinicalTrials.gov https://clinicaltrials.gov/ct2/show/NCT01655407?term=engineered+skin+substitute&draw=2&rank=1. Accessed 13 May 2020.

113. Holmes JH, Schurr MJ, King BT, Foster K, Faucher LD, Lokuta MA, et al. An open-label, prospective, randomized, controlled, multicenter, phase 1b study of StrataGraft skin tissue versus autografting in patients with deep partial-thickness thermal burns. Burns. 2019;45:1749–58. https://doi.org/10.1016/j.burns.2019.07.021.

114. Brandacher G, Gorantla VS, Lee WPA. Hand allotransplantation. Semin Plast Surg. 2010;24:11–7. https://doi.org/10.1055/s-0030-1253243.

115. Dubernard JM, Devauchelle B. Face transplantation. Lancet. 2008;372:603–4. https://doi.org/10.1016/S0140-6736(08)61252-0.

116. Morelon E, Testelin S, Petruzzo P, Badet L, Kanitakis J, Eljafari A, et al. First face allograft in human: a 2 years follow up. Transplantation. 2008;86:311. https://doi.org/10.1097/01.tp.0000331835.40669.3b.

117. Siemionow M. Face transplantation: a leading surgeon's perspective. Transplant Proc. 2011;43:2850–2. https://doi.org/10.1016/j.transproceed.2011.08.059.

118. Pomahac B, Nowinski D, Diaz-Siso JR, Bueno EM, Talbot SG, Sinha I, et al. Face transplantation. Curr Probl Surg. 2011;48:293–357. https://doi.org/10.1067/j.cpsurg.2011.01.003.

119. Tasigiorgos S, Kollar B, Krezdorn N, Bueno EM, Tullius SG, Pomahac B. Face transplantation-current status and future developments. Transpl Int. 2018;31:677–88. https://doi.org/10.1111/tri.13130.

120. Gordon JP, Zeiger HJ, Townes CH. The maser new type of microwave amplifier, frequency standard and spectrometer. Phys Rev. 1955;99:1264.

121. Nobel Foundation. The Nobel Prize in physics 1964. https://www.nobelprize.org/prizes/physics/1964/summary/. Accessed 4 July 2021.

122. Maiman TH. Stimulated optical radiation in ruby. Nature. 1960;187:493–4. https://doi.org/10.1038/187493a0.

123. Zaret MM, Breinin GM, Schmidt H, Ripps H, Siegel IM, Solon LR. Ocular lesions produced by an optical maser (laser). Science. 1961;134:1525–6. https://doi.org/10.1126/science.134.3489.1525.

124. Goldman L, Blaney DJ, Kindel DJ, Franke EK. Effect of the laser beam on the skin. Preliminary report. J Invest Dermatol. 1963;40:121–2. https://doi.org/10.1038/jid.1963.21.

125. Alster TS. Improvement of erythematous and hypertrophic scars by the 585-nm flashlamp-pumped pulsed dye laser. Ann Plast Surg. 1994;32:186–90. https://doi.org/10.1097/00000637-199402000-00015.

126. Goldman MP, Fitzpatrick RE. Laser treatment of scars. Dermatol Surg. 1995;21:685–7. https://doi.org/10.1111/j.1524-4725.1995.tb00270.x.

127. Gaston P, Humzah MD, Quaba AA. The pulsed tuneable dye laser as an aid in the management of postburn scarring. Burns. 1996;22:203–5. https://doi.org/10.1016/0305-4179(95)00112-3.

128. Bernstein LJ, Kauvar ANB, Grossman MC, Geronemus RG. Scar resurfacing with high-energy, short-pulsed and flash scanning carbon dioxide lasers. Dermatol Surg. 1998;24:101–8. https://doi.org/10.1111/j.1524-4725.1998.tb04060.x.

129. Alster TS, West TB. Resurfacing of atrophic facial acne scars with a high-energy, pulsed carbon dioxide laser. Dermatol Surg. 1996;22:151–5. https://doi.org/10.1111/j.1524-4725.1996.tb00497.x.

130. Sirithanabadeekul P, Tantrapornpong P, Rattakul B, Sutthipisal N, Thanasarnaksorn W. Comparison of fractional picosecond 1064-nm laser and fractional carbon dioxide laser for treating atrophic acne scars: a randomized split-face trial. Dermatol Surg. 2021;47:e58–65. https://doi.org/10.1097/DSS.0000000000002572.

131. Fu X, Dong J, Wang S, Yan M, Yao M. Advances in the treatment of traumatic scars with laser, intense pulsed light, radiofrequency, and ultrasound. Burns Trauma. 2019;7:1–7. https://doi.org/10.1186/s41038-018-0141-0.

132. Orentreich DS, Orentreich N. Subcutaneous incisionless (subcision) surgery for the correction

of depressed scars and wrinkles. Dermatol Surg. 1995;21:543–9. https://doi.org/10.1111/j.1524-4725.1995.tb00259.x.

133. Aust MC, Fernandes D, Kolokythas P, Kaplan HM, Vogt PM. Percutaneous collagen induction therapy: an alternative treatment for scars, wrinkles, and skin laxity. Plast Reconstr Surg. 2008;121:1421–9. https://doi.org/10.1097/01.prs.0000304612.72899.02.

134. Aust MC, Reimers K, Kaplan HM, Stahl F, Repenning C, Scheper T, et al. Percutaneous collagen induction-regeneration in place of cicatrisation? J Plast Reconstr Aesthet Surg. 2011;64:97–107. https://doi.org/10.1016/j.bjps.2010.03.038.

135. Neuber F. Bericht über die Verhandlungen der Dt Ges für Chirurgie. Berlin: Springer; 1893. p. 22–66.

136. Zielins ER, Brett EA, Longaker MT, Wan DC. Autologous fat grafting: the science behind the surgery. Aesthet Surg J. 2016;36:488–96. https://doi.org/10.1093/asj/sjw004.

137. Miller C. Cannula implants and review of implantation techniques in esthetic surgery. Chicago: The Oak Press; 1926.

138. Illouz Y. The fat cell "graft": a new technique to fill depressions (letter). Plast Recontr Surg. 1986;78:122–3.

139. Klinger M, Caviggioli F, Klinger FM, Giannasi S, Bandi V, Banzatti B, et al. Autologous fat graft in scar treatment. J Craniofac Surg. 2013;24:1610–5. https://doi.org/10.1097/SCS.0b013e3182a24548.

Recent Advances in Scar Research and Unanswered Questions

Hanna Luze, Sebastian P. Nischwitz, and Lars-Peter Kamolz

Core Messages

- Current research focuses on understanding the exact pathophysiology and the molecular abnormalities in pathological scarring.
- Scar models are essential to investigate the pathogenesis of pathological scar formation, identify new drug targets, and to test new therapeutic strategies.
- The selection of the most suitable scar model for a specific study should be based on the model's characteristics and the study goal.

Introduction

Keloids or hypertrophic scars are pathological scars that grow over time and extend beyond the initial site of injury after impaired wound healing [1]. They are aesthetically disfiguring and can cause pain, itching, discomfort as well as psycho-logical stress, often significantly impairing the patients' quality of life. The mechanisms that initiate pathological scarring are incompletely understood, which is why these scars remain a challenging problem for patients, clinicians, and researchers [2]. To date, many treatment modalities, including surgical and non-surgical, have been explored and reported to have beneficial effects. With recent advances in molecular biology and genetics, insight is being gained on the complex process of scar formation and therapeutic options are constantly evolving. However, no absolutely satisfactory or optimal treatment modality of all keloid subtypes has been defined to date [1].

The development of valuable scar models, resembling in vivo hypertrophic and keloid scar tissue not only aids the investigation of underlying mechanisms leading to pathological scarring but also benefits the development of adequate prevention and treatment strategies [3]. Besides numerous in vitro models, animal models can provide valuable translational vehicles for human treatment modalities [4]. However, as hypertrophic scarring is specific to humans, the development of adequate animal models for hypertrophic scarring or keloids is challenging [2, 4]. A major difference between laboratory animals and humans is the presence of the panniculus carnosus in many animals, a fibromuscular layer enabling the skin to slide over underlying fascia. This layer enables a rapid contraction and faster healing of wounds [4].

The lack of adequate models is a challenging obstacle for research aiming at prevention and

H. Luze (✉) · S. P. Nischwitz
Division of Plastic, Aesthetic and Reconstructive Surgery, Department of Surgery, Medical University of Graz, Graz, Austria
e-mail: hanna.luze@medunigraz.at; sebastian.nischwitz@medunigraz.at

L.-P. Kamolz
Division of Plastic, Aesthetic and Reconstructive Surgery, Department of Surgery, Medical University of Graz, Graz, Austria

COREMED - Cooperative Centre for Regenerative Medicine, JOANNEUM RESEARCH Forschungsgesellschaft mbH, Graz, Austria
e-mail: Lars.kamolz@medunigraz.at

effective therapeutic intervention. The development of improved animal models and carefully designed preclinical studies involving cells and tissue isolated from pathological scars is of utmost importance to push the field forward.

This chapter discusses the complexities of modeling hypertrophic scarring, summarizes currently available models in scar research, and describes new technologies that may improve future models. Furthermore, emerging treatment modalities for hypertrophic scars and keloids will be discussed.

Scar Models

Scar models are essential to investigate the pathogenesis of pathological scar formation, identify new drug targets, and to test new therapeutic strategies. Numerous in vitro culture and tissue-engineered models as well as in vivo models with different limitations have been created so far. The selection of the best model for a specific study should be based on the characteristics of the model and the goal of the study [5]. In vitro models can be used to identify different pathways during scar formation and for a high-throughput analysis in drug development. Preclinical, in vivo models on the other hand are often used to analyze the phenotypical scar formation and develop new treatment modalities [6]. An overview of current scar models is displayed in Fig. 1.

In Vitro Models

Early in vitro cell culture models using conventional monolayer cell cultures either compared normal and scar-derived fibroblasts or tried to

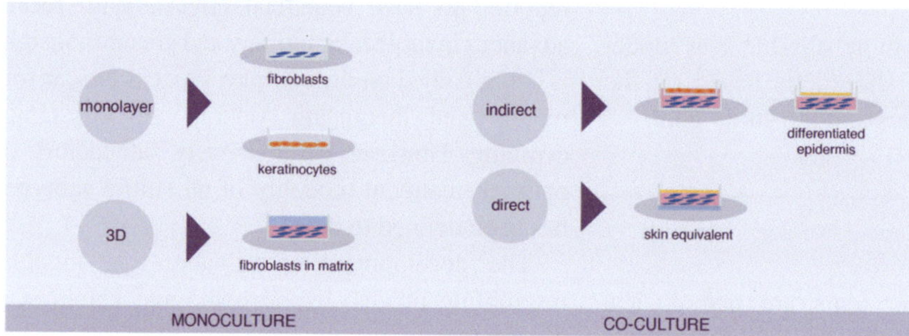

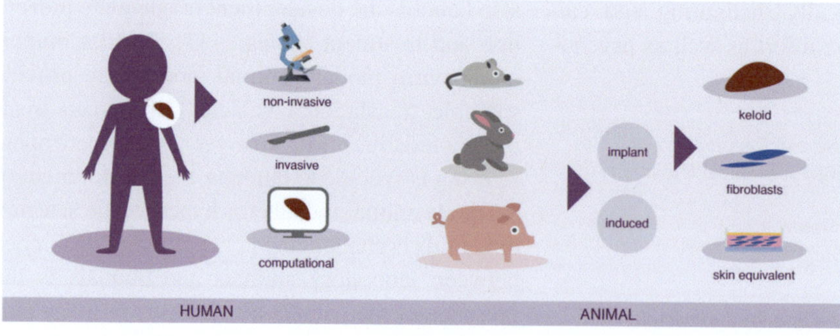

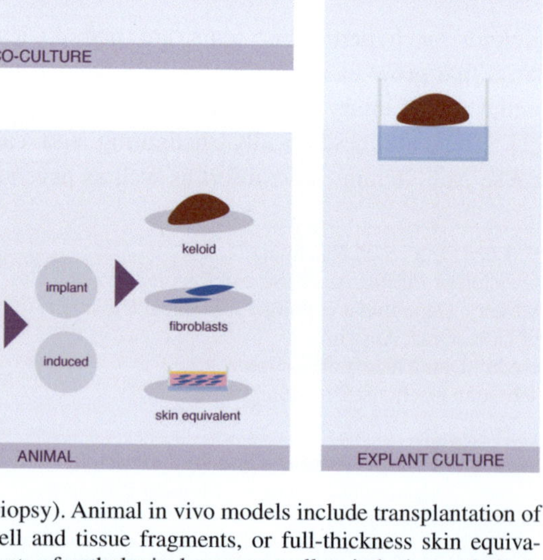

Fig. 1 Overview of current scar models. Scar models can be subdivided into human and animal in vivo and in vitro models. In vitro models range from simple monolayers to 3D structures and co-culture systems. Indirect co-culture systems include monolayer keloid fibroblasts combined with either monolayer keratinocytes or a fully differentiated epidermis. Human in vivo models include non-invasive imaging and invasive methods (e.g., serial biopsy). Animal in vivo models include transplantation of cell and tissue fragments, or full-thickness skin equivalents of pathological scars as well as inducing pathological scar development. Keloid explant models are a combination of in vivo and in vitro. [Copyright: Maike Sophie Rinder, MA (Corporate Communications, Joanneum Research Forschungsgesellschaft mbH, Graz, Austria).]

induce a scar phenotype from healthy fibroblasts. Despite this fast, simple, and inexpensive technique, pathological scarring can't exclusively be targeted via fibroblasts analysis. In indirect cocultures of keratinocytes and fibroblasts, the keratinocyte–fibroblast interactions can be investigated [7]. However, these early models are lacking physiological relevance due to the absence of any similarity with the 3D macroscopic fibrotic tissue structure typical of a scar [6]. The introduction of a more physiologically relevant 3D environment via adding collagen or fibrin gel contributed to the development of an improved, more natural scar phenotype [8]. By enabling fibroblasts to produce their own matrix, an even more in vivo-like situation can be created [9].

The realization that an extensive crosstalk between keratinocytes within the epidermis and fibroblasts within the dermis occurs to regulate the synthesis of extracellular dermal matrix led to the introduction of organotypic skin equivalents [6]. These 3D organotypic skin models using keloid fibroblasts in combination with normal skin-derived keratinocytes can be used to simulate and study keloid formation [10]. Extensive implementation of these models in the development of new treatment strategies is, however, limited due to the lack of biomarkers.

Recent developments suggest that mesenchymal stromal cells derived from subcutaneous fat can be used to construct a tissue-engineered hypertrophic scar model [11]. The model by Broek et al. for example consists of a reconstructed epidermis derived from normal healthy human keratinocytes on a dermal matrix populated with subcutaneous fat [11].

This hypertrophic scar model exhibits many characteristics of hypertrophic scars (e.g., increased collagen I secretion, contraction, and epidermal thickness; decreased epithelization, etc.) and enables relevant parameters to be identified and validated with therapeutic strategies [11]. Despite the clear advancements made in the development of these kind of models, they are only representative of hypertrophic scar formation caused by severe trauma (e.g., burns) where the adipose tissue is exposed. For simulating hypertrophic scar formation after wound closure or keloid formation developing years after relatively minor injury, these models are not suitable [11].

Keloid Explant Models

In the last years, multipotent keloid-derived mesenchymal-like stem cells have also been implicated in keloid formation [12]. Keloid explant models have been developed in the following to investigate the keloid phenotype and potential treatment modalities. These models do not necessarily require implantation into an animal model in order to survive and be used as a keloid model in and of itself; they can be maintained in cell culture after explant for up to 6 weeks [13]. Various culture methods have been investigated, but the morphology of pathological scars appears best conserved when embedded in collagen gel and cultured in an air-exposed environment [13]. While these models certainly show promising potential, they are entirely dependent on a regular supply of pathological scars that are both freshly excised and sufficiently large [6, 12]. Another important limitation of this model is the absence of a circulatory system, as is the case with all in vitro models so far [3]. Keloid explant models appear best suited for the investigation of new treatment modalities rather than studying the pathological mechanisms underlying keloid formation [3, 14, 15].

In Vivo Models

In vivo scar models are of the human or animal variety and can further be subdivided into noninvasive, invasive, and computational models. In noninvasive models, live imaging of pathological scars is usually performed to visualize certain tissue characteristics. Invasive hypertrophic scar and keloid modeling, on the other hand, vary from relatively minor procedures, e.g., by Ozawa et al. where fluorine-18-fluorodeoxyglucose injections are performed to investigate glucose metabolism [16], to serial biopsies evaluating the development of pathological scars over time [3, 17].

Despite their value especially in the clinical setting for follow-up evaluation, human in vivo models post-1962 are inherently limited in the ability to manipulate experimental variables and yield primarily observational data. While Lebeko et al. reported a particular benefit of the temporal data acquired from serial keloid biopsy analysis in their review on keloid models, [18] it is of utmost importance to emphasize the potential risk of exacerbating the existing keloid scars by continual provocation with biopsy-associated injury [3].

In animal models, pathological scars are either induced or human hypertrophic scar or keloid tissue is transplanted [3]. Despite the large number of studies describing pigs, mice, rabbits, and other animals as models to investigate hypertrophic scarring or keloid formation, the basic skin physiology, immunology, and therefore the wound healing process are markedly different with the result that animals do not develop scars which are comparable with adverse scars in humans [19–22]. The implantation of human cells or tissue fragments of pathological scars into animal models has been reported to be more successful, resulting in a palpable nodule-like mass [3, 23]. Keloid and hypertrophic scar skin (full thickness or dermis only) can directly be grafted for example in nude mice models [19]. Also the transplantation of healthy human split-thickness skin grafts has been reported for the humanization of nude mouse models [20]. The greatly reduced number of T cells in these mice results in a reduced chance of graft rejection. However, the immune component of wound healing and scar formation is severely compromised due to the immune-deficient phenotype of this mouse model [6]. While implanted scar tissue is generally able to retain the pathological scar-specific collagen even within animal models, the use of already established hypertrophic scar and keloid tissue does not allow the investigation of a de novo development [3]. To overcome this issue, Zhang et al. reported a combination of tissue culture techniques with IL-6 and IL-17 exposure for the implantation of a keloid fibroblasts-hydrogel suspension into nude mice resulting in a de novo keloidal collagen formation [21].

The most frequent model to investigate de novo keloid and hypertrophic scar formation is the rabbit ear excisional wound model; however, this model does not reflect burn injuries [22]. The red Duroc pig model may more closely reflect human hypertrophic scarring since these pigs have been shown to form robust scars with biological and anatomical similarities to human hypertrophic scars. Several modes of action after excisional wounds and burns have been developed for this model so far, which may provide an improved platform for studying the pathophysiology of burn-related hypertrophic scarring, investigating current anti-scar therapies, and developing new strategies with greater clinical benefit [24].

> **Important to Know**
> Numerous hypertrophic and keloid scar models have been developed so far. The selection of the most suitable one for a specific study should be based on the characteristics of the model and the study goal. An overview of animal in vivo models can be found in [25]

Limitations

Recent in vitro and in vivo models, aiming to identify genes and biomarkers reflecting early stages of scar formation, are simulating hypertrophic scarring already quite accurately. However, due to the complex cascade of cellular interactions involved in the development of hypertrophic scars, especially human cell culture models are still limited by their extreme simplicity.

Existing models have also a limited duration of days or weeks, whereas human scars develop over a period of several months or even years. Furthermore, the individual genetic predisposition for hypertrophic scarring, possibly influencing the whole process of scar formation, can not be incorporated in scar models yet [6]. Despite major progresses in scar research within the last years, the exact pathogenesis of hypertrophic scarring is yet to be determined. Understanding the exact pathophysiology and the molecular abnormalities is essential to develop optimal treatment and prevention strategies in the future.

Emerging Treatment Modalities

To date, various treatment concepts for pathological scars exist; however, no single treatment has proven to be the most effective [1]. Current options include surgical excision, corticosteroids, silicone-based products, pressure therapy, radiotherapy, cryotherapy, or laser therapy. More rare options include creams of Imiquimod 5% as an immune-response modifier or 5-fluorouracil as an inhibitor of fibroblast proliferation, angiogenesis, and TGF-β-induced collagen type I expression [1]. Despite multimodal approaches, the recurrence rate is very high for all modalities that have been studied to this point [26]. However, the increasing number of emerging treatment options and synergistic combinations of them is showing favorable results [27]. In the following, new therapeutic approaches currently investigated will be listed.

Ultraviolet A1 laser therapy in the spectral range of 340–400 nm induces increased collagenase activity. The existing evidence supports its use for fibrosing disorders, including localized scleroderma, lichen sclerosus et atrophicus, and graft-versus-host disease. Only a few studies have investigated UV-A1 laser therapy in the treatment of hypertrophic scars and keloids, reporting mixed results [27, 28].

Other agents that may have a potential role in keloid treatment include tamoxifen and calmodulin inhibitors. Tamoxifen citrate is a nonsteroidal antiestrogen that downregulates TFG-β, fibroblast, and collagen expression. Similarly, calmodulin inhibitors may also result in scar degradation [27].

A new alternative to topical silicone is a combination of silicone oil with hypochlorous acid as a gel or spray. Silicone oil with hypochlorous acid has an antimicrobial, antipruritic, and anti-inflammatory role by increasing oxygenation and

disrupting biofilm formation. Reports suggest that this technology performed better than 100% silicone gel in the management of keloid and hypertrophic scars [29].

Mammalian target of rapamycin (mTOR) may also be a potential therapeutic target in pathological scars. Existing evidence is suggesting that mTOR plays a role in the regulation of collagen expression. Targeting mTOR with rapamycin therefore may block excess fibroproliferation leading to abnormal scarring. In fact, in vitro studies showed blocked collagen synthesis pathways that are significantly increased in keloid scarring after rapamycin treatment of human fibroblasts [30].

TGF-β1, TGF-β2, and TGF-β3 isoforms appear to have interrelated roles in keloid pathogenesis. The TGF-β3 isoform, in particular, has been studied in clinical trials. Intradermal recombinant TGF-β3 to prophylactically improve scarring has been investigated in three double-blind, placebo-controlled, phase I/II studies [31]. However, the phase III clinical trial in 2011 did not accomplish its endpoints leading to the conclusion that this approach may not provide a significant benefit for scar revision. Efficacy of targeting other TGF-β isoforms remains to be further investigated [31].

MicroRNAs are noncoding RNAs that silence genes at the posttranscriptional level. The expression of micro RNAs in keloidal fibroblasts is expressed at different concentrations compared to normal fibroblasts. A growing body of research suggests that specific micro RNAs, such as miRNA-29 and miRNA-21-5p, appear to play key roles in keloid development providing additional targets for novel therapeutics [27].

Caution!
Numerous novel and potential therapeutic targets in pathological scars have been investigated within the last years. However, further research is required for most of them, to investigate their safety and efficacy in the treatment of hypertrophic scars.

Conclusion

Numerous in vitro culture and tissue-engineered models as well as in vivo models have been created so far. These models are essential in the elucidation of pathological scar formation and possible treatment options. However, existing models are limited in several ways and the exact pathogenesis of hypertrophic scarring is yet to be determined. The lacking elucidation of the exact pathophysiology and the molecular abnormalities leads to a variety of treatment concepts; however, no single therapy has been universally accepted as the gold standard yet.

To date, combinational therapies offer the best approach and show better efficacy with fewer side effects compared to monotherapy. A well-planned selection of treatment options, which is tailored to the patient's specific needs, is essential to enable a good clinical outcome.

Understanding the exact pathophysiology and the molecular abnormalities is definitely the focus of current research and is essential to develop optimal treatment and prevention strategies in the future. Future studies need to focus on the intersection between basic and clinical research and could especially target the efficacy of novel treatment modalities for keloid and hypertrophic scars management in an optimized scar model.

References

1. Ojeh N, Bharatha A, Gaur U, Forde AL. Keloids: current and emerging therapies. Scars Burn Health. 2020;6:205951312094049. https://doi.org/10.1177/2059513120940499.
2. Supp DM. Animal models for studies of keloid scarring. Adv Wound Care. 2019;8(2):77–89. https://doi.org/10.1089/wound.2018.0828.
3. Limandjaja GC, Niessen FB, Scheper RJ, Gibbs S. The keloid disorder: heterogeneity, histopathology, mechanisms and models. Front Cell Dev Biol. 2020;8:00360. https://doi.org/10.3389/fcell.2020.00360/full.
4. Seo BF, Lee JY, Jung S-N. Models of abnormal scarring. Biomed Res Int. 2013;2013:1–8. http://www.hindawi.com/journals/bmri/2013/423147/
5. Li J, Wang J, Wang Z, Xia Y, Zhou M, Zhong A, et al. Experimental models for cutaneous hypertrophic scar research. Wound Repair Regen. 2020;28(1):126–44. https://doi.org/10.1111/wrr.12760.
6. Broek LJ, Limandjaja GC, Niessen FB, Gibbs S. Human hypertrophic and keloid scar models: principles, limitations and future challenges from a tissue engineering perspective. Exp Dermatol. 2014;23(6):382–6. https://doi.org/10.1111/exd.12419.
7. Lim CP, Phan TT, Lim IJ, Cao X. Cytokine profiling and Stat3 phosphorylation in epithelial–mesenchymal interactions between keloid keratinocytes and fibroblasts. J Invest Dermatol. 2009;129(4):851–61. https://linkinghub.elsevier.com/retrieve/pii/S0022202X15342779
8. Derderian CA, Bastidas N, Lerman OZ, Bhatt KA, Lin S-E, Voss J, et al. Mechanical strain alters gene expression in an in vitro model of hypertrophic scarring. Ann Plast Surg. 2005;55(1):69–75. http://journals.lww.com/00000637-200507000-00013
9. Ahlfors J-EW, Billiar KL. Biomechanical and biochemical characteristics of a human fibroblast-produced and remodeled matrix. Biomaterials. 2007;28(13):2183–91. https://linkinghub.elsevier.com/retrieve/pii/S014296120700018X
10. Butler PD, Ly DP, Longaker MT, Yang GP. Use of organotypic coculture to study keloid biology. Am J Surg. 2008;195(2):144–8. https://linkinghub.elsevier.com/retrieve/pii/S0002961007008744
11. van den Broek L. Development, validation and testing of a human tissue engineered hypertrophic scar model. ALTEX. 2012;29(4):389–402. http://www.altex.org/index.php/altex/article/view/431
12. Qu M, Song N, Chai G, Wu X, Liu W. Pathological niche environment transforms dermal stem cells to keloid stem cells: a hypothesis of keloid formation and development. Med Hypotheses. 2013;81(5):807–12. https://linkinghub.elsevier.com/retrieve/pii/S0306987713004337
13. Bagabir R, Syed F, Paus R, Bayat A. Long-term organ culture of keloid disease tissue. Exp Dermatol. 2012;21(5):376–81. https://doi.org/10.1111/j.1600-0625.2012.01476.x.
14. Syed F, Bagabir RA, Paus R, Bayat A. Ex vivo evaluation of antifibrotic compounds in skin scarring: EGCG and silencing of PAI-1 independently inhibit growth and induce keloid shrinkage. Lab Investig. 2013;93(8):946–60. http://www.nature.com/articles/labinvest201382
15. Syed F, Sherris D, Paus R, Varmeh S, Pandolfi PP, Bayat A. Keloid disease can be inhibited by antagonizing excessive mTOR signaling with a novel dual TORC1/2 inhibitor. Am J Pathol. 2012;181(5):1642–58. https://linkinghub.elsevier.com/retrieve/pii/S0002944012006025
16. Ozawa T, Okamura T, Harada T, Muraoka M, Ozawa N, Koyama K, et al. Accumulation of glucose in keloids with FDG-PET. Ann Nucl Med. 2006;20(1):41–4. https://doi.org/10.1007/BF02985589.

17. Lin L, Wang Y, Liu W, Huang Y. BAMBI inhibits skin fibrosis in keloid through suppressing TGF-β1-induced hypernomic fibroblast cell proliferation and excessive accumulation of collagen I. Int J Clin Exp Med. 2015;8(8):13227–34.

18. Lebeko M, Khumalo NP, Bayat A. Multi-dimensional models for functional testing of keloid scars: in silico, in vitro, organoid, organotypic, ex vivo organ culture, and in vivo models. Wound Repair Regen. 2019;27(4):298–308. https://doi.org/10.1111/wrr.12705.

19. Ishiko T, Naitoh M, Kubota H, Yamawaki S, Ikeda M, Yoshikawa K, et al. Chondroitinase injection improves keloid pathology by reorganizing the extracellular matrix with regenerated elastic fibers. J Dermatol. 2013;40(5):380–3. https://doi.org/10.1111/1346-8138.12116.

20. Momtazi M, Kwan P, Ding J, Anderson CC, Honardoust D, Goekjian S, et al. A nude mouse model of hypertrophic scar shows morphologic and histologic characteristics of human hypertrophic scar. Wound Repair Regen. 2013;21(1):77–87. https://doi.org/10.1111/j.1524-475X.2012.00856.x.

21. Zhang Q, Yamaza T, Kelly AP, Shi S, Wang S, Brown J, et al. Tumor-like stem cells derived from human keloid are governed by the inflammatory niche driven by IL-17/IL-6 axis. PLoS One. 2009;4(11):e7798. https://doi.org/10.1371/journal.pone.0007798.

22. Domergue S, Jorgensen C, Noël D. Advances in research in animal models of burn-related hypertrophic scarring. J Burn Care Res. 2015;36(5):e259–66. https://academic.oup.com/jbcr/article/36/5/e259-e266/4568769

23. Hillmer MP, MacLeod SM. Experimental keloid scar models: a review of methodological issues. J Cutan Med Surg. 2002;6(4):354–9. https://doi.org/10.1007/s10227-001-0121-y.

24. Blackstone BN, Kim JY, McFarland KL, Sen CK, Supp DM, Bailey JK, et al. Scar formation following excisional and burn injuries in a red Duroc pig model. Wound Repair Regen. 2017;25(4):618–31. https://doi.org/10.1111/wrr.12562.

25. Rössler S, Nischwitz SP, Luze H, Holzer-Geissler JCJ, Zrim R, Kamolz LP. In Vivo Models for Hypertrophic Scars-A Systematic Review. Medicina (Kaunas). 2022;58(6):736. https://doi.org/10.3390/medicina58060736.

26. Grabowski G, Pacana MJ, Chen E. Keloid and hypertrophic scar formation, prevention, and management. J Am Acad Orthop Surg. 2020;28(10):e408–14. https://doi.org/10.5435/JAAOS-D-19-00690.

27. Ekstein SF, Wyles SP, Moran SL, Meves A. Keloids: a review of therapeutic management. Int J Dermatol. 2020;2020:15159. https://doi.org/10.1111/ijd.15159.

28. Polat M, Kaya H, Şahin A. A new approach in the treatment of keloids: UVA-1 laser. Photomed Laser Surg. 2016;34(3):130–3. https://doi.org/10.1089/pho.2015.4046.

29. Gold MH, Andriessen A, Dayan SH, Fabi SG, Lorenc ZP, Henderson Berg M-H. Hypochlorous acid gel technology-its impact on postprocedure treatment and scar prevention. J Cosmet Dermatol. 2017;16(2):162–7. https://doi.org/10.1111/jocd.12330.

30. Wong VW, You F, Januszyk M, Gurtner GC, Kuang AA. Transcriptional profiling of rapamycin-treated fibroblasts from hypertrophic and keloid scars. Ann Plast Surg. 2014;72(6):711–9. https://journals.lww.com/00000637-201406000-00021

31. Ferguson MW, Duncan J, Bond J, Bush J, Durani P, So K, et al. Prophylactic administration of avotermin for improvement of skin scarring: three double-blind, placebo-controlled, phase I/II studies. Lancet. 2009;373(9671):1264–74. https://linkinghub.elsevier.com/retrieve/pii/S0140673609603226

Part II

Scar Assessment and Prevention

Scar Assessment Scores

Dalia Barayan, Roohi Vinaik, and Marc G. Jeschke

Core Messages

- Scars can be distinguished based on several visual, palpable, and sensational features: *color, texture, thickness, pliability, surface area, pain,* and *pruritus.*
- A range of handheld devices is available to objectively measure physical scar features including pliability, firmness, color, perfusion, thickness, and 3-dimensional topography.
- Multiple subjective assessment scales, including the Vancouver Scar Scale (VSS) and the Patient and Observer Scar Assessment Scale (POSAS), have been developed to help assist in the evaluation of scar severity, progression, and response to treatment.
- While traditional scar scales are clinician/researcher-reported and focus on the physical attributes of a scar, more recently developed scales are patient-centered and measure aspects of quality of life such as pruritus, pain, and psychosocial sequelae.
- Validity, reliability, and feasibility are important clinimetric properties that must be taken into account when choosing appropriate tool(s) for scar assessments.
- The ideal assessment of scars should be non-invasive, accurate, reproducible, easy to facilitate, and include both objective and subjective scar measurements.

Introduction

Scars can lead to a wide range of functional, cosmetic, and psychological consequences [1–3]. The impact a scar has on a patient's "quality of life" is largely dependent on its location and characteristics [4]. An ideal assessment of scars should consider both objective and subjective aspects [5, 6]. The objective aspects of a scar include its physical characteristics (*color, thickness, relief, pliability,* and *surface area*) [7]. Subjective aspects of a scar, on the other hand, encompass various factors that contribute to the patient's own evaluation of the scar [8]. This includes the patient's emotional reaction to the injury and its consequences, prior and/or emergent psychiatric disorders, and changes in body image, which in turn can be more disabling than the physical sequelae because of associated emotional, social, and economic difficulties [6–9].

D. Barayan · R. Vinaik
Sunnybrook Research Institute, Toronto, ON, Canada
e-mail: Dalia.barayan@mail.utoronto.ca;
roohi.vinaik@mail.utoronto.ca

M. G. Jeschke (✉)
Sunnybrook Research Institute, Toronto, ON, Canada

Division of Plastic Surgery, Department of Surgery, University of Toronto, Toronto, Canada

Department of Immunology, University of Toronto, Toronto, Canada

Ross Tilley Burn Centre, Sunnybrook Health Sciences Centre, Toronto, Canada
e-mail: jeschke@HHSC.CA

Patients with burn scars in particular have been shown to suffer from depression and post-traumatic stress disorder, with prevalence rates ranging from 13 to 23% and 13 to 45%, respectively [3]. In fact, burn patients who reported worse body image dissatisfaction after burn injury had significantly lower psychosocial and physical adjustment even after 2 years of following up and controlling for injury severity [10]. Thus, a patient's perspective of a scar may be more important for determining overall scar morbidity outcomes than the actual physical characteristics such as total body surface area [11].

Nowadays, both subjective and objective measurements of scar features are mandatory to practice evidence-based medicine [12]. For the objective assessment of scars, a number of devices have been developed to measure their physical attributes such as *pliability*, *firmness*, *color*, *perfusion*, *thickness,* and *3-dimensional topography* (*surface area*) [13]. For the subjective evaluation of scars, different scar assessment scales are available including the Vancouver Scar Scale (VSS) and the Patient and Observer Scar Assessment Scale (POSAS) [14]. Unlike objective tools which provide quantitative measurements of a scar, these assessment scales are observer dependent and can measure other important scar parameters like *pain* and *itch* [14, 15]. Although an increasing number of subjective and objective tools have been developed, there is no general agreement as to the gold standard tool(s) for scar evaluation [15]. An optimal, universal scar scoring system is therefore still needed to better understand, evaluate, and treat pathologic scarring and its related complications.

The following chapter provides an overview of the most common scar features assessed in fundamental research and clinical practice. It then discusses the basic clinimetric principles that should be taken into account when judging scar assessment tools. Finally, currently available scar measuring devices and assessment scales are critically appraised with regard to both, scar features assessed and their clinimetric properties.

Scar Features

Grading and classifying scars are extremely important for choosing which treatment strategy will ultimately work best [7, 8]. They can be characterized as mature, immature, linear hypertrophic, widespread hypertrophic, minor keloid, or major keloid [16]. Generally, scar tissue can be distinguished based on several visual, tactile (palpable), and/or sensational characteristics [16, 17]. Several accurate and reliable tools have been developed to measure these scar features subjectively and even some objectively [17]. The most common scar features assessed are:

1. *Color:* Disturbances in the color of a scar are attributed to the amount of vascularization and pigmentation (Fig. 1a, b). Vascularization or erythema is the result of increased capillary blood flow [18]. An increase in redness during the early maturation phase is typical and a good indicator for scar activity [19]. Pigmentation (hyper/hypo) is caused by decreases or increases in melanocyte concentration and/or melanin production in the epidermis [18]. While erythema usually fades after several months or years, changes in pigmentation often remain at least to some extent [18, 19].
2. *Texture:* A clinician's overall opinion of a scar is considerably influenced by surface irregularities [20]. Relief (surface roughness) can arise in situations where a skin transplantation is required and is most common after burn treatment [21]. As illustrated in Fig. 1c, after a meshed split skin graft is applied on the burned area, the areas in between can become raised, resulting in long-lasting irregularities [21].
3. *Thickness:* Increased scar thickness (hypertrophy) is one of the most frequent and cosmetically disfiguring outcomes of scarring (Fig. 2). Hypertrophic scars can be difficult to distinguish from keloids and are regularly misdiagnosed [22]. Although both scar types involve excessive collagen deposition, keloids

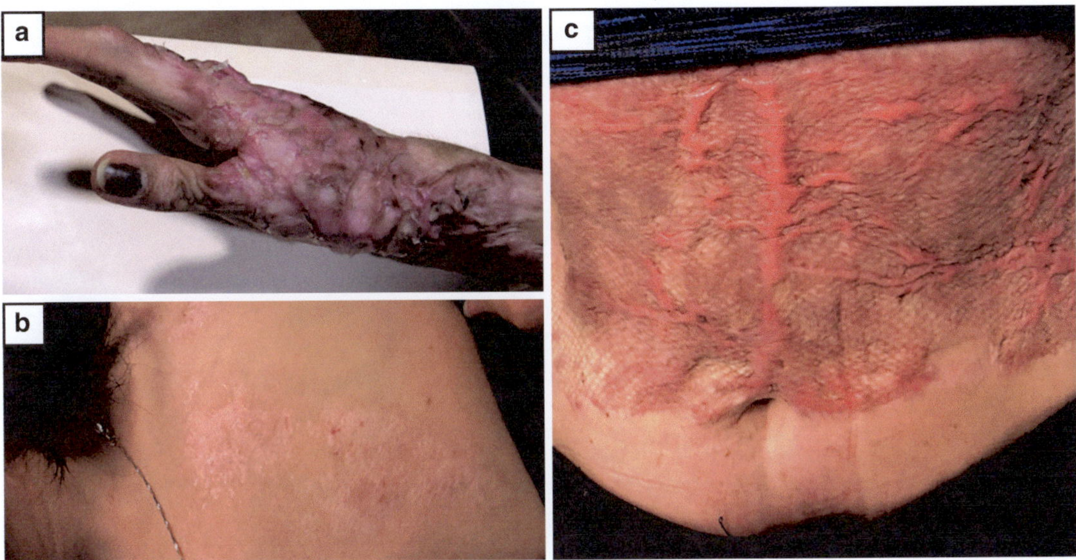

Fig. 1 (**a**) A red and raised scar after a burn injury of the hand. (**b**) Hypopigmentation of a scar on the chest wall. (**c**) Relief of a burn scar after skin transplantation of the abdomen

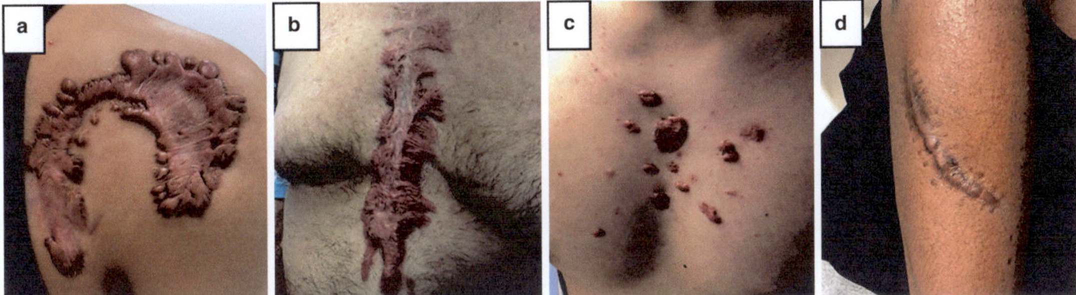

Fig. 2 Clinical appearance of (**a–c**) keloid and (**d**) hypertrophic scar formation

are characterized by their extensive proliferation beyond the borders of the original lesion [23]. In contrast, hypertrophic scars become raised but stay within their confines. Moreover, unlike keloids which show no regression and have phases of reactivation, hypertrophic scars typically decrease in thickness over time [23, 24].

4. *Pliability:* Loss of pliability is often observed in scars that become stiff and hardened due to increased collagen synthesis and/or lack of elastin in the dermal layer [25]. Increased scar stiffness will often result in a limited range of motion, especially if scars are located on or around joints (Fig. 3). This can also be a major

cause of functional impairment in the facial region, as loss of pliability can lead to asymmetry and an altered or diminished facial expression [26].

5. *Surface area:* The surface area of a scar may change over time depending on the extent of contraction or expansion in the horizontal plane [18, 25, 26]. In clinical practice, measuring scar surface area (planimetry) is useful for calculating wound size, the rate of scar contraction/expansion, as well as the percentage of a scar that becomes hypertrophic or hypopigmentated. The extent of scar contraction or expansion is also frequently used as an outcome parameter in research

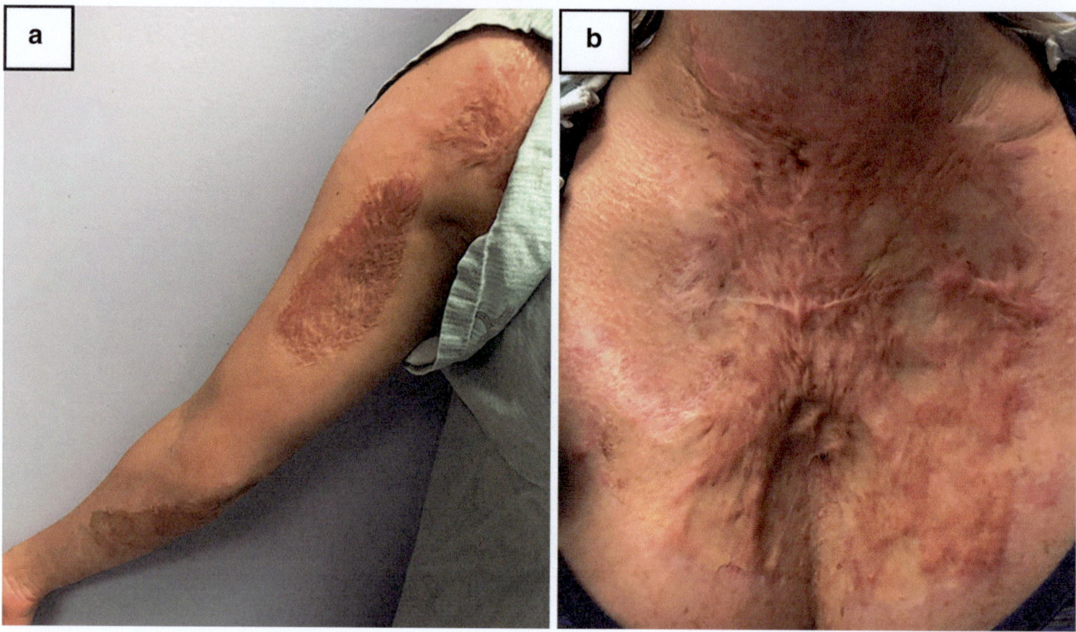

Fig. 3 Scar contracture on an upper arm (**a**) and chest and neck (**b**) after a burn injury associated with limited range of motion

studies [18]. Scar contraction is commonly observed in burn scars [27]. As shown in Fig. 3, this regularly leads to scar contracture and may require reconstructive surgery. In contrast, scar expansion (widening) is often seen in linear scarring and causes a less aesthetical result [27].

6. *Pain:* Pain is a well-recognized and often-distressing consequence of trauma and subsequent scarring. For instance, up to 30% of patients with poststernotomy scars report chronic pain along the sternal scar and in the upper extremities, which is sometimes accompanied by paresthesias [28]. The presence of pain is also common in burn scars and plays an important role in deciding whether or not to pursue treatment [3]. Patients with scar pain typically complain of neuropathic pain and describe it as a sensation of "pins and needles," "shooting," or "burning" [29]. While the underlying pathophysiology is still not known, current evidence suggests a strong relation with scar hypertrophy, itching, and psychiatric diagnoses [30].

7. *Itching/pruritus:* Itchy scars can cause significant distress for patients, particularly if they cover a large proportion of the body like burn scars. While the exact mechanisms are still unclear, this phenomenon is thought to be caused by multiple factors including friction, inflammation, stimulation of surrounding nerve endings, and increased levels of β-endorphin in scar tissue [31]. Risk predictors include a high percentage of total body surface area burned, female gender, previous surgical procedures, and early symptoms of post-traumatic stress [32]. Additionally, pruritus is often associated with hypertrophic scarring, affecting approximately 86% of keloid patients [33–36]. Another retrospective study revealed that 87% of burn victims also experience daily pruritus associated with scarring. In fact, 94% of these burn patients with chronic itch and 86% with acute itch reported pruritus to be unbearable [37]. Although it is becoming increasingly clear that factors like pain and pruritus contribute to the significant morbidity observed with pathological scarring, they are not common parameters assessed by current scar assessment tools. To date, only three of the available scar scales address both these critical issues: the modified

Vancouver Scar Scale, the Patient and Observer Scar Assessment Scale, and the University of North Carolina "4P" Scar Scale, which are discussed in detail in "Subjective Scar Assessment Scales."

Clinimetric Requirements

Scar assessment tools are paramount for evaluating scar severity, identifying risk factors (hypertrophic scarring), making a treatment plan, and monitoring scar responses to determine whether treatment is effective and successful [38, 39]. As discussed above, a number of tools have been adopted in clinical practice to evaluate scars but the use of one alone has yet been proven to be optimal [12]. In most cases, scars are assessed either with subjective assessment scales, objective measuring devices, or more recently, using a combination of both [18]. One important aspect to take into account when choosing an appropriate scar assessment tool is to ensure that it is "clinimetrically approved" [40]. The field of "clinimetrics" aims to improve the quality of assessment procedures in medicine and health care by assessing the properties of existing tools or by developing new ones [41, 42]. In the context of scar evaluation, basic clinimetric requirements for both subjective and objective measurement tools are *reliability, validity*, and *feasibility* [43–46].

Reliability is defined as "the degree to which the measurement is free from measurement error" and refers to the reproducibility and internal consistency of ratings [41, 42]. The variation that may arise between repeated measurements decreases the reliability. This measurement error cannot be attributed to true changes in the scar. Rather, it may be attributed either to the measurement tool, the persons performing the measurement, the patients undergoing the measurement, or the circumstances under which the measurements are performed [40]. Intra-observer reliability (test–retest) determines the degree to which the same result is obtained when an observer uses the instrument on the same subject for the second time [47]. This test–retest analysis should be per-

formed within a time frame that is long enough to prevent memory bias but short enough to prevent changes associated with scar maturation. Generally, 2 weeks is considered an appropriate interval. Inter-observer reliability assesses whether the same result is obtained when multiple observers use the instrument on the same subject at the same time [47]. The Intraclass Correlation Coefficient (ICC) is the most suitable parameter used to establish reliability [48]. An ICC higher than 0.7 is considered a minimum requirement for reliable results. If the single ICC (performed with a single observer) is not acceptable, multiple observers are necessary for reliable assessments and scores are averaged to calculate the final or average ICC [48].

Validity is defined as "the degree to which an instrument truly measures what it purports to measure" and can be divided into three types: content validity, construct validity, and criterion validity [40, 41]. To determine the strength of association between two scar instruments, a Pearson's Correlation or Spearman's Rank Coefficient is calculated depending on the distribution of the data [49]. A Pearson's correlation is used when the variables being studied are normally distributed and assume equal interval data [45, 49]. In contrast, Spearman's rho is used when one or both variables are skewed or ordinal and is most appropriate when extreme values are present [49]. Usually, a Pearson's/Spearman's coefficient is considered good when higher than 0.6, moderate when between 0.3 and 0.6, and weak when lower than 0.3 [45].

Currently, the lack of gold standard for comparison poses a major methodological challenge for the validation of scar scales [50]. It is also worth noting that assessment scales can consist of either nominal, ordinal, or categorical items [18]. Nominal items assign descriptive variables to groups or categories such as sex, race, etc. Although these variables are often labeled with numbers for data processing purposes, no rank ordering of the items is implied. Thus, nominal scales only provide qualitative information, rather than quantitative [18]. Ordinal scales, on the other hand, use numbers to assign a rank order of the objects assessed (e.g., first, second, third, etc.). Although ordinal scales can be used to determine which scar is better or worse, the interval between the numbers is not necessarily equal and as such does not provide absolute quantitative information [18]. Categorical scales are a combination of both nominal and ordinal scales and can either be numerical (e.g., 1, 2, 3, etc.) or quantitative (e.g., normal skin, slightly hypertrophic, hypertrophic, and keloid) [18]. Specific clinimetric parameters for these assessment scales include the Cronbach's alpha and the Cohen's Kappa or the Weighted Kappa [48, 51]. The Cronbach's alpha describes the internal consistency of a scale and is considered to be a measure of scale reliability. Results are considered reliable if Cronbach's alpha ranges between 0.7 and 0.9. Meanwhile, a high Cronbach's alpha (above 0.9) is usually an indication of redundancy, whereas a low score (below 0.7) suggests no internal consistency has been reached [48]. Cohen's Kappa or Weighted Kappa describes the level of agreement between observers, also known as interrater reliability [51]. While the Cohen's Kappa is used for nominal scales, the weighted Kappa is used for ordinal scales. Interpretation of the Kappa coefficient is based on Landis et al., where 0–0.2 indicates slight agreement; 0.21–0.4 fair agreement; 0.41–0.6 moderate agreement; 0.61–0.8 substantial agreement, and 0.81–1.0 almost perfect agreement [51].

Besides being reliable and valid, scar measurement tools should also be user friendly: *Feasibility* refers to an instrument's convenience, effectiveness, accessibility, price, and overall ease of use [41, 42]. Examples of instrument feasibility limitations include high cost, long assessment time, difficulty of clinical use, and extensive level of training or experience [18, 40]. Table 1 provides an overview of the clinimetric principles discussed above, including the parameters measured, their values as well as relative strengths. It is necessary to take all these factors into account in order to determine if the measurement tool can be used in a clinical or research setting. To date, however, none of the currently available scar evaluation tools completely satisfies the entire array of basic clinimetric requirements. In the

Table 1 Overview of clinimetric parameters and measures

Parameter	Measures	Values	Strength	References
Feasibility	Convenience; accessibility; effectiveness; assessment duration; price; ease of use; level of training/experience, etc.	–	–	[34, 35]
Reliability	Intraclass correlation coefficient	<0.40 0.40–0.75 ≥0.75	Poor Moderate to good Excellent	[40, 41]
Internal consistency	Cronbach's alpha	<0.70 0.70–0.80 ≥0.80	Low or inadequate Adequate Excellent	[41, 43]
Level of agreement	Cohen's kappa/weighted kappa	0 0.00–0.20 0.21–0.40 0.41–0.60 0.61–0.80 0.81–1.00	Poor Slight Fair Moderate Substantial Almost perfect	[43, 44]
Validity	Pearson's correlation/Spearman's rank coefficient	<0.30 0.30–0.60 ≥0.60	Weak Moderate Strong	[41, 42]

following sections, both objective measuring devices and subjective assessment scales are critically reviewed with respect to concepts of internal consistency, level of agreement, reliability, validity, and feasibility.

Objective Scar Measuring Devices

The objective assessment of scars relies on the use of several devices to measure their physical attributes described above [40]. In order for these scar-measuring tools to have clinical utility, objective data collection should ideally be non-invasive, accurate, reproducible, and easy to facilitate. Currently, available tools assess anatomical, mechanical, and physiological parameters such as *pliability, firmness, color, perfusion, thickness*, and *3-dimensional topography* [52]. Although these devices provide quantitative measurements of a scar, they are still prone to interpretation and measurement errors [38]. Thus, caution must be exercised with clinical application of these scar assessment tools.

Mechanical Parameters: Pliability, Firmness, and Elasticity

Several tools have been applied to measure pliability including the tissue tonometer, dermal torque meter, and elastometer [53]. However, the most commonly used are the pneumatonometer and cutometer [52]. The pneumatonometer is composed of a sensor, a membrane, and an airflow system that uses pressure to objectively measure skin pliability [54]. This objective scar measuring device has been applied to measure cutaneous compliance (Δ volume/Δ pressure) and demonstrated skin compliance significantly differs depending on body site. Moreover, overall compliance of burn scars was decreased in all sites as compared to normal controls, suggesting the potential use of the pneumatonometer for objectively assessing scar formation [52, 54]. In contrast, the cutometer is a noninvasive suction device that has been applied to objectively measure skin viscoelasticity by analyzing its vertical

deformation in response to negative pressure [55, 56]. It has been used to assess the effects of treatments on burn scars as well as overall scar maturation.

In addition to scar pliability, Draaijers et al. found the cutometer to also be a reliable tool for measuring other important scar features like elasticity [57]. The firmness and/or hardness of a scar are usually assessed by a durometer [52]. This device applies a vertically directed load on the scar causing indentation that is measured [58]. Although durometers were originally designed for the assessment of scleroderma, they have since been used to assess burn scars [59]. Limitations of their use include high inter- and intra-observer variability [52].

Anatomical Parameters: Color, Thickness, and 3-Dimensional Topography

Devices suitable for objectively measuring scar color include the Chromameter (Minolta, Tokyo, Japan), the DermaSpectrometer (cyberDERM, Inc., Media, PA, USA), the Mexameter (Courage-Khazaka, Cologne, Germany), and the tristimulus colorimeter [52, 60]. These devices can quantify scar pigmentation by measuring the intensity of a specific wavelength of light reflecting back from the scar to calculate erythema and melanin index (spectrophotometric color analysis) [52, 61]. Other available tools used to measure scar color are the tristimulus colorimeter, a narrow-band simple reflectance meter, and the chromameter [60]. When compared to other scar assessment tools, Draaijers et al. reported that these objective scar measuring tools assess vascularity and pigmentation better than subjective rating scales [61]. Additionally, the authors found it easier to obtain measurements with the DermaSpectrometer instead of the Chromameter; however, both devices demonstrated good reliability [52, 61].

Scar thickness (height and/or depth) can be measured by ultrasound, moulds, or dial caliper [52, 56]. Ultrasound scanners, or ultrasonography, may also include a tissue ultrasound palpation system (TULP or TUPS) [62]. Some examples of TUPS devices include PolyU, Aloka Echo Camera, and DermaScan-C and DermaScan-A [46, 62]. In terms of objectively measuring scar maturation, Fong et al. reported both ultrasonography and the cutometer to be more sensitive and specific than analysis using their own clinical rating scales for color and consistency [52, 56]. When compared to the Vancouver Scar Scale (VSS), one of the most widely applied scar assessment scales in clinical research (discussed in the following) results from TUPS demonstrated a moderate correlation in terms of reliability [52, 62]. However, TUPS requires technical training and experience in image interpretation and is relatively expensive compared to other scar-measuring modalities [52].

Surface area can be evaluated by planimetry or 3D imaging [52]. The advantages of these three-dimensional systems include their ability to capture scar surface characteristics with high definition and reproducibility [52, 63]. Roques et al. found the 3-dimensional optical profiling system (Primos imaging) to be an effective tool to generate a high-resolution topographic representation of a scar [63]. In addition, Taylor et al. applied a noncontact 3-dimensional digitizer to measure keloid volume and response to treatment [52, 64]. The authors demonstrated scanned scar volume was comparable to physical assessment as measured by the Visual Analog Scale (discussed further) with scar ranking. They also reported a statistically significant correlation between measured keloid volume and scar score [64]. Although these more advanced imaging techniques hold great promise for the objective assessment of pathologic scarring, these devices have been criticized for their high cost making them better suited for research purposes, rather than clinical assessment and treatment monitoring [38, 52].

Physiological Parameters: Blood Flow and Perfusion

Laser Doppler imaging is a well-established technique for the measurement of burn scar perfusion [52, 65]. Examples include the Laser Doppler Flowmetry (LDF), Laser Doppler Imaging (LDI), or Laser Speckle Imaging (LSI)/ Laser Speckle Perfusion Imaging (LSPI) [65, 66]. In clinical practice, laser Doppler perfusion imaging has been used for the early assessment of burn depth and subsequent treatment course [66]. These scar measuring systems have gained attention for their ability to construct color-coded maps of tissue microperfusion, thereby offering a noninvasive alternative to burn wound biopsy [52, 66]. Sarov and Stewart compared this technique to the newer laser-based method which uses photon interference patterns to map blood flow to tissues, known as a speckle decorrelation analysis [52, 67]. Statistically significant correlations were found between the two methods in terms of mapping the same relative changes in tissue blood flow [67]. The authors also found statistically significant correlations between both methods and various observed clinical parameters, mainly scar pigmentation, vascularity, pliability, and height [52, 67].

Subjective Scar Assessment Scales

Surprisingly, the subjective assessment of scars is currently more clinically useful than the objective scar-measuring devices discussed above. Scar assessment scales are questionnaires that have been developed to quantify scar appearance in response to treatment [16, 17]. They are filled out by the observer and sometimes by the patient which makes them susceptible to confounding factors [14, 15]. These factors may include (in)experience of an observer or patient as well as the psychological problems related to scarring which can highly influence the judgment of the patient [1–11]. Despite their subjective nature however, scar scales have become increasingly popular as they possess several advantages over objective scar assessment tools: they are free, easy to use, and take little time to complete which makes them very accessible in clinical practice and medical research [12–15]. Ideally, these observer-dependent scales should include the most important scar features described above

[17, 18]. In contrast, objective scar measuring devices are expensive and usually capable of measuring only one of the many scar features. Because of these drawbacks, objective scar assessment tools have only been sparsely used in medical research settings [52].

To date, no ideal scar assessment scale that is suitable for both objective and subjective purposes has emerged. In the past decades, several attempts have been made to create an appropriate scale mostly for the clinical assessment of burn scars [17, 18]. Unlike objective scar measurement tools, these scales are also frequently used in research and are particularly beneficial for studying small, linear scars. However, subjective tools are limited in their ability to assess the functional effects of scarring [11–15]. The current panel of subjective scar assessment scales is therefore insufficient to guide multimodality therapy and research for large and complex scars (Table 2) [38, 52].

Vancouver Scar Scale

Introduced by Sullivan et al. in 1990, the Vancouver Scar Scale (VSS) became the first validated scar scale adopted into clinical practice for the assessment of burn scars [68]. The VSS utilizes a semiquantitative approach to assess four physical parameters: scar height and thickness, pliability, vascularity, and pigmentation. Each variable is rated then added to generate a final score ranging from 0 to 13 [14, 68]. Although this scale set a precedent for the systematic evaluation of scars, the VSS was still far from perfect. First, the VSS did not incorporate a patient's perception of his or her respective scars and therefore lacks some important scar symptoms, like pain and itching, as well as the functional and psychological aspects of scarring [14, 38, 61]. Furthermore, not all the variables in the VSS concerned ordinal data [14, 38]. For example, the VSS pigmentation categories are scored 0 for normal, 1 for hypopigmentation, 2 for mixed pigmentation, and 3 for hyperpigmenta-

tion [68]. Based on this system, a hypopigmented scar would have a lower total VSS score than a hyperpigmented scar. Yet, there is no evidence found in the literature to support that hypopigmentation is a less severe condition than hyperpigmentation in scarring [14, 38]. Moreover, the parameters assessed do not add the same number to the final score, and thus do not contribute equally. Instead, the number of each variable appears to be a reflection of the clinical variables of that specific scar feature, suggesting a nominal scoring system [14, 52]. Therefore, although often used to quantify the absolute severity and quality of a scar, the VSS should not be used numerically [14, 38, 52]. Lastly, Forbes-Duchart et al. described poor interrater reliability with the VSS and more than two observers were required to obtain reliable data [69]. Reliability tests showed a moderate agreement with a Cohen's Kappa value of 0.5 and standard error of approximately 0.1 [38, 69]. Due to these limitations, several modifications were made to the original VSS scale, which offered a few incremental advantages.

One major modification was the replacement of the original VSS pigmentation scale with an ordinal scale that ranged from normal to severely hyper- or hypopigmented [70]. Other important modifications made include the addition of parameters such as pain and itch by Nedelec et al. as well as improvements in inter-observer reliability by Baryza et al. [70–72]. A study conducted by Truong et al. on linear scars reported an inadequate internal consistency (Cronbach's alpha = 0.71) and an excellent inter-observer reliability (ICC = 0.78) [73]. While Cohen's Kappa values of the variables improved, the overall nominal nature of this scale still remained [73, 74]. Additionally, other subjective parameters beyond itch and pain are absent in both the original and modified VSS. Extending the clinical use of such a scale to other types of scars is therefore difficult [38, 74]. Nevertheless, the modified version of the VSS remains the most commonly used scale to evaluate scar therapy and outcome in burn studies worldwide [74].

Table 2 Comparison of scar assessment scales

Scar scale	VAS	DLQI	mVSS	Seattle	MSS	Hamilton	POSAS (2.0)	MAPS	SBSES	UNC4P
Year	1921	1994	1995	1997	1998	1998	2004	2005	2007	2012
Scoring system	0–100	0–30	0–13	−4 to −16	4–14	0–14	6–60	3–12	0–5	0–12
Scar type	Mix	Mix	Burns	Burns	Mix	Mix	Mix	Burns	Mix	Burns
Features										
Erythema			✓				✓			
Pigmentation			✓	✓	✓	✓	✓	✓	✓	
Relief					✓	✓	✓	✓		
Thickness/height			✓	✓	✓	✓	✓	✓	✓	
Pliability			✓		✓		✓			✓
Surface area				✓			✓		✓	
Comorbidities										
Pain	✓	✓	✓				✓	✓		✓
Pruritus		✓	✓				✓	✓		✓
Functional		✓					✓			✓
Psychosocial		✓								
Validity	✓	✓	✓		✓		✓		✓	

This table was published in *Seminars in cutaneous medicine and surgery*, 34, Nguyen TA, Feldstein SI, Shumaker PR, Krakowski AC, A review of scar assessment scales, 28–36. Copyright Frontline Medical Communications (2015)

Not all items included in the scales are scored in this table

DLQI Dermatology Life Quality Index, *MAPS* Matching Assessment of Scars and Photographs, *MSS* Manchester Scar Scale, *PSOAS* Patient and Observer Scar Assessment Scale, *SBES* Stony Brook Scar Evaluation Scale, *UNC4P* University of North Carolina "4P" Scar Scale, *VAS* Visual Analog Scale, *mVSS* Modified Vancouver Scar Scale

Seattle Scale

In 1997, Yeong et al. designed the Seattle Scale for photographic scar assessment with improved interrater reliability [75]. The Seattle Scale utilizes a numeric-rating system in which several scar parameters, including surface area, thickness, border height, and pigmentation, are assessed based on 24 standardized color pictures. While this scale improved interrater reliability, a major flaw of its design is that it allows for certain parameters, such as hypopigmentation or atrophy, to be assigned negative values [14, 38]. Although these negative values helped differentiate between scar types, they also resulted in "improved" total scores and poor interpretation of scar severity [76]. This limitation coupled with the lack of consideration to symptoms has hindered wide adoption of the Seattle Scale [14].

Manchester Scar Scale

In 1998, Beausang et al. proposed the Manchester Scar Scale (MSS) to quantitatively assess scarring: (1) clinically, by developing a comprehensive rating scale, (2) photographically, using an image capture system and a scar assessment panel, and (3) histologically following scar excision [77]. This scale evaluates individual scar parameters, including color, contour, radiance, texture, and distortion, which are then combined with a visual analog scale (VAS) (discussed below) to determine an overall score proportional to scar severity [14, 38, 52, 77]. It is important to note that this scale uses one parameter for color mismatching rather than dividing it into two parameters: pigmentation and vascularity [77]. While considered to be more complete compared to the VSS, the MSS has been criticized for being better suited to the assessment of linear scars and for a lack of accounting for the patient's own judgment and symptoms [76]. Additionally, multiple observers were necessary for the scale to have an accepted reliability (more than nine observers) [77]. Nevertheless, the authors found a statistically significant correlation between the MSS-generated assessment and the histologic findings within the scar itself (0.87 for the total score and 0.83 for texture/stiffness) [77]. Although these findings suggest that the total score and height are indicative of histological abnormalities, approximately 90% of the histological assessment only included collagen fiber characteristics such as orientation, density, and maturity [14, 38]. Other important scar features like angiogenesis and melanin concentration were excluded and as such, it cannot be considered a gold standard [76].

Hamilton Scale

In the same year, Crowe et al. introduced another photographic scar assessment tool referred to as the Hamilton Scale [78]. This lesser-known scale asks observers to rate several scar features including surface irregularities, thickness, color, and vascularity based on photographs alone [14, 18, 77]. One advantage of the Hamilton scale is its good reliability; interrater reliability ranged from 0.66 to 0.90 and test–retest reliability ranged from 0.73 to 0.89 [78]. It was shown to have a "substantial" to "almost perfect" reliability even when used by novice therapists indicating that training was not a necessity [14, 18, 76, 78]. Despite this promising reliability, the assessment process used by the Hamilton Scale relies on photographs rather than actual scars and thus, an observer's interpretation may potentially be distorted [76]. Moreover, similar to the scales preceding it, the Hamilton Scale fails to assess subjective symptoms [14].

Patient and Observer Scar Assessment Scale

Until 2000, all developed scales were clinician reported, focusing on visual and physical scar characteristics [76]. Finally, in 2004, the Patient and Observer Scar Assessment Scale (POSAS) was introduced as the first reliable and feasible tool designed for a subjective evaluation of various scar formation [20]. The POSAS was the first scale to take into account both the patient and provider perspective and consists of 2 numeric scales: A Patient Scar Assessment Scale (P-SAS) and the Observer Scar Assessment Scale (O-SAS). In addition to assessing physical features of scars (vascularity, pigmentation, thickness, relief, pliability, and surface area), the POSAS also incorporates patient assessments of pain, itching, color, stiffness, thickness, and relief which are rated on a 1–10 ordinal scale [20]. While the POSAS became the only scale that considers subjective features, it was still limited to pain and pruritus, and lacked functional and psychological aspects and the overall impact on quality of life [76]. In 2005, the original POSAS was modified by van de Kar et al. to provide additional subjective assessment of the impact of the scar on the activities of daily life [79]. When compared to the VSS, the most frequently used scar assessment scale to date, the POSAS was found to be more consistent, reliable, and feasible for single observers, making it a more useful subjective evaluation tool [73, 76]. In terms of validity, Truong et al. reported a moderate (Spearman's Rho = 0.52) and weak (Spearman's Rho = 0.25) correlations between the VSS total score and the total score of the O-SAS and the P-SAS, respectively [73]. However, a good correlation (Spearman's Rho = 0.89) between the VSS and the O-SAS was found on burn scars, suggesting that these scales are more appropriate for burn scar evaluation [79].

Matching Assessment of Scars and Photographs

Developed in 2005, the Matching Assessment of Scars and Photographs (MAPS) is a modification of the previously mentioned Seattle Scale designed to aid in the photographic assessment of the long-term progression of a scar and its follow-up [80]. Similar to the Seattle Scale, this assessment scale is based on five scar parameters: border height, thickness, color/pigmentation, surface, and localization. The MAPS improved on the Seattle Scale by introducing set reference photographs and a localization technique to improve interrater reliability during follow-up

[80]. Interrater reliability demonstrated good agreement when assessing border height, thickness, and color (0.55–0.81), but only fair when considering surface texture (0.25–0.40) [74, 80]. The authors also found that extensive training of the observers was not necessary. However, the negative scoring system used in the Seattle Scale also persisted in the MAPS, making it impossible to calculate an overall score by adding the different components [80]. Thus, while the MAPS offers significant improvements over the Seattle Scale, it suffers from some of the same limitations [14].

Stony Brook Scar Evaluation Scale

Developed in 2007 by Singer et al. the Stony Brook Scar Evaluation Scale (SBSES) is a dichotomous five-item ordinal scale specifically aimed at measuring the long-term appearance of scars [81]. The five parameters assessed are scar width, elevation or depression, color, suture or staple marks, and overall appearance. Each variable is individually rated on a scale from 0 (worst) to 5 (best), which is then added to create a final score [81]. The authors found good interrater reliability (ranging from 0.73 to 0.85). Furthermore, a significant correlation between the SBSES total score and the visual analog cosmetic scale (Spearman's Rho 0.75–0.92) was also demonstrated, suggesting that the SBSES is able to distinguish between better and worse scars [81]. However, small scaling systems (i.e., a total score of maximum five points) reduce the sensitivity and responsiveness to minimal changes that may be clinically important for the comparison of different treatments [76]. Additionally, the SBSES lacks a subjective parameter which further limits its clinical utility [14, 52].

University of North Carolina "4P" Scar Scale

The University of North Carolina "4P" Scar Scale (UNC4P) was designed with the goal of increasing the breadth of qualitative assessment in conjunction with existing scar scales [82, 83]. The UNC4P covers the patient's subjective perception of the scar and evaluates pain, pruritus, paresthesia, and pliability. These "4Ps" are rated on a scale from 0 (worst) to 3 (best), for a combined maximum score of 12 [82, 83]. In studies conducted by Hultman et al. comparing scar characteristics before and after laser resurfacing, the UNC4P was utilized as an adjunct to the traditional VSS. Prior to the start of laser therapy, patients reported an average of 6.0 on this scale. However, patient scores decreased to a mean of 2.2 by the end of the study [82, 83]. Although the UNC4P stresses the importance of subjective input from patients throughout treatment phases, it was not designed to be used alone. Moreover, the reliability of UNC4P has yet to be independently validated [14, 76].

Visual Analog Scale

The Visual Analog Scale (VAS) is frequently used to evaluate the severity in scars and other dermatologic disorders. While not originally designed for scar evaluation, the VAS is often used in clinical assessment as a simple and quick tool to assess patients' subjective experiences of pain [84]. This multidimensional scale utilizes a photograph-based system in which standardized digital photographs are evaluated based on four dimensions (pigmentation, vascularity, acceptability, and observer comfort) plus contour. Patients are asked to rate the intensity of their pain, from no pain to the worst pain imaginable, by placing a mark on a 100 mm line [84]. Individual scores are then added to get a single overall score ranging from "excellent" to "poor." The VAS has been validated in several studies and demonstrated high observer reliability and internal consistency when compared to expert panel evaluation and other pain assessment scales such as the fixed interval scale and the verbal rating scale [85–88]. However, it has shown only moderate reliability when used among lay panels [89].

Dermatology Life Quality Index

Like the VAS, the Dermatology Life Quality Index (DLQI) was not specifically designed for scars but is commonly used in clinical practice for assessing the impact of a scar on a patient's psychosocial health and quality of life [90]. The DLQI was introduced in 1994 as the first dermatology-specific questionnaire that evaluates quality of life based on parameters like pain, itch, embarrassment or social impairment, and functional impairment [90]. It has also been shown to have good reliability and validity in multiple studies [90–92]. The wide adoption of both the VAS and the DLQI in conjunction with other scar assessment scales highlights the importance of incorporating subjective input from patients in determining overall scar morbidity and its impact on quality of life.

Burn Objective Scar Scale

The subjective scar scales VSS and POSAS are widely used because of their ease of use [65]. However, these scales have low interrater reliability and are primarily optimal for comparison of scar changes for the same individual rather than different patients [93]. In contrast, objective assessments of burn scars represent an attractive alternative and are not observer dependent. There are several objective scar measurement tools that may be employed, and these measurements can be incorporated to form a global objective scar assessment scale [94]. These include the DSM II colormeter, the Dermascan 20 MHz high-frequency ultrasound, and the cutometer elasticity probe.

The DSM II colormeter is a handheld device that can quantify color using two primary methods, narrow-band spectrophotometry and tristimulus reflectance colorimetry, combining the results into a single measurement [95]. Dermascan C USB is a high-frequency ultrasound scanner that allows for high-resolution imaging of soft tissue using a computer with software for skin thickness measurement [96]. Skin thickness is calculated as the distance between the stratum corneum and the inner dermal surface of the burn scar. The cutometer elasticity probe is an instrument that can assess skin elasticity. The probe generates a negative pressure over the area of interest, drawing tissue into an aperture in the center of the probe. A laser is then used to estimate the amount of skin displacement and reports "R-parameters (R0 and R2)," or maximum deformation of the skin (R0) and ratio of final retraction and maximum deformation (R2) [96]. We next discuss the correlation between subjective and objective values below, focusing on color and scar thickness, and pliability.

Color

A comparison of subjective erythema scores measured with a modified VSS (mVSS) vascularity subscale can be made with the DSM II colormeter narrow band (erythema) and trismus colorimetry (a*) [94]. Narrowband erythema measurements and the a* parameter have a weak but positive correlation with the mVSS vascularity [94]. With regard to pigmentation, adjustments to the mVSS pigmentation subscale were made by converting hypopigmentation into a negative value (−1), while normal skin is considered "0" and other scores were adjusted down accordingly. This allows for comparison to the DSM II pigmentation parameters—narrow band melanin and tristimulus colorimetry (L*) [94]. Both parameters are weakly but significantly correlated with the mVSS pigmentations subscale [94]. Taken together, objective scar color assessment is weakly correlated with mVSS subjective scales but is statistically significant.

Thickness and Pliability

Dermascan can be used to determine scar thickness, and this tool demonstrates a moderate but statistically significant correlation with the mVSS height subscale [94]. The Cutometer R0 and R2 subscales can be used to assess scar pliability. However, while the R0 subscale has a moderate and statistically significant correlation

with the mVSS pliability scale, the R2 subscale has no significant correlation [94]. Additionally, while the Dermascan scar thickness scores discussed previously are not a direct measure of pliability, values obtained correlate significantly with mVSS pliability values [94]. Likely, this is attributable to the fact that scar tissue pliability is affected by thickness, suggesting that Dermascan values can be used as an indirect measure to determine pliability.

Conclusion

Reliable assessment and measurements of scarring are increasingly important in research and clinical practice. In particular, this is the case in wound healing studies in which the effectiveness of surgical procedures and other medical interventions is assessed by long-term scarring outcomes, necessitating a reliable longitudinal assessment strategy. As illustrated in this chapter, there are a variety of assessment tools that can be based on subjective and/or objective qualities of scar tissue, and ideally both should be incorporated into scar assessment. Subjective qualities include the patient's own evaluation of the scar and pending psychological and social impact, while objective qualities are primarily focused on physical characteristics including color, thickness, pliability, etc.

In order to assess the effectiveness of subjective and objective measurements, multiple scar scales and assessment parameters have been developed. Here, we outline several subjective measures including VSS and the POSAS, discussing shortcomings (e.g., observer-dependent variability), which introduce the need for objective measures and devices (e.g., DSM II colorimeter). The utility of these devices includes standardized and measurable parameters such as scar color, thickness, and pliability among other features. Recent studies focusing on objective scales such as BOSS compare objective parameter outcomes to subjective scales, allowing for the development of objective scar assessment panels that could serve as alternatives to traditional scales such as VSS.

Importantly, while we discuss the utility of objective versus subjective parameters and compare the various scar scales, we cannot unequivocally claim one to be superior over another. It is important to note that there currently is not an agreement with regard to the "gold standard" for assessing scars. While studies provide a basis for the creation of disease-specific tools (e.g., BOSS), further multi-center verification of effectiveness is important to ensure global applicability.

Acknowledgments RV is a recipient of the Frederick Banting and Charles Best Canada Graduate Scholarship (CGS-D). This work was supported by grants from the Canadian Institutes of Health Research (#123336), the Canada Foundation for Innovation Leaders Opportunity Fund (Project #25407), and the National Institutes of Health (R01GM133961).

References

1. Van Loey NE, Van Son MJ. Psychopathology and psychological problems in patients with burn scars: epidemiology and management. Am J Clin Dermatol. 2003;4(4):245–72.

2. van Baar ME, Essink-Bot ML, Oen IM, Dokter J, Boxma H, van Beeck EF. Functional outcome after burns: a review. Burns. 2006;32(1):1–9.

3. Rumsey N, Clarke A, White P. Exploring the psychosocial concerns of outpatients with disfiguring conditions. J Wound Care. 2003;12(7):247–52.

4. Bock O, Schmid-Ott G, Malewski P, Mrowietz U. Quality of life of patients with keloid and hypertrophic scarring. Arch Dermatol Res. 2006;297(10):433–8.

5. Reish RG, Eriksson E. Scars: a review of emerging and currently available therapies. Plast Reconstr Surg. 2008;122(4):1068–78.

6. Powers PS, Sarkar S, Goldgof DB, Cruse CW, Tsap LV. Scar assessment: current problems and future solutions. J Burn Care Rehabil. 1999;20(1 Pt 1):54–60.

7. Falder S, Browne A, Edgar D, Staples E, Fong J, Rea S, Wood F. Core outcomes for adult burn survivors: a clinical overview. Burns. 2009;35(5):618–41.

8. Baur KM, Hardy PE, Van Dorsten B. Posttraumatic stress disorder in burn populations: a critical review of the literature. J Burn Care Rehabil. 1998;19(3):230–40.

9. Gilboa D, Bisk L, Montag I, Tsur H. Personality traits and psychosocial adjustment of patients with burns. J Burn Care Rehabil. 1999;20(4):340–6.

10. Fauerbach JA, Heinberg LJ, Lawrence JW, et al. Effect of early body image dissatisfaction on subsequent psychological and physical adjustment after disfiguring injury. Psychosom Med. 2000;62(4):576–82.

11. Lawrence JW, Mason ST, Schomer K, Klein MB. Epidemiology and impact of scarring after burn injury: a systematic review of the literature. J Burn Care Res. 2012;33(1):136–46.

12. Nguyen DQ, Potokar T, Price P. A review of current objective and subjective scar assessment tools. J Wound Care. 2008;17(3):101–2.

13. Brusselaers N, Pirayesh A, Hoeksema H, Verbelen J, Blot S, Monstrey S. Burn scar assessment: a systematic review of objective scar assessment tools. Burns. 2010;36(8):1157–64.

14. Nguyen TA, Feldstein SI, Shumaker PR, Krakowski AC. A review of scar assessment scales. Semin Cutan Med Surg. 2015;34(1):28–36.

15. van Zuijlen PP, Angeles AP, Kreis RW, Bos KE, Middelkoop E. Scar assessment tools: implications for current research. Plast Reconstr Surg. 2002;109(3):1108–22.

16. Mustoe TA, Cooter RD, Gold MH, Hobbs FD, Ramelet AA, Shakespeare PG, Stella M, Téot L, Wood FM, Ziegler UE. International advisory panel on scar management. International clinical recommendations on scar management. Plast Reconstr Surg. 2002;110(2):560–71.

17. Idriss N, Maibach HI. Scar assessment scales: a dermatologic overview. Skin Res Technol. 2009;15(1):1–5.

18. Verhaegen PDHM, van der Wal MBA, Middelkoop E, van Zuijlen PPM. Scar assessment. In: Handbook of burns: reconstruction and rehabilitation, vol. 2. Berlin: Springer; 2012. p. 69–89. https://doi.org/10.1007/978-3-7091-0315-9_6.

19. Chadwick S, Heath R, Shah M. Abnormal pigmentation within cutaneous scars: a complication of wound healing. Indian J Plast Surg. 2012;45(2):403–11.

20. Draaijers LJ, Tempelman FR, Botman YA, Tuinebreijer WE, Middelkoop E, Kreis RW, van Zuijlen PP. The patient and observer scar assessment scale: a reliable and feasible tool for scar evaluation. Plast Reconstr Surg. 2004;113(7):1960–5.

21. Herd AN, Hall PN, Widdowson P, Tanner NS. Mesh grafts—an 18 month follow-up. Burns Incl Therm Inj. 1987;13(1):57–61.

22. Finnerty CC, Jeschke MG, Branski LK, Barret JP, Dziewulski P, Herndon DN. Hypertrophic scarring: the greatest unmet challenge after burn injury. Lancet. 2016;388(10052):1427–36.

23. Peacock EE Jr, Madden JW, Trier WC. Biologic basis for the treatment of keloids and hypertrophic scars. South Med J. 1970;63(7):755–60.

24. O'Sullivan ST, O'Shaughnessy M, O'Connor TP. Aetiology and management of hypertrophic scars and keloids. Ann R Coll Surg Engl. 1996;78(3 (Pt 1)):168–75.

25. Bayat A, McGrouther DA, Ferguson MW. Skin scarring. BMJ. 2003;326(7380):88–92.

26. Brissett AE, Sherris DA. Scar contractures, hypertrophic scars, and keloids. Facial Plast Surg. 2001;17(4):263–72.

27. Goel A, Shrivastava P. Post-burn scars and scar contractures. Indian J Plast Surg. 2010;43(Suppl):S63–71.
28. van Leersum NJ, van Leersum RL, Verwey HF, Klautz RJ. Pain symptoms accompanying chronic poststernotomy pain: a pilot study. Pain Med. 2010;11(11):1628–34.
29. Schneider JC, Harris NL, El Shami A, Sheridan RL, Schulz JT 3rd, Bilodeau ML, Ryan CM. A descriptive review of neuropathic-like pain after burn injury. J Burn Care Res. 2006;27(4):524–8.
30. Bijlard E, Uiterwaal L, Kouwenberg CA, Mureau MA, Hovius SE, Huygen FJ. A systematic review on the prevalence, etiology, and pathophysiology of intrinsic pain in dermal scar tissue. Pain Physician. 2017;20(2):1–13.
31. Zhu J, Cheng B, Liu H, Tang J, Xiang X, Peng Y. Expression of beta-endorphin in hypertrophic scar and its relationship with pruritus. Zhongguo Xiu Fu Chong Jian Wai Ke Za Zhi. 2012;26(6):731–4.
32. Van Loey NE, Bremer M, Faber AW, Middelkoop E, Nieuwenhuis MK. Itching following burns: epidemiology and predictors. Br J Dermatol. 2008;158(1):95–100.
33. Ward RS, Tuckett RP, English KB, Johansson O, Saffle JR. Substance P axons and sensory threshold increase in burn-graft human skin. J Surg Res. 2004;118(2):154–60.
34. Scott JR, Muangman PR, Tamura RN, Zhu KQ, Liang Z, Anthony J, Engrav LH, Gibran NS. Substance P levels and neutral endopeptidase activity in acute burn wounds and hypertrophic scar. Plast Reconstr Surg. 2005;115(4):1095–102.
35. Tredget EE, Shankowsky HA, Pannu R, Nedelec B, Iwashina T, Ghahary A, Taerum TV, Scott PG. Transforming growth factor-beta in thermally injured patients with hypertrophic scars: effects of interferon alpha-2b. Plast Reconstr Surg. 1998;102(5):1317–28.
36. Lee SS, Yosipovitch G, Chan YH, Goh CL. Pruritus, pain, and small nerve fiber function in keloids: a controlled study. J Am Acad Dermatol. 2004;51(6):1002–6.
37. Parnell LK, Nedelec B, Rachelska G, LaSalle L. Assessment of pruritus characteristics and impact on burn survivors. J Burn Care Res. 2012;33(3):407–18.
38. Roques C, Teot L. A critical analysis of measurements used to assess and manage scars. Int J Low Extrem Wounds. 2007;6(4):249–53.
39. Thompson CM, Sood RF, Honari S, Carrougher GJ, Gibran NS. What score on the Vancouver Scar Scale constitutes a hypertrophic scar? Results from a survey of North American burn-care providers. Burns. 2015;41(7):1442–8.
40. Jaspers MEH, Moortgat P. Objective assessment tools: physical parameters in scar assessment. In: Téot L, Mustoe TA, Middelkoop E, Gauglitz GG, editors. Textbook on scar management. Cham: Springer; 2020. p. 150–7. https://doi.org/10.1007/978-3-030-44766-3_17.
41. Mokkink LB, Terwee CB, Patrick DL, Alonso J, Stratford PW, Knol DL, Bouter LM, de Vet HC. The COSMIN study reached international consensus on taxonomy, terminology, and definitions of measurement properties for health-related patient-reported outcomes. J Clin Epidemiol. 2010;63(7):737–45.
42. De Vet HCW, Terwee CB, Mokkink LB, Knol DL, Measurement in medicine. A practical guide. 1st ed. Cambridge: Cambridge University Press; 2011.
43. Andresen EM. Criteria for assessing the tools of disability outcomes research. Arch Phys Med Rehabil. 2000;81(12 Suppl 2):S15–20.
44. van de Ven-Stevens LA, Munneke M, Terwee CB, Spauwen PH, van der Linde H. Clinimetric properties of instruments to assess activities in patients with hand injury: a systematic review of the literature. Arch Phys Med Rehabil. 2009;1:151–69.
45. Fitzpatrick R, Davey C, Buxton MJ, Jones DR. Evaluating patient-based outcome measures for use in clinical trials. Health Technol Assess. 1998;2(14):1–74.
46. Terwee CB, Bot SD, de Boer MR, van der Windt DA, Knol DL, Dekker J, Bouter LM, de Vet HC. Quality criteria were proposed for measurement properties of health status questionnaires. J Clin Epidemiol. 2007;60(1):34–42.
47. Streiner DL, Norman GR. Reliability. Health measurement scales. 4th ed. Oxford: Oxford University Press; 2008. p. 167–210.
48. Nunnaly JC. Psychometric theory. 2nd ed. New York: McGraw-Hill; 1978.
49. Streiner DL, Norman GR. Validity. Health measurement scales. 4th ed. Oxford: Oxford University Press; 2008. p. 247–76.
50. Patrick DL, Chiang YP. Measurement of health outcomes in treatment effectiveness evaluations: conceptual and methodological challenges. Med Care. 2000;9(Suppl):214–25.
51. Landis JR, Koch GG. The measurement of observer agreement for categorical data. Biometrics. 1997;33(1):159–74.
52. Fearmonti R, Bond J, Erdmann D, Levinson H. A review of scar scales and scar measuring devices. Eplasty. 2010;10:e43.
53. Perry DM, McGrouther DA, Bayat A. Current tools for noninvasive objective assessment of skin scars. Plast Reconstr Surg. 2010;126(3):912–23.
54. Spann K, Mileski WJ, Atiles L, Purdue G, Hunt J. The 1996 clinical research award. Use of a pneumatonometer in burn scar assessment. J Burn Care Rehabil. 1996;17(6 Pt 1):515–7.
55. Enomoto D, Mekkes J, Bossuyt P, et al. Quantification of cutaneous sclerosis with a skin elasticity meter in patients with generalized scleroderma. J Am Acad Dermatol. 1996;35:381–7.
56. Fong S, Hung L, Cheng J. The cutometer and ultrasonography in the assessment of postburn hypertrophic scar: a preliminary study. Burns. 1997;23(1):S12–8.
57. Draaijers LJ, Botman YA, Tempelman FR, Kreis RW, Middelkoop E, van Zuijlen PP. Skin elasticity meter

or subjective evaluation in scars: a reliability assessment. Burns. 2004;30(2):109–14.

58. Falanga V, Bucalo B. Use of the durometer to assess skin hardness. J Am Acad Dermatol. 1993;29(1):47–51.

59. Magliaro A, Romanelli M. Skin hardness measurement in hypertrophic scars. Wounds. 2003;15:66–70.

60. Haudenschild DR, Nguyen B, Chen J, D'Lima DD, Lotz MK. Rho kinase-dependent CCL20 induced by dynamic compression of human chondrocytes. Arthritis Rheum. 2008;58(9):2735–42.

61. Draaijers LJ, Tempelman FR, Botman YA. Colour evaluation in scars: tristimulus colorimeter, narrowband simple reflectance meter or subjective evaluation? Burns. 2004;30:103–7.

62. Lau JC, Li-Tsang CW, Zheng YP. Application of tissue ultrasound palpation system (TUPS) in objective scar evaluation. Burns. 2005;31:445–52.

63. Roques C, Téot L, Frasson N, Meaume S. PRIMOS: an optical system that produces three-dimensional measurements of skin surfaces. J Wound Care. 2003;12(9):362–4.

64. Taylor B, McGrouther D, Bayat A. Use of a non-contact 3D digitizer to measure the volume of keloid scars: a useful tool for scar assessment? JPRAS. 2007;60:87–94.

65. Lee KC, Dretzke J, Grover L, Logan A, Moiemen N. A systematic review of objective burn scar measurements. Burns Trauma. 2016;4:14.

66. Bray R, Forrester K, Leonard C, McArthur R, Tulip J, Lindsay R. Laser Doppler imaging of burn scars: a comparison of wavelength and scanning methods. Burns. 2003;29:199–206.

67. Sarov M, Stewart AF. The best control for the specificity of RNAi. Trends Biotechnol. 2005;23:446–8.

68. Sullivan T, Smith J, Kermode J, McIver E, Courtemanche DJ. Rating the burn scar. J Burn Care Rehabil. 1990;11(3):256–60.

69. Forbes-Duchart L, Marshall S, Strock A, Cooper JE. Determination of inter-rater reliability in pediatric burn scar assessment using a modified version of the Vancouver Scar Scale. J Burn Care Res. 2007;28(3):460–7.

70. Nedelec B, Correa JA, Rachelska G, Armour A, LaSalle L. Quantitative measurement of hypertrophic scar: intrarater reliability, sensitivity, and specificity. J Burn Care Res. 2008;29(3):489–500.

71. Nedelec B, Shankowsky HA, Tredget EE. Rating the resolving hypertrophic scar: comparison of the Vancouver Scar Scale and scar volume. J Burn Care Rehabil. 2000;21(3):205–12.

72. Baryza MJ, Baryza GA. Vancouver scar scale: an administration tool and its inter-rater reliability. J Burn Care Rehabil. 1995;16:535–8.

73. Truong PT, Lee JC, Soer B, Gaul CA, Olivotto IA. Reliability and validity testing of the patient and observer scar assessment scale in evaluating linear scars after breast cancer surgery. Plast Reconstr Surg. 2007;119:487–94.

74. Tyack Z, Simons M, Spinks A, Wasiak J. A systematic review of the quality of burn scar rating scales for clinical and research use. Burns. 2012;38(1):6–18.

75. Yeong EK, Mann R, Engrav LH, et al. Improved burn scar assessment with use of a new scar-rating scale. J Burn Care Rehabil. 1997;18(4):353–5.

76. van der Wal MB, Verhaegen PD, Middelkoop E, van Zuijlen PP. A clinimetric overview of scar assessment scales. J Burn Care Res. 2012;33(2):e79–87.

77. Beausang E, Floyd H, Dunn KW, Orton CI, Ferguson MW. A new quantitative scale for clinical scar assessment. Plast Reconstr Surg. 1998;102(6):1954–61.

78. Crowe JM, Simpson K, Johnson W, Allen J. Reliability of photographic analysis in determining change in scar appearance. J Burn Care Rehabil. 1998;19(2):183–6.

79. Fearmonti RM, Bond JE, Erdmann D, Levin LS, Pizzo SV, Levinson H. The modified patient and observer scar assessment scale: a novel approach to defining pathologic and nonpathologic scarring. Plast Reconstr Surg. 2011;127(1):242–7.

80. Masters M, McMahon M, Svens B. Reliability testing of a new scar assessment tool, matching assessment of scars and photographs (MAPS). J Burn Care Rehabil. 2005;26(3):273–84.

81. Singer AJ, Arora B, Dagum A, Valentine S, Hollander JE. Development and validation of a novel scar evaluation scale. Plast Reconstr Surg. 2007;120(7):1892–7.

82. Hultman CS, Friedstat JS, Edkins RE, Cairns BA, Meyer AA. Laser resurfacing and remodeling of hypertrophic burn scars: the results of a large, prospective, before after cohort study, with long-term follow-up. Ann Surg. 2014;260(3):519–29.

83. Hultman CS, Edkins RE, Lee CN, Calvert CT, Cairns BA. Shine on: review of laser- and light-based therapies for the treatment of burn scars. Dermatol Res Pract. 2012;2012:243651.

84. Scott J, Huskisson EC. Graphic representation of pain. Pain. 1976;2(2):175–84.

85. Joyce CR, Zutshi DW, Hrubes V, Mason RM. Comparison of fixed interval and visual analogue scales for rating chronic pain. Eur J Clin Pharmacol. 1975;8(6):415–20.

86. Ohnhaus EE, Adler R. Methodological problems in the measurement of pain: a comparison between the verbal rating scale and the visual analogue scale. Pain. 1975;1(4):379–84.

87. Carlsson AM. Assessment of chronic pain. I. Aspects of the reliability and validity of the visual analogue scale. Pain. 1983;16(1):87–101.

88. Jensen MP, McFarland CA. Increasing the reliability and validity of pain intensity measurement in chronic pain patients. Pain. 1993;55(2):195–203.

89. Bae SH, Bae YC. Analysis of frequency of use of different scar assessment scales based on the scar condition and treatment method. Arch Plast Surg. 2014;41(2):111–5.

90. Finlay AY, Khan GK. Dermatology Life Quality Index (DLQI)—a simple practical measure for routine clinical use. Clin Exp Dermatol. 1994;19(3):210–6.

91. Mazharinia N, Aghaei S, Shayan Z. Dermatology Life Quality Index (DLQI) scores in burn victims after revival. J Burn Care Res. 2007;28(2):312–7.

92. Balci DD, Inandi T, Dogramaci CA, Celik E. DLQI scores in patients with keloids and hypertrophic scars: a prospective case control study. J Dtsch Dermatol Ges. 2009;7(8):688–92.

93. Brusselaers N, Pirayesh A, Hoeksema H, Verbelen J, Blot S, Monstrey S. Burn scar assessment: a systematic review of different scar scales. J Surg Res. 2010;164(1):e115–23.

94. Lee KC, Bamford A, Gardiner F, Agovino A, Ter Horst B, Bishop J, Grover L. Burns objective scar scale (BOSS): validation of an objective measurement devices based burn scar scale panel. Burns. 2020;46(1):110–20.

95. van der Wal M, Bloeman M, Verhaegen P, Tuinebreijer W, de Vert H, van Zuijlen P, et al. Objective color measurements: clinimetric performance of three devices on normal skin and scar tissue. J Burn Care Res. 2013;34(3):e187–94.

96. Van den Kerchove E, Staes F, Flour M, Stappaerts K, Boeckx W. Reproducibility of repeated measurements on post-burn scars with Dermascan C. Skin Res Technol. 2003;9(1):81–4.

Measuring Postoperative SCAR Quality

SCAR Cosmesis Assessment and Rating (SCAR) Scale

Jean-Phillip Okhovat and Jonathan Kantor

Core Messages

- The Scar Cosmesis Assessment and Rating (SCAR) scale is a reliable assessment tool specifically designed as an outcomes measure for postoperative scars.
- The SCAR scale has excellent intrarater and interrater reliability and can be used equivalently on both live patients and photographs for the assessment of postsurgical scars.

Introduction

Historically, there have been many unique challenges in objectively assessing postoperative scar quality (see previous chapter). Initially, the

J.-P. Okhovat
Department of Dermatology, University of Maryland, Baltimore, MD, USA

J. Kantor (✉)
Center for Global Health, University of Pennsylvania Perelman School of Medicine, Philadelphia, PA, USA

Center for Clinical Epidemiology and Biostatistics, University of Pennsylvania Perelman School of Medicine, Philadelphia, PA, USA

Department of Dermatology, University of Pennsylvania Perelman School of Medicine, Philadelphia, PA, USA

Florida Center for Dermatology, St. Augustine, FL, USA

Beth Israel Deaconess Medical Center, Boston, MA, USA

Vancouver Scar Scale (VSS) was used to assess scarring even though this four-item scar was initially developed to assess burn scars as opposed to postoperative linear scars [1]. This scar assessment tool was based on several physical parameters, including pigmentation, vascularity, pliability, and scar height, with an increasing score given to a greater pathologic condition, and normal skin having a score of 0. Subsequently, a Patient and Observer Scar Assessment Scale (POSAS) was developed for burn scars, which was then reliably tested for linear scars as well [2, 3]. The POSAS was developed to assess linear surgical scars based on vascularity, pigmentation, thickness, and surface area [3]. Other scales that have been utilized for assessment of scars have included the Hamilton Scale, Seattle Scar, the Manchester Scar Scale, the Stony Brook Scar Evaluation Scale, and the University of North Carolina 4P Scar Scale, among others [4–8].

Until more recently, however, there was no psychometrically rigorous scale that existed specifically designed to assess the evolution of postoperative linear scar cosmesis and function. The Scar Cosmesis Assessment and Rating (SCAR) scale was developed for precisely this purpose—as a rating scale for postoperative linear scars that could be used with both live patients and photographs, while capturing change in a particular scar component over time (Table 1) [9]. Building upon the foundations of prior work, the SCAR scale was developed to differentially weigh scar

S. P. Nischwitz et al. (eds.), *Scars*, https://doi.org/10.1007/978-3-031-24137-6_8

Table 1 The Scar Cosmesis Assessment and Rating (SCAR) scale

Clinician items	Scale ratings
Scar spread	0, None to near-invisible
	1, Pencil-thin line
	2, Mild spread, noticeable on close inspection
	3, Moderate spread, obvious scarring
	4, Severe spread
Erythema	0, None
	1, Light pink, some telangiectasias may be present
	2, Red, many telangiectasias may be present
	3, Deep red or purple
Dyspigmentation (includes hyperpigmentation and hypopigmentation)	0, Absent
	1, Present
Track marks or suture marks	0, Absent
	1, Present
Hypertrophy/atrophy	0, None
	1, Mild: palpable, barely visible hypertrophy or atrophy
	2, Moderate: clearly visible hypertrophy or atrophy
	3, Severe: marked hypertrophy or atrophy or keloid formation
Overall impression	0, Desirable scar
	1, Undesirable scar
Patient items	
Have you been bothered by any itch from the scar in the past 24 h?	0, No 1, Yes
Have you been bothered by any pain from the scar in the past 24 h?	0, No 1, Yes
Total score range	0 (Best possible scar) to 15 (worst possible scar)

hypertrophy, spread, and erythema when assessing scar quality—it is unique in that the items are weighted based on the degree of clinical importance assigned by multispecialty validity committees, as well as patients.

SCAR Assessment Scale

The initial study introducing the SCAR assessment scale sought to assess whether high-quality clinical photographs may be used in lieu of live assessments by raters and to assess both the interrater and intrarater reliability of the SCAR scale on a range of postoperative scars [9]. Twenty patients were analyzed for photographic equivalency (both live scar and photographs were examined) while 60 photographs of 60 other patients were analyzed by 5 raters—of the latter 60 patients, 10 of these were rated utilizing the SCAR scale, POSAS, and VSS, and 10 were assessed twice by the same rater at different time intervals to assess intrarater reliability.

In order to assess interrater reliability, a group of five clinicians (four board-certified dermatologists and one physician's assistant) scored a separate set of 60 high-quality scar photographs of scars reflecting a broad range of patient ages, skin types, and severity. As mentioned above, to assess for intrarater reliability, 10 patients were assessed twice by each rater, and raters were not informed beforehand that selected scars would be rated twice in order to minimize recall bias. Assessed scars included a wide variety of outcomes, ranging from nearly undetectable scars to large keloids, in patients ranging from 18 to 96 years and skin types ranging from Fitzpatrick types I–VI.

With respect to photographs and live patients, there was near equivalence with the use of the SCAR scale. The intraclass correlation coefficiency (ICC) for each of two raters on a separate 20-scar set of live patients and photographs was

0.99 (95% CI 0.96–0.99) and 0.98 (95% CI 0.96–0.99) suggesting clinical equivalence between the SCAR scale use on live patients and high-quality photographs. Furthermore, using a two-sample random effects model, the interrater reliability was found to be 0.95—this was equal to or better than previously reported scale, suggesting remarkable agreement between different clinicians when scoring the SCAR scale. Similarly, intrarater reliability was also high with one-sample random effects model ICCs ranging from 0.96 to 0.99 for each rater using a 1-way random effects model—suggesting that the same observer is likely to rate the same scar with the same overall score when assessed a second time. With regard to generalizability to different skin types, the interrater reliability of the SCAR scale in patients with Fitzpatrick type IV–VI demonstrated an ICC of 0.93 (95% CI 0.86–0.98), and the ICC for the erythema component was 0.92 (95% CI 0.84–0.96)—suggesting that the SCAR scale can reliably be used for patients with different skin types.

Advantages Over Other Tools

Overall, the SCAR scale represents a reliable outcome measure for assessing linear scars that can be utilized for both live patients and high-quality scar photographs. It includes six observer components and two patient components, adding to its feasibility. As opposed to other scar assessment tools which may utilize a broad range of scores for individual items, most of the SCAR scale components are graded as either binary (yes or no) outcomes or linked to clinically objective outcomes—this allows raters to distinguish between the presence or absence of specific objective clinical findings, as opposed to an assessor's overall impression of a scar, which may lead to poor interrater reliability.

Furthermore, the SCAR scale has to its advantage the incorporation of a multidisciplinary team in its developments, as specialists from dermatology, plastic surgery, surgical oncology, physiatry, and emergency medicine were involved in the

validation and reliability assessments. A unique advantage of this tool is the incorporation of separate scores for erythema and dyspigmentation, which allows investigators to capture improvement in one or both components as scars evolve over time or treated with different approaches.

In terms of the benefits of the SCAR scale when compared to the POSAS and other scar assessment tools for post-reconstructive surgery photographic scar assessment, the SCAR has several advantages. First, the SCAR scale was specifically designed for the assessment of postsurgical scars, whereas earlier tools were originally developed for burn scars. Second, other prior scar assessment tools are composite scales with equal weightings of a number of different measures, and they do not differentially weight those of greatest concern to surgeons and patients. Limitations with respect to the POSAS tool include the removal of pliability, potentially altering the psychometric properties of the scale, including dimensionality, validity, and reliability. Further, reliability testing in POSAS predominantly included centrofacial scars in patients with fair skin, thus limiting its use and generalizability to a broader range of scars. The SCAR scale represents a more meaningful and adaptable assessment tool that is more feasible to use, relies more on objective measures, is clinically meaningful given that items are weight-based depending on their impact on appearance, and is patient centered; in addition it employs clearer terminology.

Conclusion

The SCAR scale is a feasible and reliable instrument designed to rate postsurgical scars with a high degree of interrater and intrarater reliability. It assigns weighted measurements to individual components of a scar that change over time and takes into account both patient and physician assessments in the overall score. It is an easy tool to use with clear language and features attributes that minimize one's overall impression of a scar when using the scoring system, but rather focuses on clinically objective findings.

References

1. Sullivan T, Smith J, Kermode J, McIver E, Courtemanche DJ. Rating the burn scar. J Burn Care Rehabil. 1990;11(3):256–60.
2. Draaijers LJ, Tempelman FR, Botman YA, et al. The patient and observer scar assessment scale: a reliable and feasible tool for scar evaluation. Plast Reconstr Surg. 2004;113(7):1960–5.
3. van de Kar AL, Corion LU, Smeulders MJ, Draaijers LJ, van der Horst CM, van Zuijlen PP. Reliable and feasible evaluation of linear scars by the patient and observer scar assessment scale. Plast Reconstr Surg. 2005;116(2):514–22.
4. Crowe JM, Simpson K, Johnson W, Allen J. Reliability of photographic analysis in determining change in scar appearance. J Burn Care Rehabil. 1998;19(2):183–6.
5. Yeong EK, Mann R, Engrav LH, et al. Improved burn scar assessment with use of a new scar-rating scale. J Burn Care Rehabil. 1997;18(4):353–5.
6. Beausang E, Floyd H, Dunn KW, Orton CI, Ferguson MW. A new quantitative scale for clinical scar assessment. Plast Reconstr Surg. 1998;102(6):1954–61.
7. Singer AJ, Arora B, Dagum A, Valentine S, Hollander JE. Development and validation of a novel scar evaluation scale. Plast Reconstr Surg. 2007;120(7):1892–7.
8. Hultman CS, Friedstat JS, Edkins RE, Cairns BA, Meyer AA. Laser resurfacing and remodeling of hypertrophic burn scars: the results of a large, prospective, before-after cohort study, with long-term follow-up. Ann Surg. 2014;260(3):519–29.
9. Kantor J. Reliability and photographic equivalency of the SCAR cosmesis assessment and rating (SCAR) scale, an outcome measure for postoperative scars. JAMA Dermatol. 2017;153(1):55–60.

Scar Prevention

Surgical and Nonsurgical Aspects to Reduce Scar Formation, Including Early Therapies

Alejandra Monte-Soldado and Juan P. Barret

Core Messages

- Avoid skin tension during wound closure by an optimal planning of surgical incision line location, within or parallel to the relaxed skin tension lines. Use a layered closure to reduce tension in the superficial dermis and epidermis. Consider the use of adhesive tapes.
- Avoid postoperative movements that stretch the wound. Use thigh brassieres and/or abdominal bands as an adjunctive measure to reduce skin-stretching tension in thorax or abdominal wounds.
- Prevent surgical site infection by meticulous attention to aseptic technique, removal of foreign bodies and devitalized tissues, and antibiotic prophylaxis when indicated.
- Recognize and manage factors that hamper and delay wound healing such as smoking, alcoholism, malnutrition, or poor glycemic control.
- Consider silicone gel sheeting or topical silicone gel as a first-line prophylactic therapy in non-burn surgical scars.
- Consider pressure garments as a first-line prophylactic therapy in burn scars and scars resulting from chronic or extensive wounds.
- Consider silicone gel sheeting and pressure garments as a combined prophylactic therapy in high-risk, more complex cases.
- Consider the use of steroid injections in high-risk individuals or in keloid excision surgery to avoid recurrence.

Introduction

The wound healing and scar formation process involves a set of changes in skin structure that differentiate it from the surrounding skin. It includes color, thickness, elasticity, and texture changes. In addition, some degree of skin contraction and functional impairment can be present in case of joint involvement. Abnormal scars can be pruritic and painful and may have unpleasant aesthetic, functional, and psychosocial implications, leading to severe emotional distress and impairment of quality of life.

The pathogenesis of hypertrophic scars and keloids is complex and continues to be under investigation. Multiple contributing factors have been proposed: infection, persistent inflammation, hypoxia, endocrine factors, mechanical tension, and an individual genetic predisposition are described [1]. However, there is no clear evidence to support a single, unified theory that explains the pathogenesis of excessive scarring.

Given the multiple etiologic factors involved in abnormal scar formation, a wide range of pro-

A. Monte-Soldado · J. P. Barret (✉)
Department of Plastic Surgery and Burns, Vall
d'Hebron Barcelona Hospital Campus, Universitat
Autònoma de Barcelona, Barcelona, Spain
e-mail: amonte@vhebron.net; jpbarret@vhebron.net

phylactic and therapeutic options are also available. Nevertheless, to date, there is no therapy with clearly proven and consistent efficacy, and treating a pathological scar, once established, can be complex and frustrating. For this reason, it is particularly important to establish preventive strategies in order to minimize scar formation early in the event of any injury, either in case of accidental trauma or elective surgery.

Prevention Strategies to Reduce Scar Formation

Surgical Aspects to Prevent Excessive Scar Formation

Preoperative Considerations

Before any elective surgical procedure, a thorough history of excessive scar formation should be obtained from the patient. Patients with a known personal or family history of keloids should be advised to avoid body piercing and nonessential surgical procedures, especially at anatomic sites that are at higher risk of keloid formation such as the shoulders, upper back, and anterior chest [2].

Preventive measures to reduce scar formation should be applied even before starting any surgical procedure. A meticulous planning of the skin incision line location and orientation is fundamental. Incisions should be designed parallel to the relaxed skin tension lines or Langer's lines whenever feasible. A Z-plasty wound closure technique may be designed and used in case of incisions that have to cross relaxing skin tension lines. Z-plasty technique involves the creation of two transposition triangular flaps of equal dimensions to achieve a more favorable reorientation of the incision line (Fig. 1).

Exposure of scars to ultraviolet irradiation has been shown to negatively impact cosmetic outcomes by worsening erythema, pigmentation, and scar size. For this reason, patients should be advised to avoid sunlight exposure a few days prior to surgery and during the whole scar maturation process to avoid hyperpigmentation. Postoperatively, sunscreen should be used as primary protection when skin is exposed to direct sunlight.

Risk factors that promote the development of excessive scars and that can be avoided or limited by the surgeon are skin stretching tension on wound edges and excessive or prolonged inflammation caused by surgical site infection, foreign bodies, and delayed wound healing.

Mechanical Tension (Skin Stretching)

There is evidence that increased mechanical tension during early phases of wound healing is a major factor involved in hypertrophic scar and keloid formation. Mechanical stress strongly modulates cellular behavior and has demonstrated to decrease fibroblast apoptosis, which leads to fibroblast accumulation and pathological scar formation [3–5]. Based on this theory, the

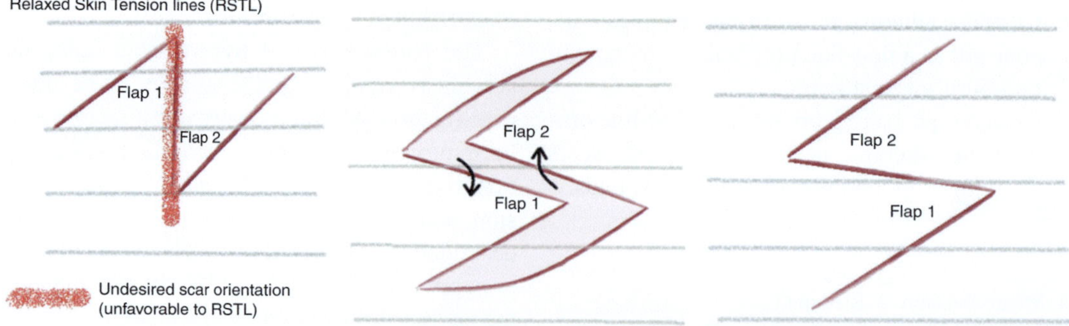

Fig. 1 Basic z-plasty flaps are created using an angle of 60° on each side, which can theoretically reorient the direction of the wound by 90°. Length and angle of the flaps must be the same in order to avoid mismatches that may hamper closure of the wound

surgeon must focus efforts on minimizing mechanical stress on wound edges during and after the surgical procedure. Main recommendations are summarized as follows:

1. Incisions must be designed parallel to the relaxed skin tension lines. It is highly recommended that wounds do not cross joint spaces and that shoulder, upper back, and midchest incisions are avoided whenever feasible. These areas all share the common characteristic of being frequently subjected to increased skin tension or recurrent stretching.
2. A layered skin closure should be applied in deep wounds (Fig. 2). Placement of absorbable sutures into the fascial layer (when needed) and deep dermal layer both eliminate dead space and relieve tension on the superficial dermis and epidermis. Furthermore, a meticulous layered suture can achieve a precise approximation and eversion of skin edges.
3. The use of adjunctive measures immediately following skin suture such as adhesive tapes and/or skin glue may strengthen the wound closure and limit skin stretching during healing [6].
4. The surgeon must pay careful attention to postoperative wound care. Patients should be advised to avoid postoperative movements in the body region where the surgical wound is located, especially if it is near a joint or in a highly mobile area. In the case of abdominal wounds, an elastic abdominal band may be worn during the healing process to reduce skin stretching. In female patients with chest wounds, tight brassieres are recommended.

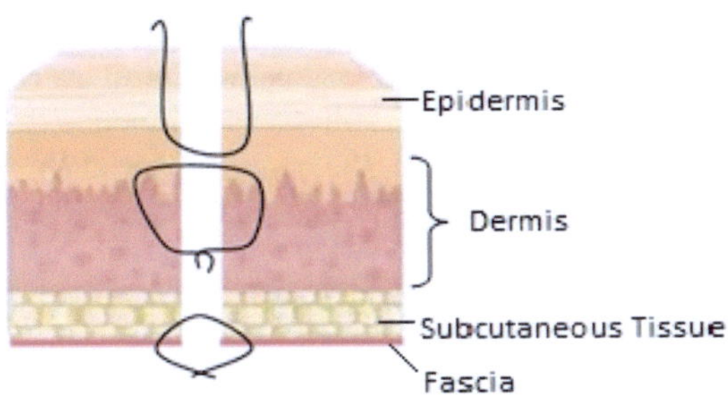

Fig. 2 Schematic representation of the layered skin closure

Inflammation

Inflammation is also a well-known contributing factor to pathologic scarring by affecting fibroblast biological processes of proliferation, differentiation, and abnormal collagen deposition [7–11]. For this reason, every attempt to minimize inflammation during and after surgery must be done.

Both infection and foreign body reaction lengthen the inflammatory response associated with wound healing. In order to avoid an excessive and/or prolonged inflammatory response, surgical management must be performed under strict sterile conditions to minimize the risk of bacterial contamination and wound infection. Surgical antibiotic prophylaxis should be administered within 120 min before incision when indicated. Wound dressings applied after skin closure provide protection from external contamination and absorb exudate from the wound, keeping it dry and clean [12].

The use of the most inert suture materials is also advisable. Absorbable sutures placed in subcutaneous tissue are less likely to cause significant foreign body inflammatory response in comparison with non-absorbable sutures. Monofilament sutures have been reported to cause less inflammation than braided sutures [13–17].

Traumatic wounds should be properly irrigated to reduce tissue contamination. Debridement of devitalized tissues and the removal of foreign bodies are mandatory. Antibiotic prophylaxis is recommended in traumatic contaminated wounds [18, 19].

A delayed healing also lengthens the inflammatory process associated with excessive scar formation. For this reason, special care should be taken to ensure the fast healing of wounds by understanding and managing critical factors that influence wound healing in a negative manner, such as preexisting malnutrition, diabetes, obesity, alcoholism, smoking, and infection. Physicians should be able to recognize these factors in both elective surgery and traumatic wound healing by secondary intention, offering early intervention. Optimizing the patient's nutritional status and blood sugar levels, encouraging the patient to stop smoking, and implementing measures to prevent wound infection, as mentioned earlier, are key points [20, 21].

Nonsurgical Scar Prevention Strategies

There is general consensus among researchers and authors that prevention of excessive scarring is preferable and much more efficient than treatment. For this reason, it is recommended that immature scars are managed early by one or more of the nonsurgical preventive therapies available, especially in individuals considered at higher risk for pathologic scar formation: patients who have individual or familiar history of excessive scarring, patients who undergo surgery in high-risk areas such as the breast and thorax or upper back, and particularly, burn patients. In terms of timing, the scar maturation process takes 12–18 months. Preventive strategies should be applied during this time period, when the scar is still immature, and as early as possible after wound closure. As a general rule, scars should be evaluated every 4 weeks to decide whether additional preventive interventions should be applied.

Most of the conventional nonsurgical therapies to prevent or treat excessive scars act by reducing inflammation (e.g., corticosteroid injections, radiation, tapes, and compression therapy, 5-fluorouracil therapy) and/or by reducing the mechanical tension that contributes to hypertrophic scar formation (e.g., tapes and compression therapy, silicone sheeting). Many of these options have shown their potential through extensive use; nevertheless, there is still a lack of large, high-quality clinical trials on this topic. Taking into account the need for a more consistent scientific evidence, there is a set of preventive therapies widely available and commonly used that have some evidence in support of their efficacy and can be recommended [22–24]:

Silicone-Based Products

Clinical evidence supports the use of silicone sheeting or gel as first-line prophylaxis on high-risk wounds or whenever there is a concern regarding the future scar appearance. Silicone-based products have proven effective in scar management, by preventing and reducing the thickness, redness, hardness, pain, and itching associated with hypertrophic scars. Their noninvasive character makes them easily acceptable for patients as a prophylactic measure to avoid excessive scarring [25–28].

The exact mechanism of action of silicone-based products in the prevention and management of excessive scars has not been completely determined, although hydration and occlusion seem to be the principal mode of action. Mechanisms that have been described to explain their positive impact on scar remodeling include:

Skin Hydration Effects After the reepithelization period, the immature stratum corneum allows high levels of transepidermal water loss due to a compromised water barrier function. There is evidence that the injured epidermis plays a key function in the activation of inflammatory mediators—immediately and long term after the injury—trying to achieve a rapid restoration of barrier function and homeostasis. As mentioned earlier, prolonged or excessive inflammatory responses directly contribute to excessive scarring. It is believed that skin occlusion with silicone-based products affects the stratum corneum by decreasing water epidermal loss and therefore increasing hydration, producing an earlier restoration of homeostasis and a reduction of inflammatory and proliferative signals from keratinocytes to dermal fibroblasts [29–32].

Increased Temperature Skin surface temperature under the silicone sheets can increase up to 1.7 °C. The temperature rise is thought to have a significant effect on collagenase kinetics by increasing its activity and therefore producing collagen breakdown [33–36].

Tensile Reduction Effects Silicone gel sheeting (SGS) may produce a slight compression on scar tissue that can be effective in reducing the tension at the border between the scar and normal skin [37, 38].

Polarization It has been hypothesized that the negative static electric field generated by friction with SGS causes polarization of the charged components of biological fluids, thus producing collagen realignment that may result in the involution of hypertrophic scars [25, 39, 40].

Silicone gel sheeting should be applied shortly after the incision or the wound has fully epithelialized and it should be maintained for at least 2 months to 1 year. To achieve optimal results, a 24-h daily wear time is recommended, with daily washing to prevent complications such as infection, skin maceration, or rash. Despite its effectiveness, patient compliance can be low when scars are located on mobile areas and visible regions as the face or joints. Accurate and detailed information to the patient can lead to a better treatment compliance and, therefore, a better scar outcome [41].

Topical silicone gel (formulated in a tube) is a treatment modality that can be used as an alternative to SGS. Silicone gel dries after spreading as an ultra-thin, invisible, flexible, and water-impermeable sheet and may be preferable to SGS for mobile and large areas (where the sheets will not conform), hot humid climates, and bare and visible areas like the face or neck, hence increasing patient compliance. There is enough evidence supporting that SGS and topical silicone gel have equivalent efficacy in the management of abnormal scarring [42, 43].

Pressure Therapy

Pressure therapy has become one of the main noninvasive prophylactic and therapeutic options in the management of scars, particularly those related to burn injuries. Prevention and treatment of unsightly and functionally disabling hypertrophic burn scars continue to remain a major challenge in burn care, and their successful management depends on early and aggressive preventive management. Pressure garments, either custom-made or commercially available, are a widely used and clinically accepted modality well sustained in literature. Its application during the scar maturation process can reduce the thickness, rigidity, and redness associated with hypertrophic scars [44–47].

Pressure garments are indicated as the first-line prophylactic therapy in patients who sustained deep burns requiring burn wound excision and grafting or in wounds taking longer than 15 days to heal. Furthermore, they are the best option in extensive scar tissue areas (like those affecting a whole extremity) difficult to treat with other noninvasive therapies [48].

The main hypothesized mechanisms of action of pressure garments are

1. Restriction in blood flow, which creates a hypoxic environment. Pressure-induced local hypoxia leads to fibroblast apoptosis and subsequent decrease in collagen production. Blanching of an immature scar after applying compression is the most visible and immediate indicator of decreased blood flow in the area [49].
2. Experimental studies have demonstrated that pressure significantly reduces the secretion and concentration of TGF-β1. This inhibits the differentiation and proliferation of fibroblasts, resulting in a decrease in collagen fiber deposition [50–52].
3. An increase in collagenase activity and therefore collagen breakdown by inhibiting α-macroglobulins has also been described. It is suggested that α-macroglobulins may play an important role in locally controlling the activity of collagenases [55].
4. Remodelation and realignment of collagen bundles, which change from nodular to parallel orientation with the skin surface, have also been documented [51].
5. Constant compression helps to reduce the edema associated with immature scars. This may prevent blistering and alleviate pruritus.

Pressure therapy must be used in the early phase of the maturation scar process once the wounds are fully closed and able to tolerate pressure. If pressure is applied immediately after wound healing, it may suppress the abnormal neovascularization process that has been involved in the development of hypertrophic scars and keloids [56].

To ensure optimal scar remodeling, an adequate and sustained use of pressure garments should be maintained. This involves wearing the pressure garments for at least 23 h a day, until the scars are mature. The required amount of pressure that should be applied to achieve optimal results remains unclear. Nevertheless, an experimental study showed that the growth of cultured fibroblasts and TGF-1 secretion were significantly decreased under a pressure system of at least 20 mmHg for 18 h [50]. Other studies [44, 46] have demonstrated that the thickness of hypertrophic scars significantly reduced after pressure loading, proportionally as the pressure level increased; most authors agree that the minimum pressure loading that produces remarkable reduction in scar thickness is 15 mmHg [45, 47]. Pressures less than 15 mmHg may appear to have poor/no effect. It has also been suggested that theoretically the effective pressure level should be equal to or exceed the capillary pressure, which is normally quoted as 25 mmHg [57].

These results may support the idea that higher pressure would be more effective to further reduce scar thickness. However, in the clinical scenario, pressures over 25 mmHg might be uncomfortable and difficult to tolerate for the patient. For this reason, the standard recommended pressure is between 20 and 25 mmHg. Physician must be aware of the gradual pressure loss of the garments over the wearing period, consequence of stress relaxation in the fabric material. Pressure loss can lead to treatment failure; for this reason, change of the pressure garment every 6 months is recommended [58].

A major obstacle to pressure therapy is low compliance due to patient discomfort and problems related to their use like erosions, sweating, itching, pain, or difficulty performing normal movements. A lack of perceived benefits and emotional distress with wearing visible garments are other factors related to low treatment compliance. This remains an important issue, as duration of pressure therapy seems to be directly related to efficacy: the optimal duration required to achieve permanent remodeling of scars is on average 12 months, as scar maturation is a 12–18-month process. Social support and a good doctor–patient relationship, together with detailed and motivational medical instructions may improve patient adherence to treatment [59, 60].

Corticosteroid Therapy

There is a broad consensus that intralesional corticosteroids injections are an effective treatment for excessive scars, being considered as a first-line therapy in the treatment of keloids and a second-line therapy in the treatment of hypertrophic scars when other therapies have not been efficacious. Steroid injections produce improvement in unpleasant symptoms and in scar appearance by reducing thickness, increasing pliability, reducing vascularity and erythema, reducing pain and itching, and even producing a complete regression of the pathologic scar.

Furthermore, steroid injections may be considered as a prophylactic therapy in combination with elective surgery in high-risk individuals or after keloid excision surgery.

The exact mechanism of action remains unclear but is thought to act by

1. reducing the inflammatory process in the immature scar and suppressing mediators such as transforming growth factor (TGF)-β1,
2. producing vasoconstriction, thus creating a hypoxic environment that promotes fibroblast apoptosis,
3. decreasing fibroblast proliferation and function: steroids bind to glucocorticoid receptors on fibroblasts and downregulate its function, and
4. producing a reduction of protease inhibitors like alpha2-macroglobulin, thereby activating collagenases and increasing collagen degradation [61–64].

Triamcinolone acetonide is the most commonly used intralesional steroid. The concentration of triamcinolone injection may be 10–40 mg/mL, depending on the characteristics of the scar, its size, and location. The steroid vial should be shaken before its use and immediately injected after transferring it into the syringe to avoid settling of the medication. Lidocaine (1%) can be used to dilute triamcinolone to reduce the pain associated with injection. Pretreatment with topical lidocaine can also help prevent pain.

In terms of scar prevention, it has been widely demonstrated that surgical excision of keloids combined with intradermal injection of triamcinolone is effective in preventing recurrence of keloids. In this case, lower concentrations such as 5–10 mg/mL may be preferred. Triamcinolone injection must be done immediately after surgical excision. Postoperatively, the wound should be monitored periodically, and injections may be repeated every 4–6 weeks and discontinued if the scar remains stable after 6 months or if side effects develop (Fig. 3). An experimental study [65] demonstrated that postsurgical wounds treated with triamcinolone immediately after surgical removal of keloid expressed decreased pro-α1(I) type I collagen gene expression when compared with those not treated. The collagen bundles were also thinner and less dense.

Furthermore, healing of the wound is not apparently compromised by inhibition of type I collagen gene expression [61, 66–69].

Despite its proven effectiveness, intradermal steroid injections can produce adverse effects in approximately half of the patients treated. Most common adverse side effects are hypopigmentation, skin and subcutaneous atrophy, and telangiectasia formation. Infection, ulceration, and skin necrosis are uncommon local complications. Injection in the normal adjacent skin must be avoided to prevent perilesional skin complications. Systemic effects are rare but can be possible in case of repeated use and higher concentrations.

An alternative to injection is the use of topical steroids or steroid tapes. Methylprednisolone cream can help prevent hypertrophic scar formation after superficial dermal lesions, such as those

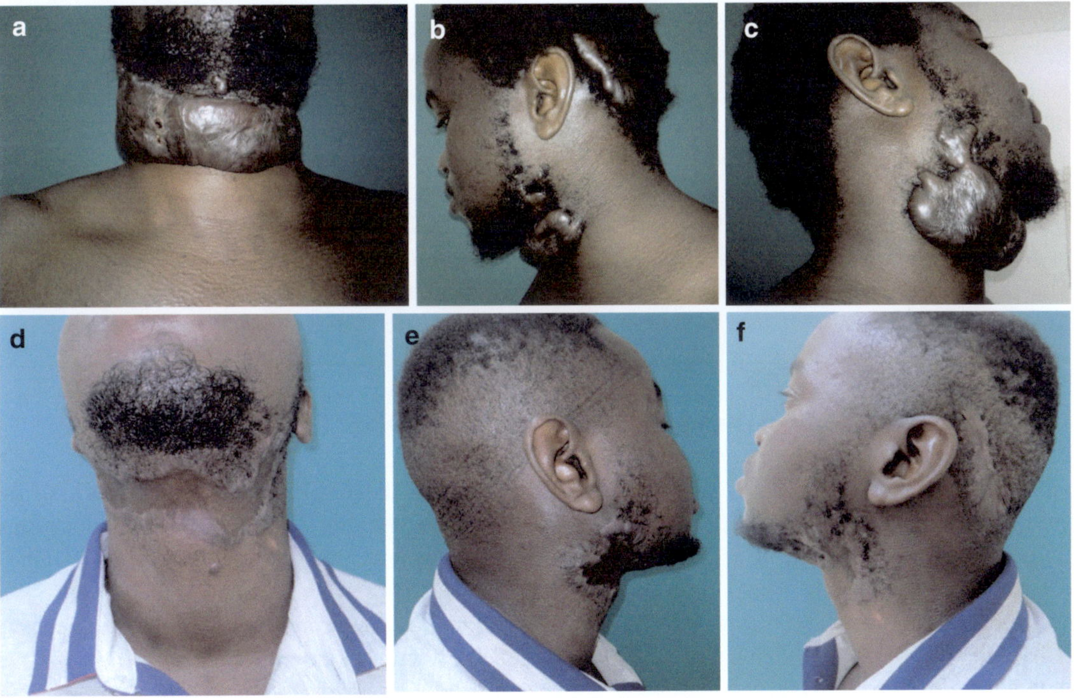

Fig. 3 (**a–c**) Preoperative view of a massive neck keloid involving submandibular area. The lesion caused a limited range of motion; (**d–f**) postoperative view of the same patient 2 years after excision of the keloid tissue. The defect was covered by a dermal substitute and a partial-thickness skin graft. Intradermal triamcinolone injections were intraoperatively applied on the wound edges. Postoperatively, the patient was monitored periodically, and injections were repeated every 4–6 weeks during the first 6 months. After this time period, injections are repeated every 4–6 months

produced by dermabrasion or laser therapy. Nevertheless, there is a lack of evidence to support their use in deeper wounds of other etiologies.

Physical Therapy

Physical therapies are a group of conservative techniques that may be used as an adjunct in the treatment and prevention of excessive scars. Physical therapy includes manual and mechanical massage, thermal therapy, physiotherapy, and shock wave therapy.

Massage

Massage, either manual or mechanical, is a popular and widely used technique in the management of scars. It has been reported that massage therapy reduces itching, pain, and anxiety levels associated with burn scars, thus having a positive impact on mental health state [70, 71]. Nevertheless, evidence quality is poor due to a lack of consistent and objective scar assessment tools; therefore, data to support the use of scar massage is inconclusive, both in the treatment and in the prevention of excessive scarring [72]. Despite the paucity of consistent evidence, it is a frequently recommended technique due to its noninvasive character in an effort to improve scar-related symptoms such as pain and itch and as an intervention to treat psychological stress frequently associated with scars [73, 74].

Extracorporeal Shock Wave Therapy

Extracorporeal shock wave therapy (ESWT) is an emerging noninvasive therapy to treat both wounds and scars, especially those related to burn injuries. It seems to be a safe and well-tolerated therapy, easy to apply in an outpatient setting, and with a low complication rate [75].

Besides its promising role in acute and chronic wound healing [76–79], there is a growing body of evidence suggesting that ESWT is also effective in treating hypertrophic scars and keloids. Studies showed that ESWT produces a significant decrease of burn scar thickness measured by ultrasonography [80], a significant improvement in scar elasticity [81], a significant improvement in Vancouver Scar Scale [80, 82], and a signifi-

cant decrease in pain [84] and pruritus score after a 3-week treatment [82, 84, 85].

Shockwaves are acoustic waves of great amplitude characterized for a fast alternation between positive and negative pressures. As a mechanotherapy, mechanotransduction is the working mechanism behind shock wave therapy: this is the molecular mechanism by which many cell types convert mechanical stimuli into biological and physiological cell responses, thus producing changes in biological processes such as migration, proliferation, differentiation, and apoptosis [86]. It has been demonstrated that shock waves have an important role in modulating function and physiology of fibroblasts. Preclinical evidence from a controlled in vitro study conducted on fibroblasts obtained from human hypertrophic scars showed that one application of ESWT produced a decrease on TGF-β1, a-SMA, vimentin, collagen I, fibronectin, and N-cadherin, and a reduction in the migration of fibroblasts; thereby inducing extracellular matrix remodeling and a reduction in fibrous tissue [87].

Although further investigation is needed to determine the exact role of ESWT in reducing the formation of excessive fibrous tissue and preventing pathological scars, there is enough evidence to suggest that ESWT applied in early stages of wound healing can be a valuable noninvasive prophylactic therapy.

Conclusion

Preventing the development of excessive scarring can be challenging, particularly in patients with a known history of excessive scarring, wounds located at high-risk corporal regions, and burn wounds. Furthermore, there is still no consensus in literature regarding the optimal preventive therapy to avoid excessive scar formation.

A personalized multimodal approach, based on an optimal surgical planification and surgical technique, added to physical and pharmacological therapy if needed, can significantly improve functional and aesthetic outcomes even in those patients at high risk to develop excessive scarring. The type of preventive measures to be applied depends on the type of wound, the individual risk factors, and his or her aesthetic concerns.

References

1. Butzelaar L, Ulrich MMW, Mink van der Molen AB, Niessen FB, Beelen RHJ. Currently known risk factors for hypertrophic skin scarring: a review. J Plast Reconstr Aesthet Surg. 2016;69(2):163–9.
2. Ogawa R. Keloid and hypertrophic scarring may result from a mechanoreceptor or mechanosensitive nociceptor disorder. Med Hypotheses. 2008;71:493–500.
3. Aarabi S, Bhatt KA, Shi Y, Paterno J, Chang EI, Loh SA, et al. Mechanical load initiates hypertrophic scar formation through decreased cellular apoptosis. FASEB J. 2007;21(12):3250–61.
4. Ogawa R, Okai K, Tokumura F, Mori K, Ohmori Y, Huang C, et al. The relationship between skin stretching/contraction and pathologic scarring: the important role of mechanical forces in keloid generation. Wound Repair Regen. 2012;20(2):149–57.
5. Akaishi S, Akimoto M, Ogawa R, Hyakusoku H. The relationship between keloid growth pattern and stretching tension: visual analysis using the finite element method. Ann Plast Surg. 2008;60:445–62.
6. Atkinson JA, McKenna KT, Barnett AG, McGrath DJ, Rudd M. A randomized, controlled trial to determine the efficacy of paper tape in preventing hypertrophic scar formation in surgical incisions that traverse Langer's skin tension lines. Plast Reconstr Surg. 2005;116:1648–56.
7. Wang J, Hori K, Ding J, Huang Y, Kwan P, Ladak A, et al. Toll-like receptors expressed by dermal fibroblasts contribute to hypertrophic scarring. J Cell Physiol. 2011;226(5):1265–73.
8. Ogawa R. Keloid and hypertrophic scars are the result of chronic inflammation in the reticular dermis. Int J Mol Sci. 2017;18(3):606.
9. Chen Y, Jin Q, Fu X, Qiao J, Niu F. Connection between T regulatory cell enrichment and collagen deposition in keloid. Exp Cell Res. 2019;383(2):111549.
10. Wang J, Jiao H, Stewart TL, Shankowsky HA, Scott PG, Tredget EE. Increased TGF-beta-producing CD4+ T lymphocytes in postburn patients and their potential interaction with dermal fibroblasts in hypertrophic scarring. Wound Repair Regen. 2007;15(4):530–9.
11. Wang ZC, Zhao WY, Cao Y, Liu YQ, Sun Q, Shi P, Cai JQ, Shen XZ, Tan WQ. The roles of inflammation in keloid and hypertrophic scars. Front Immunol. 2020;4(11):603187.
12. Tziotzios C, Profyris C, Sterling J. Cutaneous scarring: pathophysiology, molecular mechanisms and scar reduction therapeutics part II. Strategies to reduce scar formation after dermatologic procedures. J Am Acad Dermatol. 2012;66(1):13–24.
13. Niessen FB, Spauwen PH, Kon M. The role of suture material in hypertrophic scar formation: monocryl vs. vicryl-rapide. Ann Plast Surg. 1997;39:254–60.
14. Fowler JR, Perkins TA, Buttaro BA, Truant AL. Bacteria adhere less to barbed monofilament than braided sutures in a contaminated wound model. Clin Orthop Relat Res. 2013;471(2):665–71.
15. Lilly GE, Cutcher JL, Jones JC, Armstrong JH. Reaction of oral tissues to suture materials IV. J Oral Surg. 1972;33:152–7.
16. Masini BD, Stinner DJ, Waterman SM, Wenke JC. Bacterial adherence to suture materials. J Surg Educ. 2011;68(2):101–4.
17. Reid LA, Cahoon N, Stewart KJ. A prospective randomized control trial comparing one monofilament absorbable suture to a braided absorbable suture in children. J Plast Reconstr Aesthet Surg. 2009;62(2):270–2.
18. World Health Organization. Global guidelines for the prevention of surgical site infection. Geneva: World Health Organization; 2022.
19. Berríos-Torres SI, et al. Centers for Disease Control and Prevention guideline for the prevention of surgical site infection, 2017. JAMA Surg. 2017;152(8):784–91.
20. Arnold M, Barbul A. Nutrition and wound healing. Plast Reconstr Surg. 2006;117(7 suppl):42S–58S.
21. Guo S, DiPietro LA. Factors affecting wound healing. J Dent Res. 2010;89(3):219–29.
22. Mustoe TA, Cooter RD, Gold MH, Hobbs FD, Ramelet AA, Shakespeare PG, et al. International clinical recommendations on scar management. Plast Reconstr Surg. 2002;110(2):560–7.
23. Shih R, Waltzman J, Evans GR. Review of over-the-counter topical scar treatment products. Plast Reconstr Surg. 2007;119:1091–5.
24. Morganroth P, Wilmot AC, Miller C. Over-the-counter scar products for postsurgical patients: disparities between online advertised benefits and evidence regarding efficacy. J Am Acad Dermatol. 2009;61:e31–47.
25. Mustoe TA. Evolution of silicone therapy and mechanism of action in scar management. Aesthet Plast Surg. 2008;32(1):82–92.
26. Maján JI. Evaluation of a self-adherent soft silicone dressing for the treatment of hypertrophic postoperative scars. J Wound Care. 2006;15:193–6.
27. Gold MH, Foster TD, Adair MA, Burlison K, Lewis T. Prevention of hypertrophic scars and keloids by the prophylactic use of topical silicone gel sheets following a surgical procedure in an office setting. Dermatol Surg. 2001;27:641–4.
28. O'Brien L, Pandit A. Silicon gel sheeting for preventing and treating hypertrophic and keloid scars. Cochrane Database Syst Rev. 2006;1:CD003826.
29. Suetake T, Sasai S, Zhen YX, Ohi T, Tagami H. Functional analyses of the stratum corneum in scars. Sequential studies after injury and comparison among keloids, hypertrophic scars, and atrophic scars. Arch Dermatol. 1996;132:1453–e8.

30. Suetake T, Sasai S, Zhen YX, Tagami H. Effects of silicone gel sheet on the stratum corneum hydration. Br J Plast Surg. 2000;13:157–9.
31. Sawada Y, Sone K. Hydration and occlusion treatment for hypertrophic scars and keloids. Br J Plast Surg. 1992;45:599–603.
32. Mustoe TA, Gurjala A. The role of the epidermis and the mechanism of action of occlusive dressings in scarring. Wound Repair Regen. 2011;19(01):s16–21.
33. Musgrave MA, Umraw N, Fish JS, Gomez M, Cartotto RC. The effect of silicone gel sheets on perfusion of hypertrophic burn scars. J Burn Care Rehabil. 2002;23(3):208–14.
34. Borgognoni L. Biological effects of silicone gel sheeting. Wound Repair Regen. 2002;10(2):118–21.
35. Lyle WG. Silicone gel sheeting. Plast Reconstr Surg. 2001;107:272–5.
36. Krieger LM, Pan F, Doong H, Lee RC. Thermal response of the epidermis to surface gels. Surg Forum. 1993;44:738–42.
37. Akaishi S, Akimoto M, Hyakusoku H, Ogawa R. The tensile reduction effects of silicone gel sheeting. Plast Reconstr Surg. 2010;126(2):109e–11e.
38. Yagmur C, Akaishi S, Ogawa R, Guneren E. Mechanical receptor-related mechanisms in scar management: a review and hypothesis. Plast Reconstr Surg. 2010;126(2):426–34.
39. Hirshowitz B, Lindenbaum E, Har-Shai Y, Feitelberg L, Tendler M, Katz D. Static-electric field induction by a silicone cushion for the treatment of hypertrophic and keloid scars. Plast Reconstr Surg. 1998;101(5):1173–83.
40. Har-Shai Y, Lindenbaum E, Tendler M, Gamliel-Lazarovich A, Feitelberg L, Hirshowitz B. Negatively charged static electricity stimulation as a possible mechanism for enhancing the involution of hypertrophic and keloid scars. Isr Med Assoc J. 1999;1(3):203–5.
41. So K, Umraw N, Scott J, Campbell K, Musgrave M, Cartotto R. Effects of enhanced patient education on compliance with silicone gel sheeting and burn scar outcome: a randomized prospective study. J Burn Care Rehabil. 2003;24:411–7.
42. Chan KY, Lau CL, Adeeb SM, Somasundaram S, Nasir-Zahari M. A randomized, placebo-controlled, double-blind, prospective clinical trial of silicone gel in prevention of hypertrophic scar development in median sternotomy wound. Plast Reconstr Surg. 2005;116:1013–20.
43. Kim SM, Choi JS, Lee JH, Kim YJ, Jun YJ. Prevention of postsurgical scars: comparison of efficacy and convenience between silicone gel sheet and topical silicone gel. J Korean Med Sci. 2014;29(Suppl 3):S249–53.
44. Li JQ, Li-Tsang CW, Huang YP, Chen Y, Zheng YP. Detection of changes of scar thickness under mechanical loading using ultrasonic measurement. Burns. 2013;39(1):89–97.
45. Van den Kerckhove E, Stappaerts K, Fieuws S, Laperre J, Massage P, Flour M, et al. The assess-ment of erythema and thickness on burn related scars during pressure garment therapy as a preventive measure for hypertrophic scarring. Burns. 2005;31(6):696–702.
46. Candy LH, Cecilia LT, Ping ZY. Effect of different pressure magnitudes on hypertrophic scar in a Chinese population. Burns. 2010;36(8):1234–41.
47. Ai JW, Liu J, Pei SD, Liu Y, Li DS, Lin H, Pei B. The effectiveness of pressure therapy (15–25 mmHg) for hypertrophic burn scars: a systematic review and meta-analysis. Sci Rep. 2017;7:40185.
48. Bloemen MC, van der Veer WM, Ulrich MM, Van Zuijlen PM, Niessen FB, Middelcoop E. Prevention and curative management of hypertrophic scar formation. Burns. 2009;35(4):463–75.
49. Lynam EC, Xie Y, Dawson R, Mcgovern J, Upton Z, Wang X. Severe hypoxia and malnutrition collectively contribute to scar fibroblast inhibition and cell apoptosis. Wound Repair Regen. 2015;23(5):664–71.
50. Chang LW, Deng WP, Yeong EK, Wu CY, Yeh SW. Pressure effects on the growth of human scar fibroblasts. J Burn Care Res. 2008;29:835–41.
51. Kischer CW, Shetlar MR, Shetlar CL. Alteration of hypertrophic scars induced by mechanical pressure. Arch Dermatol. 1975;111:60–4.
52. Li-Tsang CW, Feng B, Huang L, Liu X, Shu B, Chan YT. A histological study on the effect of pressure therapy on the activities of myofibroblasts and kerati-nocytes in hypertrophic scar tissues after burn. Burns. 2015;41(5):1008–16.
53. Atiyeh BS, El Khatib AM, Dibo SA. Pressure garment therapy (PGT) of burn scars: evidence-based efficacy. Ann Burns Fire Disasters. 2013;26(4):205–12.
54. Munro KJG. Treatment of hypertrophic and keloid scars. J Wound Care. 1995;4(5):243–5.
55. Sottrup-Jensen L, Birkedal-Hansen H. Human fibroblast collagenase-α-macroglobulin interactions: localization of cleavage sites in the bait regions of five mammalian α-macroglobulins. J Biol Chem. 1989;264(1):393–401.
56. Amadeu T, Braune A, Mandarim-de-Lacerda C, Porto LC, Desmoulière A, Costa A. Vascularization pattern in hypertrophic scars and keloids: a stereological analysis. Pathol Res Pract. 2003;199(7):469–73.
57. Ward RS. Pressure therapy for the control of hypertrophic scar formation after burn injury. A history and review. J Burn Care Rehabil. 1991;12:257–62.
58. Sau-Fun Ng F. Medical clothing: the stress relaxation and shrinkage of pressure garments. Int J Cloth Sci Technol. 1994;6:17–27.
59. Macintyre L, Baird M. Pressure garments for use in the treatment of hypertrophic scars—a review of the problems associated with their use. Burns. 2006;32:10–5.
60. Ripper S, Renneberg B, Landmann C, Weigel G, Germann G. Adherence to pressure garment therapy in adult burn patients. Burns. 2009;35(5):657–64.

61. Roques C, Téot L. The use of corticosteroids to treat keloids: a review. Int J Low Extrem Wounds. 2008;7(3):137–45.

62. Butler P, Longaker M, Yang G. Current progress in keloid research and treatment. J Am Coll Surgeons. 2008;208:731–41.

63. Coppola MM, Salzillo R, Segreto F, Persichetti P. Triamcinolone acetonide intralesional injection for the treatment of keloid scars: patient selection and perspectives. Clin Cosmet Investig Dermatol. 2018;11:387–96.

64. Garg AM, Shah YM, Garg A, Zaidi S, Saxena K, Gupta K. The efficacy of intralesional triamcinolone acetonide (20 mg/mL) in the treatment of keloid. Int Surg J. 2018;5(3):868–72.

65. Kauh YC, Rouda S, Mondragon G, Tokarek R, diLeonardo M, Tuan RS, Tan EM. Major suppression of pro-α1(I) type I collagen gene expression in the dermis after keloid excision and immediate intra-wound injection of triamcinolone acetonide. J Am Acad Dermatol. 1997;37:586–9.

66. Donkor P. Head and neck keloid: treatment by core excision and delayed intralesional injection of steroid. J Oral Maxillofac Surg. 2007;65:1292–6.

67. Chowdri NA, Masarat M, Mattoo A, Darzi MA. Keloids and hypertrophic scars: results with intraoperative and serial post-operative corticosteroid injection therapy. Aust N Z J Surg. 1999;69(9):655–9.

68. Jung JY, Roh MR, Kwon YS, Chung KY. Surgery and perioperative intralesional corticosteroid injection for treating earlobe keloids: a Korean experience. Ann Dermatol. 2009;21:221–5.

69. Park TH, Seo SW, Kim JK, Chang CH. Clinical characteristics of facial keloids treated with surgical excision followed by intra- and postoperative intralesional steroid injections. Aesthet Plast Surg. 2012;36(1):169–73.

70. Field T, Peck M, Hernandez-Rief M, Krugman S, Burman I, Ozment-Schenk L. Postburn itching: pain, and psychological symptoms are reduced with massage therapy. J Burn Care Rehabil. 2000;21(3):189–93.

71. Parlak Gürol A, Polat S, Nuran AM. Itching, pain, and anxiety levels are reduced with massage therapy in burned adolescents. J Burn Care Res. 2010;31(3):429–32.

72. Shin TM, Bordeaux JS. The role of massage in scar management: a literature review. Dermatol Surg. 2012;38:414–23.

73. Ault P, Plaza A, Paratz J. Scar massage for hypertrophic burns scarring—a systematic review. Burns. 2018;44(1):24–38.

74. Anthonissen M, Daly D, Janssens T, Van den Kerckhove E. The effects of conservative treatments on burn scars: a systematic review. Burns. 2016;42(3):508–18.

75. Moortgat P, Anthonissen M, Van Daele U, Meirte J, Vanhullebusch T, Maertens K. Shock wave therapy for wound healing and scar treatment. In: Téot L, Mustoe TA, Middelkoop E, Gauglitz GG, editors. Textbook on scar management. Cham: Springer; 2020.

76. Ottomann C, Stojadinovic A, Lavin PT, Gannon FH, Heggeness MH, Thiele R, Schaden W, Hartmann B. Prospective randomized phase II trial of accelerated reepithelialization of superficial second-degree burn wounds using extracorporeal shock wave therapy. Ann Surg. 2012;255:23–9.

77. Arnó A, García O, Hernán I, Sancho J, Acosta A, Barret JP. Extracorporeal shock waves, a new non-surgical method to treat severe burns. Burns. 2010;36:844–9.

78. Antonic V, Mittermayr R, Schaden W, Stojadinovic A. Evidence supporting extracorporeal shock wave therapy for acute and chronic soft tissue wounds. Wounds Compend Clin Res Pract. 2011;23:204–15.

79. Aguilera-Sáez J, Muñoz P, Serracanta J, Monte A, Barret JP. Extracorporeal shock wave therapy role in the treatment of burn patients. A systematic literature review. Burns. 2019;19:30211–6.

80. Fioramonti P, Cigna E, Onesti MG, Fino P, Fallico N, Scuderi N. Extracorporeal shock wave therapy for the management of burn scars. Dermatol Surg. 2012;38(5):778–82.

81. Moortgat P, Anthonissen M, Van Daele U, Vanhullebusch T, Maertens K, De Cuyper L, et al. The effects of shock wave therapy applied on hypertrophic burn scars: a randomised controlled trial. Scars Burn Health. 2020;6:1–10.

82. Taheri P, Khosrawi S, Mazaheri M, Parsa MA, Mokhtarian A. Effect of extracorporeal shock wave therapy on improving burn scar in patients with burnt extremities in Infahan. Iran J Res Med Sci. 2018;23:81.

83. Saggini R, Saggini A, Spagnoli AM, Dodaj I, Cigna E, Maruccia M, et al. Extracorporeal shock wave therapy: an emerging treatment modality for retracting scars of the hands. Ultrasound Med Biol. 2016;42:185–95.

84. Cho YS, Joo SY, Cui H, Cho SR, Yim H, Seo CH. Effect of extracorporeal shock wave therapy on scar pain in burn patients: a prospective, randomized, single-blind, placebo controlled study. Medicine (Baltimore). 2016;95(32):e4575.

85. Joo SY, Cho YS, Seo CH. The clinical utility of extracorporeal shock wave therapy for burn pruritus: a prospective, randomized, single-blind study. Burns. 2018;44(3):612–9.

86. d'Agostino MC, Craig K, Tibalt E, Respizzi S. Shock wave as biological therapeutic tool: from mechanical stimulation to recovery and healing, through mechanotransduction. Int J Surg. 2015;24(Pt B):147–53.

87. Cui HS, Hong AR, Kim JB, Yu JH, Cho YS, Joo SY, et al. Extracorporeal shock wave therapy alters the expression of fibrosis-related molecules in fibroblast derived from human hypertrophic scar. Int J Mol Sci. 2018;19(1):124.

Further Reading

Kerwin LY, El Tal AK, Stiff MA, Fakhouri TM. Scar prevention and remodeling: a review of the medical, surgical, topical and light treatment approaches. Int J Dermatol. 2014;53(8):922–36.

Mari W, Alsabri SG, Tabal N, Younes S, Sherif A, Simman R. Novel insights on understanding of keloid scar: article review. J Am Coll Clin Wound Spec. 2016;7(1–3):1–7.

Perez JL, Rohrich RJ. Optimizing postsurgical scars. A systematic review on best practices in preventative scar management. Plast Reconstr Surg. 2017;140(6):782e–93e.

Pérez-Bustillo A, González-Sixto B, Rodríguez-Prieto MA. Surgical principles for achieving a functional and cosmetically acceptable scar. Actas Dermosifiliogr. 2013;104(1):17–28.

Trace AP, Enos CW, Mantel A, Harvey VM. Keloids and hypertrophic scars: a spectrum of clinical challenges. Am J Clin Dermatol. 2016;17(3):201–23.

Part III

Scar Treatment

Intralesional Therapy

Christian Tschumi and Jan A. Plock

Core Messages

- Intralesional therapy is a key element in the treatment of hypertrophic scars and keloids.
- Use intralesional glucocorticoids, 5FU, and cryosurgery alone or in combination.
- Intralesional therapy is a good option in the prophylactic and therapeutic setting.
- Nano- and microfat grafting improves the appearance and quality of atrophic and non-hypertrophic scars.

Introduction

Intralesional scar treatment can be divided into two groups depending on the type, age, and phase of maturity of a scar. Therefore, a profound understanding of physiological and pathological scar evolution is a prerequisite in scar care. Intralesional applications are one of the main pillars in the treatment of pathological scars. Another important modality is the use of minimally invasive treatments like micro- and nanofat grafting, PRP, and fillers, which are reliable tools especially in the care of atrophic and non-hypertrophic scars.

It is important to note that in pathological scars, none of the available methods for scar treatment guarantees a scar reduction or improvement of the functional and aesthetic outcome, which has to be communicated to the patient beforehand.

There is no standard pathway for intralesional scar treatment mainly because there are many variables influencing the development and regression of a hypertrophic scar or keloid.

Thus, the chosen option should lead to significant improvement within 3–6 months or 3–6 therapeutic cycles. A significant improvement is a 50% reduction of the symptoms, decreasing of volume of more than 30–50%, or sufficient patient satisfaction [1].

> **Caution!**
> Add or change treatment modality of hypertrophic scars or keloids if there is no significant improvement in 3–6 months or 3–6 therapeutic cycles.

The therapeutic objective should be individualized based on each patients' symptoms. A combination of different methods is often indicated.

Three intralesional therapeutic methods have enough evidence in the current literature to be recommended for the treatment of hypertrophic scars and keloids.

- Corticosteroids (triamcinolone acetonide).
- Cryosurgery.
- 5-Fluorouracil and bleomycin.

C. Tschumi · J. A. Plock (✉)
Department of Plastic Surgery and Hand Surgery,
Cantonal Hospital Aarau, Aarau, Switzerland
e-mail: Jan.Plock@ksa.ch

Indications for intralesional therapy are active, aesthetically not acceptable hypertrophic scars without impairment in function. In keloids, intralesional therapy is always part of the treatment strategy, either as the sole method or in combination with other modalities (surgery, radiation).

Intralesional Therapeutic Options

Corticosteroids

Intralesional corticosteroids in the management of pathological scars are by far the most used method. It has sufficient obviousness to make evidence-based recommendations [2]. Most commonly used is triamcinolone acetonide (TAC).

Mechanism of action: Corticosteroids reduce the excessive scar development through the reduction of collagen and glycosaminoglycan synthesis and inhibit the proliferation of fibroblasts. In addition to the known anti-inflammatory effect, there is an inhibition of the iNOS-transcription with a decrease in the synthesis of collagen in fibroblasts and alpha2-macroglobulin, an inhibitor of the collagenase [3].

Adverse effects: Painful injection. Infiltration too deep can lead to atrophy of the subcutis and widening of the scar. An infiltration too superficial to delayed wound healing, telangiectasia, and pigment disorder. Overdosing can lead to an exogenous Cushing's syndrome.

Therapeutic application: Most commonly used is triamcinolone acetonide (TAC) 10–40 mg, maximal 5 mg/cm^2, injected undiluted or 1:2–1:4 diluted with sodium chloride 0.9% or with short- and long-lasting local anesthetics for more treatment comfort. Alternatively, use short cryosurgery before injection (see cryosurgery). Use a Luer Lock syringe, inject strictly intralesionally, and stop injecting as soon as a blanching effect occurs (Figs. 1 and 2).

Repeat the treatment five times in 2 weeks intervals and pause treatment for 3 months before you reevaluate and consider a second therapy cycle.

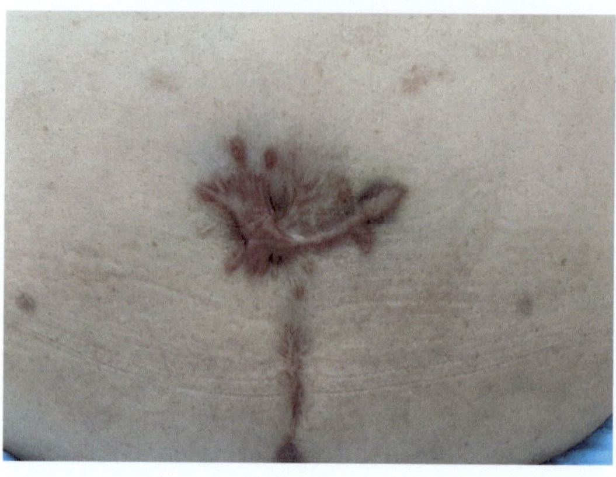

Fig. 1 Periumbilical hypertrophic scar after abdominal surgery

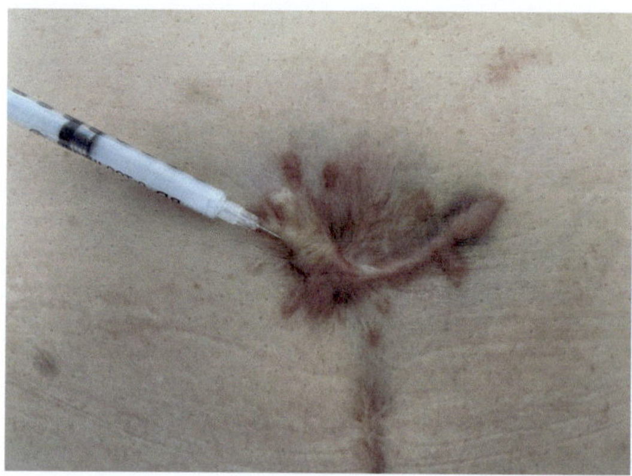

Fig. 2 First-line therapy with intralesional corticosteroids. The blanching effect can be seen here and is the endpoint for the intralesional injection

A good alternative mode of application is using a Derma Jet injection instrument. This is a good method especially in larger scars and keloids.

In the prophylactic setting, 1 mg per cm wound margin injected intraoperatively has a good efficacy without side effects [4].

> **Clinical Tip**
> Use intralesional corticosteroids after surgical treatment of hypertrophic scars and keloids.

Add 5 FU to the treatment regime if glucocorticoid injections do not have the desired effect after 3 cycles.

Mix intralesional corticosteroids with anesthetics:

TAC 1 mL/40 mg + 3 mL bupivacaine 0.5% + 3 mL mepivacaine 1%.

Important to Know

Therapy of hypertrophic scars and keloids with corticosteroids, 5-FU or bleomycin should always be strictly intralesional.

Cryosurgery of hypertrophic scars and keloids is recommended, and can be combined with triamcinolone acetonide.

The remission of a keloid after intralesional cryosurgery takes between 4 and 6 months, with blisters and oozing wounds for 4 weeks.

The off-label use of 5 FU in the therapy of hypertrophic scars and keloids requires adequate informed consent of the patients.

5-Fluorouracil and Bleomycin

The treatment with 5-FU and bleomycin shows good results, especially in combination with other therapy options. The tendency to less adverse reactions than with glucocorticoids makes it ideal for use in corticosteroid sensible areas [5, 6].

Mechanism of action: 5-FU, a pyrimidine analog, inhibits the proliferation of fibroblasts. Bleomycin decreases collagen production and increases its degradation due to regulation of lysyl oxidase and a cross-linking enzyme related to maturation of collagen and TGF-β1 [7].

Adverse effects: Burning pain during injection. Hyperpigmentation. Skin irritation and ulceration.

Therapeutic application: Treatment with 50 mg/mL and maximum doses of 50–150 mg per session is usually repeated every 4 weeks.

The injection should be strictly intralesional. A combination with TAC at a ratio of 1–3 or 1–9 seems to have better results than the particular monotherapy. Compared with TAC, 5-FU has less unwanted side effects. It makes a good alternative for the treatment in corticosteroid-vulnerable areas [5, 8].

Bleomycin can be used as an alternative with a lower risk of skin ulcers. This makes it a preferable choice for the treatment of scars in intensely pigmented skin to avoid hypopigmentation. Bleomycin is injected at a concentration of 1.5 IU/mL intralesionally.

Cryosurgery

Thirty years ago, Zouboulis and Orfanos showed a beneficial effect of surface/spray cryosurgical sessions with high remission rates and almost no recurrence [9]. They were also the first to describe intralesional cryotherapy for keloids and hypertrophic scars [10]. Gupta and Kumar showed their experience with intralesional cryosurgery in large keloids not responding to intralesional corticosteroid application [11] (Fig. 3). Compared to surface cryotherapy, intralesional cryotherapy has the main advantage of a larger volume of frozen scar tissue and minimal surface destruction. Thus, significantly less therapy cycles are neces-

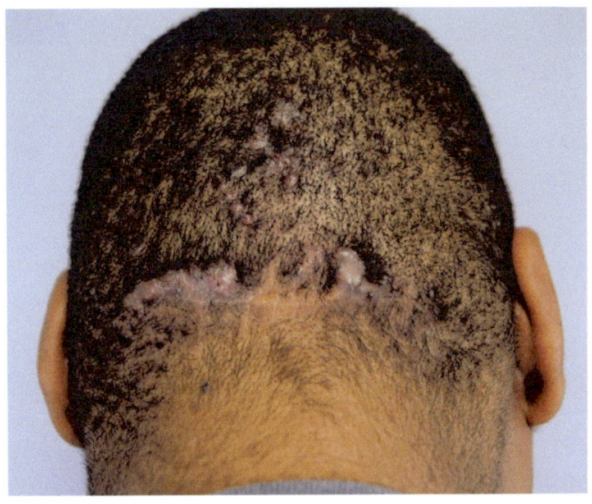

Fig. 3 Patient with acne keloidalis nuchae before cryosurgery as a second-line option. Previous cycles with TAC without satisfying results

sary. The cryoneedle methods available are simple to operate and safe to use [12, 13].

Mechanism of action: The effect of cryosurgery is based on changes in the microcirculation induced by the low temperature, thrombosis, and cell death [14]. Histological and immunobiological studies indicate that cryosurgery can induce tissue rejuvenation changes in keloids. In the treated scars, collagen structure as well as the presence of type III collagen tends to normalize [12].

Adverse effects: Healing time is up to 6 weeks with possible pigment disorder, especially in dark-colored skin. Oozing wounds.

Therapeutic application: There are two different approaches.

1. Short cryosurgery which makes the administration of TAC easier and less painful.
2. Complete cryosurgery involves freezing the entire lesion, including 3–5 mm of the neighboring tissue under local anesthesia (Fig. 4).

The intralesional cryosurgery is performed with a double-barreled cannula using liquid nitrogen. Depending on the size of the keloid multiple syringes are necessary to achieve complete freezing of the tissue.

Remission of the treated keloid takes up to 4–6 months (Fig. 5), and the initial oozing wounds should be dressed with antiseptic dressings. Additional treatment (cryosurgery or others) should be postponed until the wound has completely healed [15].

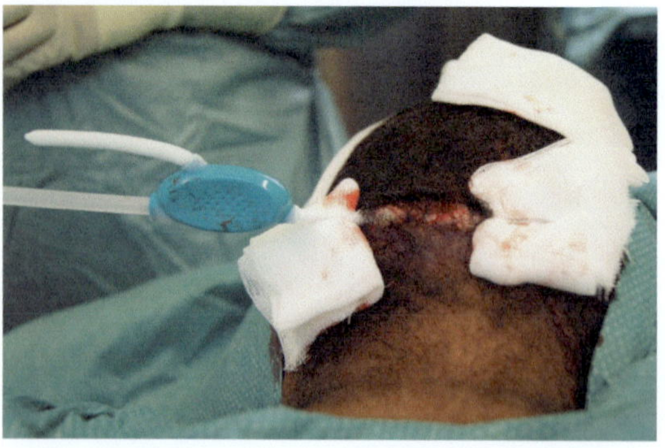

Fig. 4 Cryosurgery using a double-barreled cannula and liquid nitrogen. Complete freezing of the keloids including a halo of neighboring tissue

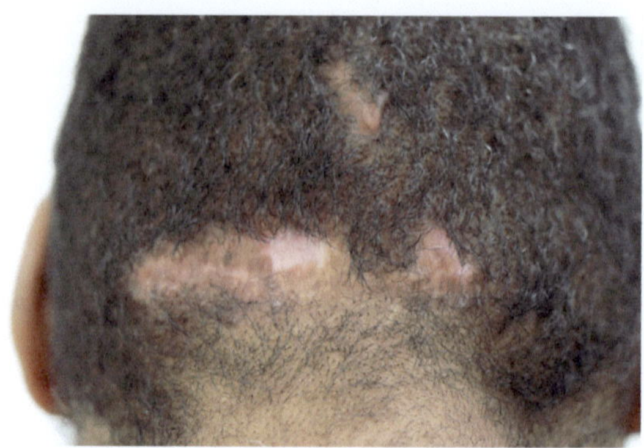

Fig. 5 Postoperative figures 1 year after one application of complete cryosurgery with complete remission of the keloids and no recurrences. (With courtesy of the Department of Plastic Surgery and Hand Surgery Inselspital Bern, Switzerland in collaboration with Prof. Y. Har-Shai, Unit of Plastic Surgery, Carmel Medical Center, Haifa, Israel)

Clinical Tip
Intralesional cryosurgery should always exceed the border of the keloids by 5 mm (halo) to have the best therapeutic success.

Microfat and Nanofat Grafting

The atrophic stage is the end of scar maturation. Atrophic, depressed scars or—when there is also loss of subcutaneous tissue—lipoatrophic scars benefit from lipofilling with good and predictable outcomes using recent techniques with finer components (nanofat) [16, 17]. Microfat grafting has been used successfully for a long time in treating ulcers and scars ensuing from radiotherapy [18].

The advantage of lipofilling is the supply of adipose-tissue-derived stem cells (ADSC), which are multipotent, undifferentiated, and self-renewing progenitor cells resembling mesenchymal stem cells [19]. Their ability to differentiate into a variety of different cell lines and their anti-apoptotic, anti-inflammatory, immunomodulatory, proangiogenic, and anti-scarring properties have made lipofilling a key element in regenerative medicine [20, 21].

Mechanism of action: Microfat grafting increases the number of adipocytes in the grafted area. The mechanically emulsified autologous fat referred to as nanofat contains no vivid adipocytes. It retains its regenerative potential because the stromal vascular fraction (SVF) that survives the emulsification process contains fibroblasts, endothelial cells, pre-adipocytes, vascular smooth muscle cells, lymphocytes, monocytes, and ADSCs [20] that are responsible for the proliferative, and subsequent filling effects of nanofat [22]. It has shown remarkable effects in skin regeneration after injection [23] (Figs. 6, 7, and 8).

Adverse effects: Donor site hematoma and irregularities. Oil cysts and calcifications. Variable retention rate and unpredictability of effect.

Therapeutic application: Use tumescent anesthesia with standard aseptic precaution. The fat harvesting can be done with one-way harvesting cannulas or a triport Colemans cannula with Luer Lock syringes. Leave the aspirate undisturbed in a vertical position for 15 min. Discard the tumescent fluid separating on the bottom of the syringe. The aspirated fat can now be emulsified using a Luer Lock single or 3-way connector passing between two syringes 30 times (microfat) or 60 times (nanofat). Sieve the emulsion through a two-layered moist saline surgical gauze to remove all solid elements to ensure free flow through a 27 G needle.

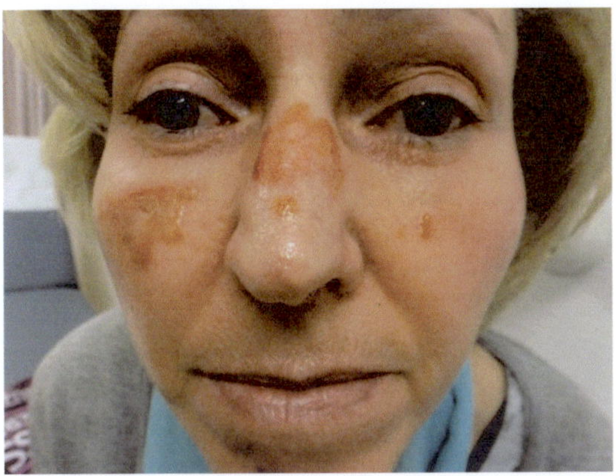

Fig. 6 Deep dermal burn injury at day 7 after mishandled laser rejuvenation therapy of the face

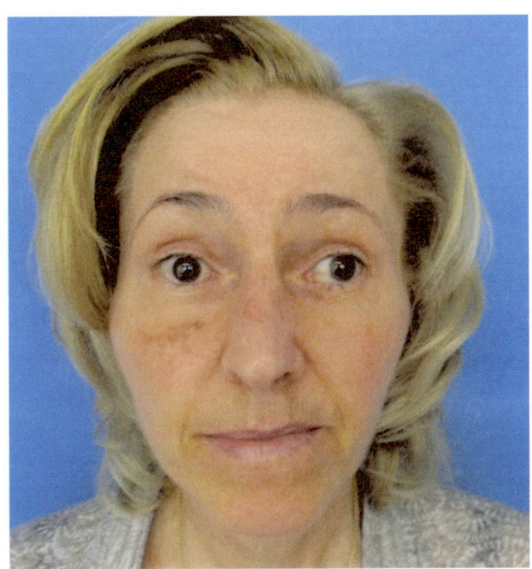

Fig. 7 Hyperpigmentation and scarring of the skin in this patient as a residuum of the burn injury 6 months after the trauma

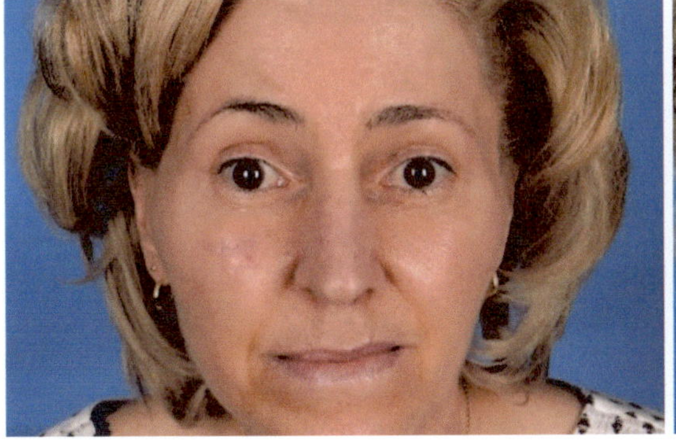

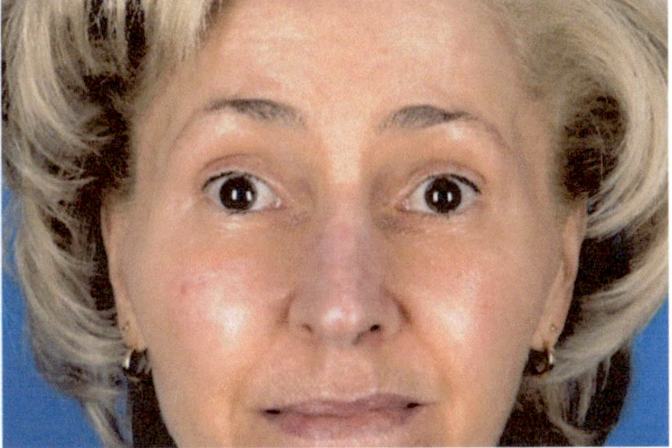

Fig. 8 Post-therapeutic result after 1 cycle of nanofat 1.5. year after the initial injury. Improved quality of the skin and reversed hyperpigmentation

Inject intralesionally into the scar using a 27 G needle. Yellowish blanching of the scar marks the end point of injection [17].

> **Clinical Tip**
> Use nanofat grafting with PRPs in combination with needling or other resurfacing procedures to achieve best outcomes.

Platelet-Rich Plasma (PRP) and Related Treatments

PRP consists of plasma that is enriched with a high concentration of platelets. The effect of PRP on scars, atrophic scars in particular, is understood through the release of growth factors. Furthermore, PRP generates hyaluronic acid, which is also a promotor of cell proliferation and extracellular matrix formation in addition to the known effect of drawing water into the matrix, causing swelling, volume, and skin turgor. PRP has been studied mostly as adjunctive therapy to other treatment modalities like micro-needling and fractional ablative laser [16].

Conclusion

Intralesional therapy is an established key component in the treatment of abnormal scarring with proven good results. It can be used in a prophylactic setting or in active hypertrophic scars. In keloids, a combination of several intralesional treatments or a multimodal approach can lead to better results. Always reassess therapeutic success and consider a change or addition to the treatment in the absence of satisfactory results.

In non-hypertrophic and atrophic scars, autologous intralesional therapy plays an important and effective role in the correction of contour and improvement of scar quality and pigmentation.

References

1. 013-030l_S2k_Therapie-pathologischer-Narben-hypertrophe-Narben-Keloide_2020-11.pdf (awmf.org).
2. Mustoe TA, Cooter RD, Gold MH, et al. International clinical recommendations on scar management. Plast Reconstr Surg. 2002;110(2):560–71. https://doi.org/10.1097/00006534-200208000-00031.
3. Schäffer MR, Efron PA, Thornton FJ, Klingel K, Gross SS, Barbul A. Nitric oxide, an autocrine regulator of wound fibroblast synthetic function. J Immunol. 1997;158(5):2375–81.
4. Danielsen PL, Rea SM, Wood FM, et al. Verapamil is less effective than triamcinolone for prevention of keloid scar recurrence after excision in a randomized controlled trial. Acta Derm Venereol. 2016;96(6):774–8. https://doi.org/10.2340/00015555-2384.
5. Hietanen KE, Järvinen TA, Huhtala H, Tolonen TT, Kuokkanen HO, Kaartinen IS. Treatment of keloid scars with intralesional triamcinolone and 5-fluorouracil injections—a randomized controlled trial. J Plast Reconstr Aesthet Surg. 2019;72(1):4–11. https://doi.org/10.1016/j.bjps.2018.05.052.
6. Kim WI, Kim S, Cho SW, Cho MK. The efficacy of bleomycin for treating keloid and hypertrophic scar: a systematic review and meta-analysis. J Cosmet Dermatol. 2020;19(12):3357–66. https://doi.org/10.1111/jocd.13390.
7. Trisliana Perdanasari A, Lazzeri D, Su W, et al. Recent developments in the use of intralesional injections keloid treatment. Arch Plast Surg. 2014;41(6):620–9. https://doi.org/10.5999/aps.2014.41.6.620.
8. Gupta S, Kalra A. Efficacy and safety of intralesional 5-fluorouracil in the treatment of keloids. Dermatology. 2002;204(2):130–2. https://doi.org/10.1159/000051830.
9. Zouboulis CC, Blume U, Büttner P, Orfanos CE. Outcomes of cryosurgery in keloids and hypertrophic scars. A prospective consecutive trial of case series. Arch Dermatol. 1993;129(9):1146–51.
10. Zouboulis CC. Principles of cutaneous cryosurgery: an update. Dermatology. 1999;198(2):111–7. https://doi.org/10.1159/000018084.
11. Gupta S, Kumar B. Intralesional cryosurgery using lumbar puncture and/or hypodermic needles for large, bulky, recalcitrant keloids. Int J Dermatol. 2001;40(5):349–53. https://doi.org/10.1046/j.1365-4362.2001.01117.x.
12. Har-Shai Y, Amar M, Sabo E. Intralesional cryotherapy for enhancing the involution of hypertrophic scars and keloids. Plast Reconstr Surg. 2003;111(6):1841–52. https://doi.org/10.1097/01.PRS.0000056868.42679.05.

13. Har-Shai Y, Brown W, Labbé D, et al. Intralesional cryosurgery for the treatment of hypertrophic scars and keloids following aesthetic surgery: the results of a prospective observational study. Int J Low Extrem Wounds. 2008;7(3):169–75. https://doi.org/10.1177/1534734608322813.

14. Hoffmann NE, Bischof JC. Cryosurgery of normal and tumor tissue in the dorsal skin flap chamber: part II—injury response. J Biomech Eng. 2001;123(4):310–6. https://doi.org/10.1115/1.1385839.

15. van Leeuwen MC, Bulstra AE, Ket JC, Ritt MJ, van Leeuwen PA, Niessen FB. Intralesional cryotherapy for the treatment of keloid scars: evaluating effectiveness. Plast Reconstr Surg Glob Open. 2015;3(6):e437. https://doi.org/10.1097/GOX.0000000000000348.

16. Gupta A, Kaur M, Patra S, Khunger N, Gupta S. Evidence-based surgical management of post-acne scarring in skin of color. J Cutan Aesthet Surg. 2020;13(2):124–41. https://doi.org/10.4103/JCAS.JCAS_154_19.

17. Bhooshan LS, Devi MG, Aniraj R, Binod P, Lekshmi M. Autologous emulsified fat injection for rejuvenation of scars: a prospective observational study. Indian J Plast Surg. 2018;51(1):77–83. https://doi.org/10.4103/ijps.IJPS_86_17.

18. Sardesai MG, Moore CC. Quantitative and qualitative dermal change with microfat grafting of facial scars. Otolaryngol Head Neck Surg. 2007;137(6):868–72. https://doi.org/10.1016/j.otohns.2007.08.008.

19. Zuk PA, Zhu M, Mizuno H, et al. Multilineage cells from human adipose tissue: implications for cell-based therapies. Tissue Eng. 2001;7(2):211–28. https://doi.org/10.1089/107632701300062859.

20. Frese L, Dijkman PE, Hoerstrup SP. Adipose tissue-derived stem cells in regenerative medicine. Transfus Med Hemother. 2016;43(4):268–74. https://doi.org/10.1159/000448180.

21. Coleman SR, Katzel EB. Fat grafting for facial filling and regeneration. Clin Plast Surg. 2015;42(3):289–97. https://doi.org/10.1016/j.cps.2015.04.001.

22. Rigotti G, Marchi A, Galiè M, et al. Clinical treatment of radiotherapy tissue damage by lipoaspirate transplant: a healing process mediated by adipose-derived adult stem cells. Plast Reconstr Surg. 2007;119(5):1409–22. https://doi.org/10.1097/01.prs.0000256047.47909.71.

23. Tonnard P, Verpaele A, Peeters G, Hamdi M, Cornelissen M, Declercq H. Nanofat grafting: basic research and clinical applications. Plast Reconstr Surg. 2013;132(4):1017–26. https://doi.org/10.1097/PRS.0b013e31829fe1b0.

Further Reading

Ren Y, Zhou X, Wei Z, Lin W, Fan B, Feng S. Efficacy and safety of triamcinolone acetonide alone and in combination with 5-fluorouracil for treating hypertrophic scars and keloids: a systematic review and meta-analysis. Int Wound J. 2017;14(3):480–7. https://doi.org/10.1111/iwj.12629.

Tonnard P, Verpaele A, Peeters G, Hamdi M, Cornelissen M, Declercq H. Nanofat grafting: basic research and clinical applications. Plast Reconstr Surg. 2013;132(4):1017–26. https://doi.org/10.1097/PRS.0b013e31829fe1b0.

Wong TS, Li JZ, Chen S, Chan JY, Gao W. The efficacy of triamcinolone acetonide in keloid treatment: a systematic review and meta-analysis. Front Med (Lausanne). 2016;3:71. https://doi.org/10.3389/fmed.2016.00071.

Lasers and Energy-Based Devices in Scar Therapy: A Practical Use

Hugues Cartier [ID], Francois Will, Thierry Fusade, and Hans-Joachim Laubach [ID]

Abbreviations

2940 nm, Er:YAG	Erbium:YAG (yttrium-aluminum-garnet) laser
AFL	Ablative fractional laser
BED	Biologically effective dose
DCD	Dynamic cooling device
EBD	Energy-based devices (EBD)
HIFU	High-intensity focused ultrasound
IPL	Intense pulsed light
Ktp	Crystal titanyl phosphate de potassium
LADD	Laser-assisted drug delivery
LEDs	Light-emitting diodes
LIOB	Laser-induced optical breakdown
MMPs	Collagenase-type metalloproteinases
MMPs	Metalloproteinases
MRN, MRF	Radiofrequency micro needling
MTZ	Microthermal zone
NAFL	Non-ablative fractional laser
Nm	Nanometer
Ns, nano	Nanosecond
PDL = LCP	Pulsed dye laser (p135, switch LCP French wording for PDL)
PIH	Post-inflammatory pigmentation
Ps, pico	Picosecond
QS	Q-switched
RF	Radiofrequency
SOC	Skin of color type
TAC	Acetate of triamcinolone
tca	Trichloroacetic acid
UV	Ultraviolet
VSSS	Vancouver scar scale score

The original version of the chapter has been revised. A correction to this chapter can be found at https://doi.org/10.1007/978-3-031-24137-6_18

H. Cartier (✉)
Arras, France

F. Will
Brumath, France

T. Fusade
Paris, France

H.-J. Laubach
Strasbourg, France

Introduction

Each scar is unique; it is this diversity that makes the issue so complex and so simple to manage! In most cases, the evolution of a process is normal, and it is necessary to explain to the patient that it takes time, generally from 6 to 18 months.

The analysis of the scar profile according to its form and evolution, its mode of occurrence, its topography and on whom it forms, and much more like the habits of sporting life are so much data to be considered as a challenge for the laserist doctor.

Lasers and all other available devices are only one way to improve a scar. But they are part of a combination with the other techniques developed in the other chapters.

The psychological experience of a scar must also be considered, especially as the "miracle of the laser" can sometimes disappoint the patient. Therefore, "Primum non nocere," not all scars should be treated by laser.

We wish to be as synthetic and practical as possible in the development of this chapter with a certain bias that may be subject to discussion. Thus, we will review the available devices and the therapeutic proposals for scars of less than 100 days and more than 100 days and of course acne scars. Why 100 days or around 3 months is a bias but also a clinical observation beyond which a healing is on the right way or not and when patients usually wish to intervene because the scar does not disappear as they would like. Of course, it is possible to intervene at other times in the life of a scar because in most cases, everything happens according to the normal evolution of a healing process.

Laser and Other Electromagnetic Devices

A distinction is made between photonic devices and other devices that deliver a direct heat source without targeting a particular tissue.

A LASER is defined by its wavelength, which is monochromatic photon emission (Light Amplification by Stimulated Emission of Radiation). The laser emits light that is absorbed by three essential skin targets: pigment, vascular, i.e., everything that is red, and water. The beam of photons emitted by the laser, like all other electromagnetic sources, is converted into heat or thermal effect by the target. Nevertheless, there are radiation effects: photocoagulation, photo thermolysis, photoacoustic, and photoablation.

It is important to remember that the thermal energy released will alter the skin tissue and induce its remodeling and structural modification. In this respect, the ratio of delivered energy, wave penetration, and duration of the thermal effect is also important to obtain the desired result.

It should also be kept in mind that a laser or other sources penetrate deeply into the skin. This is an essential element to consider because if you have a thick scar and the photons remain on the surface, there will be a minor impact in the long term. But this penetrance must be correlated to its absorption in the tissues that stop and absorb the waves. This is the anisotropy that is very variable according to the nature of the scar tissue and the color of the skin.

Laser

Ablative Laser, Ablative Fractional Laser (AFL)

There are two possible wavelengths CO_2 (10,600 nm Fig. 1) and Erbium:YAG laser (2940 nm, Er:YAG = yttrium-aluminum-garnet). These two lasers have the function of vaporizing, coagulating, and remodeling skin tissue. Depending on their mode of operation, they can abrade a surface for a classic mode-locked mode for a resurfacing or in a fractional mode but with a variable density of MTZ (microthermal zone) to create thermal columns whose density, size of the points, and depth of penetration are function of each indication: retractile or mature scar, drug delivery (laser-assisted drug delivery = LADD).

The difference between these two wavelengths and their use is a matter of debate for the respec-

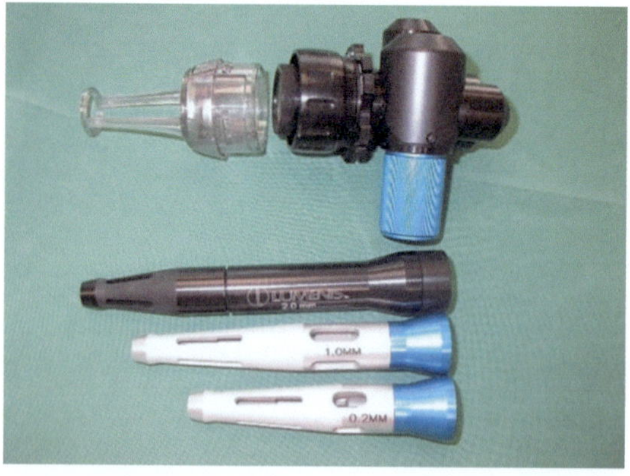

Fig. 1 CO_2 handpieces: continuous wave with 3 spot sizes and scanner system (spot size 120 microns, density 3–5–10%, energy 10–150 mJ, variable emission time). Courtesy of Hugues Cartier

tive users. Simply put, the CO_2 laser induces greater and more penetrating thermal damage while the Er: YAG laser induces a gentler and more precise dermabrasion.

In fractional mode, the dots or spot size of a CO_2 laser can vary in diameter from 120 microns (max depth 3.5 mm) to 1.3 mm (max depth 0.3 mm). You can use both for a remodeling and a resurfacing combination in the same session but with a higher risk of side effects (Fig. 2).

The Er: YAG laser is not very coagulant, even though its emission time can be modulated to 1500 µs. It is also possible to stack the shots with variable fluence or time emission to combine thermal and penetrating effects (max depth 1.5–2 mm).

These two lasers abrade or reshape scars profile by breaking the collagen fibers. The resurfacing mode with these two lasers is also possible, which leaves no space in the healthy skin and is particularly effective, but with variable effects in terms of healing, from 5 to 10 days.

In fractional mode, as a creation of spaced skin wells, healing is faster than in resurfacing mode (Fig. 3). This often requires several sessions to obtain a result, but they also allow the penetration of active ingredients such as corticoids, which are particularly useful for highly inflammatory, hypertrophic, or even keloid scars. The procedure is called laser-assisted drug delivery (LADD) [1].

The optimal depth is difficult to determine because studies report that drug deposition depends on both the anisotropy of the scars and skin areas, the laser sequences, the type of AFL and the drugs. The increasing laser fluence and irradiation time will increase cellular uptake of large molecules through the skin in a dose-dependent manner, but it is not that simple. If the barrier of the thermal columns is too coagulated, or if the drug applied is too late after the session, the drugs will not be able to penetrate. Similarly, drugs diffusion is also variable depending on their intrinsic nature.

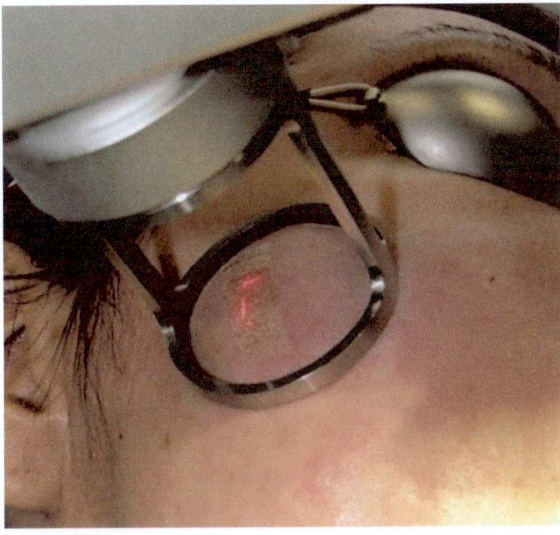

Fig. 2 Fractional emission for a laser CO_2 with microbeams spot size 180 microns, and 0.4 mm between each MTZ. Courtesy of Hugues Cartier

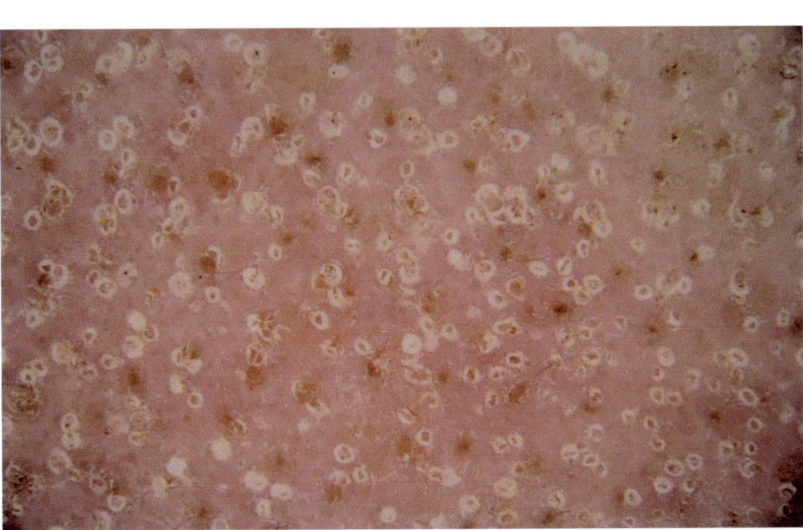

Fig. 3 Microbeams of AFL irradiation induce MTZ rankings from classically 100 to 300 µm but until 1.25 mm diameter. Holes can extend down to the deep reticular dermis. Courtesy of Hugues Cartier

The parameters of these devices vary, and we can only advise you to follow the settings of the laboratories or those of the publications which refer to them. To reshape a scar, it is necessary to penetrate to an estimated depth of 50–75% into the thickness of the scar 4a, b and 5a–d.

There are no standardized settings but Matteo Clementoni recommends to keep the following in mind:
- The thicker the lesion, the higher the energy will be.
- The higher the energy is, the lower the density will be.
- In a thick retractive bundle, consider different directions of the shots.
- Consider multiple passes instead of increasing the density of the shots.

- A pinpoint bleeding is a good endpoint (if the time emission of a CO_2 is less than 1 ms).
- For a collagen remodeling and to avoid a surrounding burn to the scar, reduce energy if you see a skin contraction.
- Consider a superficial fractional ablation to improve the aesthetic appearance.
- With a superficial handpiece use very low energy and high frequency to sculpt the superficial irregularities or prefer the use of Er: YAG to CO_2.

When applicable, the combined-mode Er: YAG + CO_2 can offer synergistic benefit of ablative and coagulation effect. However, it is difficult to determine superiority between modalities due to the clinical heterogeneity, settings, combination, and lack of comparative study design.

Case 1 Post Hemangioma Scar of the Upper Lip
See Fig. 4a, b.

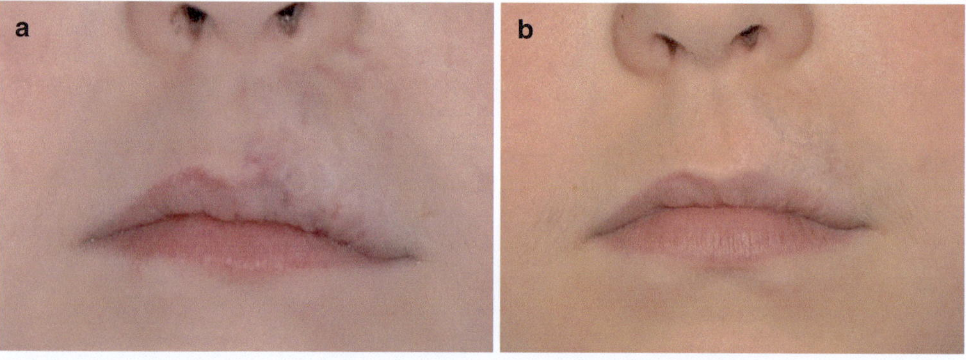

Fig. 4 (**a**) CO_2 resurfacing of hemangioma sequelae in a single session. (**b**) Outcome maintained 3 years after. Courtesy of Thierry Fusade

Case 2 Atrophic and Pox Scars with Large Pores

See Fig. v.

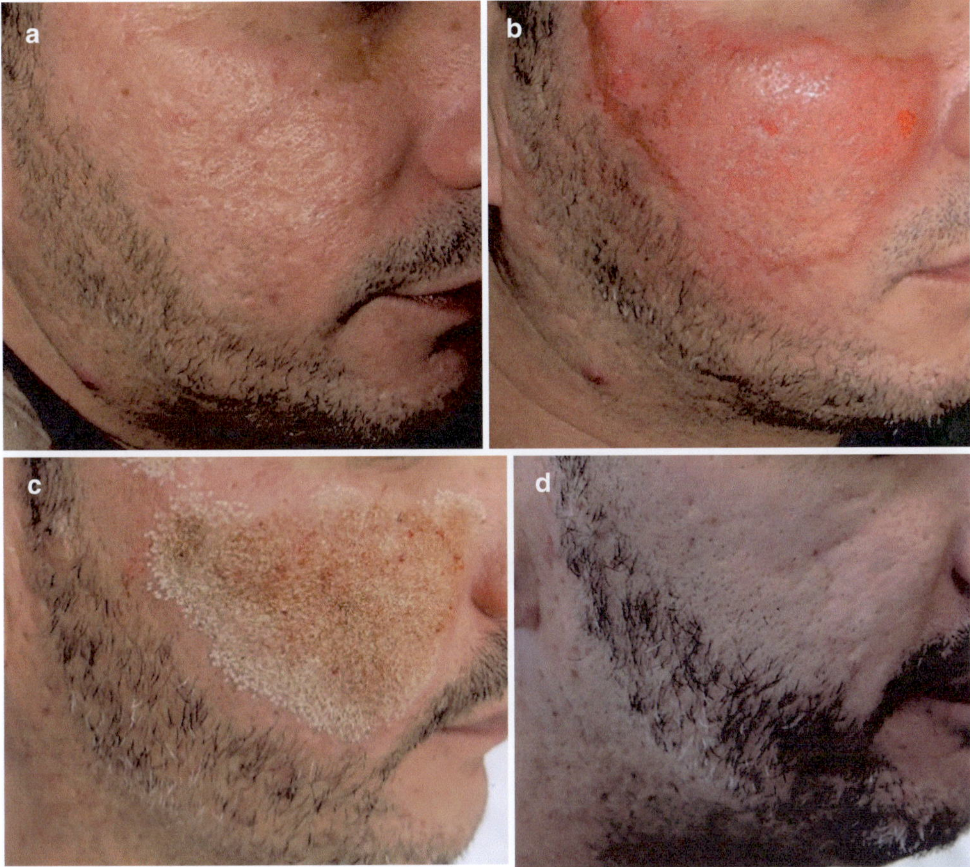

Fig. 5 (**a**) Acne scars with large pores. (**b**) Just after a first session ablative Er:YAG 10 J/cm², 1000 μs. The epidermis and dermis are completely removed down to the base of the scars. Of course, it is necessary to evaluate this depth visually in order not to obey the healing process. Bleeding is a sign that the papillary dermis has been touched. (**c**) Just after the fractional CO_2: 150 mJ-200 Hz-density 5/9-spot size 1.25 mm. Although this is a fractional mode, the impacts are wider (1.25 mm) and not as deep (120 μm estimated depth) as the classic fractional mode with small MTZ mode (120–300 μm). In this case, the skin debris is not wiped off, but left as is by applying a protective healing ointment such as Vaseline. (**d**) Final result 4 years after 3 sessions of ablative fractional and two non-fractional laser (CO_2 + Er:YAG). Courtesy of Hugues Cartier

Comments

There were clear improvements in the textural differences but it needed numerous sessions to reduce scars and dilated pores. The risk of permanent hypochromia must also be taken into account. And too high a fluence, too long a shooting time, and too high a density can induce this secondary effect. The debate is open to consider that one or two aggressive sessions are better than several accumulated sessions. It is a balance between the variable healing effects of thermal aggression and the risk of causing hypochromic scars.

Non-ablative Lasers

Non-ablative Fractional Laser (NAFL)

The modeling of NAFLs is described in the Princeps Publication [2].

There are two main types of laser: the erbium-glass, 1540–1550–1565 nm, and the Nd: YAP laser, 1340 nm. They act in a fractionated mode with a variable pulse time, density, and size of points. Due to the thermal columns they induce, the photons penetrate between 1 and 2 mm, allowing scar remodeling without creating skin vaporization. Unlike ablative lasers, there is therefore no scar desiccation phase (Fig. 6). There is no crust, and the healing time is short, less than 48–72 h with slight skin swelling and redness for a few days (Fig. 7a, b).

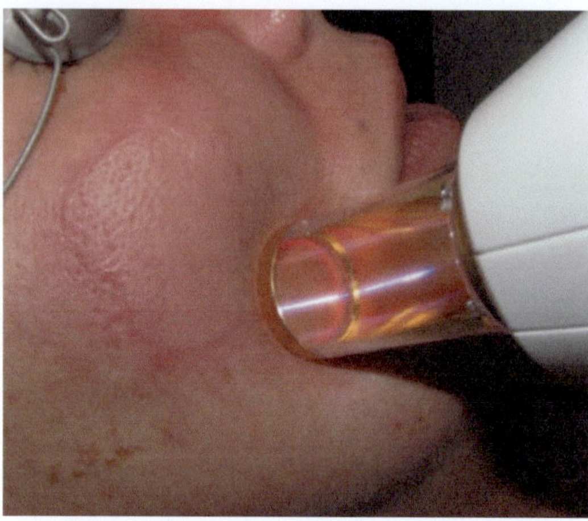

Fig. 6 Laser beam emission by a scanning procedure of a NAFL, Er:glass 1565 nm with variable settings (fluence 70 mJ maximum, time of emission variable function of the spot density, density 100–500 MTZ/cm²). A slight swelling is already visible. Courtesy of Hugues Cartier

Case 3 Mature Hypertrophic Acne Scars

See Fig. 7a, b.

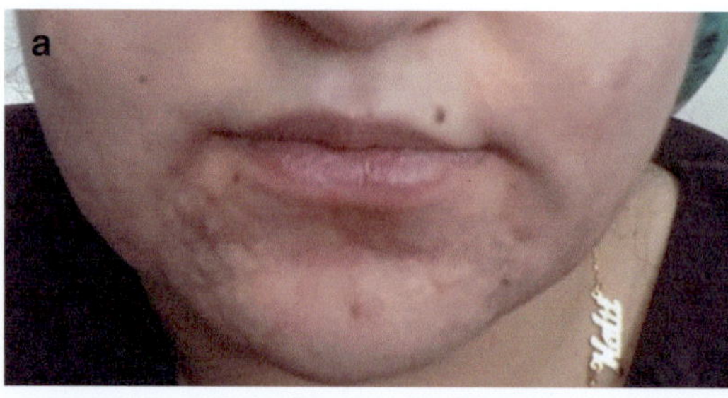
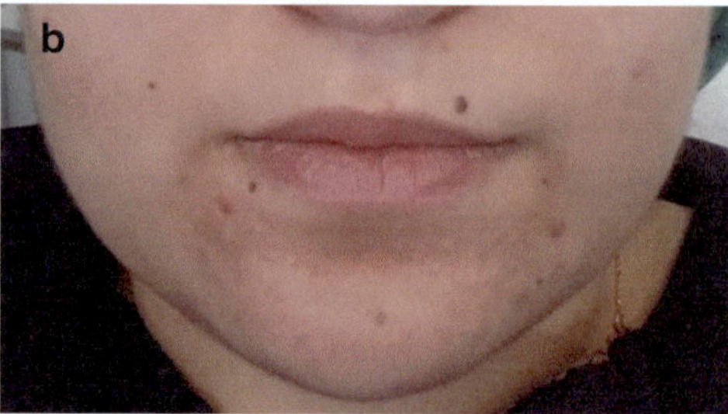

Fig. 7 (**a**) Hypertrophic mature acne scars of the chin. (**b**) After three sessions, 6 weeks apart, of NAFL, Nd: YAP 1340 nm (100 MTZ/cm², 130 mJ, 3–5 ms). Reduction of skin surface with low downtime, no crust. Courtesy of Hugues Cartier

Comments

Non-ablative fractional lasers have the advantage of minimal postoperative effects with light swelling and redness for a few days. There is no crusting and the risk of infection is minimal. They are increasingly proposed before ablative lasers even if the result is much more progressive and sometimes in plateau after a few sessions. New device combines AFL and NAFL in the same session, by example CO_2 plus 1570 nm and ultrasound but we need more data to conclude.

Non-ablative, Non-fractional Laser

The 1210 nm diode laser is the main one. To our knowledge, it is the only one in its category developed and used immediately after a surgical suture. Its particularity is its portability (750 g), and the complete automation of its settings to heat a skin surface of 2 cm^2 per shot always at the same temperature (maximum 53 °C) automatically matching the skin heat in contact with the handpiece.

The wavelength allows us to treat all skin colors. It is advisable to use only colorless threads under the skin (external threads are not, however, contraindicated) so as not to concentrate the photons on colored threads, particularly black ones. Indeed, this can create heat points that are harmful to a fresh scar.

Vascular Lasers

The so-called vascular lasers focus on the vascular network. Apart from a hypochromic and atrophic scar, these lasers are useful alone or combined to reduce an inflammatory process or a scar that remains red, the result of a dilated vascular network.

Pulsed Dye Laser 595 nm (PDL)

The first pulsed dye laser emitted at 585 nm, systematically inducing purpura, i.e., photothermolysis of the vascular network. The latest generations emit 595 nm for a higher penetration (estimated 1–2 mm) and can vary the emission time in photothermolysis or photocoagulation. In the first case, the privileged target remains the vascular pattern. The purpura is caused by damaged vascular walls. The settings range is in between 0.5 and 6 ms: 6 and 10 J/cm^2, with variable spot size 5–10 mm, considered as an intermediate sub-purpuric mode.

In the second case, as the emission time is longer (beyond 6 ms), there is no or very little purpura but a thermal effect which can be interesting also in a scarring process in progress or for vessels of diameter greater than 1 mm (Fig. 8a, b).

It is necessary to integrate the adjustment of the delivered energy which varies the target effect, the thermal effect, and the penetrance of the photons. The aim of vascular lasers and particularly the pulsed dye laser is to destroy capillary destruction, generate hypoxemia, and reduce collagen production. In fact, it is not so simple because these lasers promote the production of neocollagenesis, break fibrous bridges by the intrinsic photonic effect, and release collagenase-type metalloproteinases (MMPs). What is paradoxical is that eventually, despite the inflammatory cascade that it provokes, the scar does not suffer from a laser burn [3].

Case 4 Hypertrophic Scar of the Upper Lip

See Fig. 8a, b.

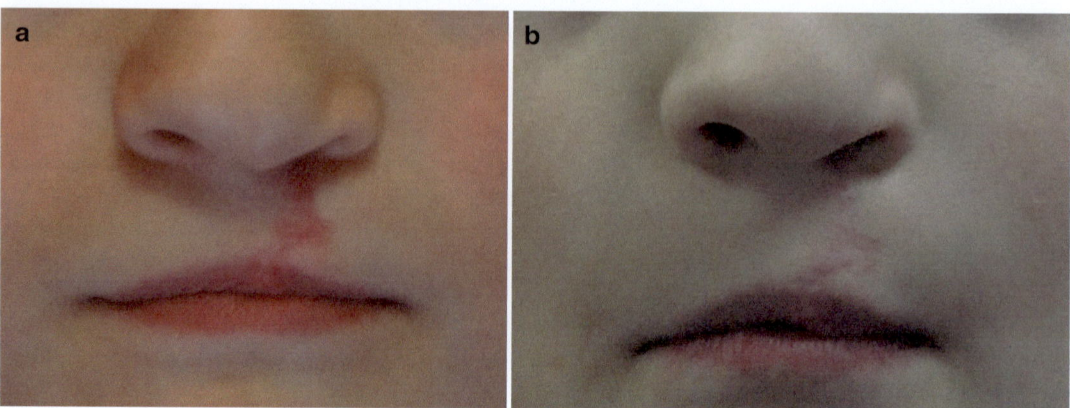

Fig. 8 (a) Hypertrophic scar after cleft palate repair. (b) Result 1 year after 2 PDL treatments, 6 weeks apart (6 J/cm², 1.5 ms), associated with 10 days of corticoids cream and silicone tape fixed during the night for 3 months. Courtesy of Hugues Cartier

Comments

- *The pulsed dye laser is the gold standard of vascular lasers. Initially used for angiomas from birth, it can be equally useful for vascular or inflammatory scars with a minimal risk of burning.*
- *For skin of color type (SOC), patients have more melanin in their epidermis. This melanin can act as a competing target chromophore for hemoglobin, causing an increased risk of adverse effects. Higher fluence may be necessary to produce the expected clinical endpoint.*

For a diffuse redness in SOC, a non-purpuric approach (e.g., 5 J/cm^2, 12 mm spot size, 0.45 ms, DCD 40 ms before/20 ms post cooling cryogenic system) is recommended for an immediate vessel disappearance without purpura.

For large vessel in SOC: large spot, 10/15 J/cm^2, 10 ms, DCD 40/20 ms for a same clinical endpoint.

KTP 532 nm

The KTP 532 laser is the competitor of the pulsed dye laser. The short wave penetrates only slightly less than the pulsed dye laser. It has an affinity for both the vascular network and the pigment. It is therefore necessary to be careful when using it on tanned skin or on skin with a phototype above III on the Fitzpatrick scale. The new generations of this type of laser also allow photocoagulation and photothermolysis modes.

Yellow Laser 577 nm and 589 nm

These two wavelengths are those best absorbed by hemoglobin. They are therefore an intermediate between the KTP laser and the pulsed dye laser. And even if there are few publications for the treatment of scars, there is no reason to believe that they cannot reduce vascular redness. However, they do not cause purpura.

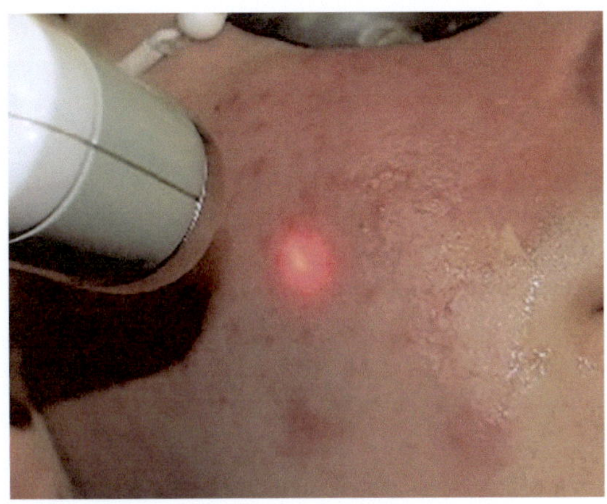

Fig. 9 Laser beam of a Nd-YAG 1064 nm, classic settings to treat active acne scar or inflammatory scar: 0.3–0.5 ms, 3–5 J/cm^2, fast motion of a laser beam scanning procedure to obtain a thermal effect close from 52 °C. Courtesy of Hugues Cartier

Nd: YAG 1064 nm Long Pulse and Nd: YAG 1319 nm

These two lasers do not emit the same wavelengths but are still in the infrared range. Nevertheless, their indications are in the same range. They aim to remodel scar tissue, even if it is more than 3–4 mm thick, and have a significant thermal effect. The Nd-YAG laser, however, has the characteristic of being able to photocoagulate large vessels beyond the millimeter. It can be used point by point or in scanning mode to accumulate this thermal effect to promote red scar or remodeling to give for flexibility. For Nd: YAG, a low fluence less than 5 J/cm^2 and an emission time between 0.3 and 0.5 ms are recommended for skin tightening (Fig. 9). Devices have a thermal sensor that continuously calculates the skin surface temperature, which should be stable at around 52 °C, but it is difficult to know for how long you should maintain this thermal level.

A more classic setting is also possible but variable according to the publications by example for hypertrophic and red scars: spot diameter

5–10 mm, time per pulse 25–60 ms, energy density between 10 and 75 J/cm^2 and two to three passes every 2–4–6 weeks between each session until an efficacy [4, 5].

The decision between the two modes is empirical but it is important to avoid accumulating too much energy which will cause immediate whitening, signaled by a thermal burn.

Q-Switched Nanosecond and Picosecond Laser

Several wavelengths are available: 532, 755, 585–650–694, and 1064 nm. The characteristic of these lasers is that they emit phenomenal photoacoustic energy in an extremely short time, 300 picoseconds to 50 ns depending on the device. Initially used for tattoo removal, they are also an indication for pigmented scars, to a certain extent post-inflammatory or post-inflammatory pigmentation (PIH), collagen remodeling in scanning mode or a fractional MLA mode as the LIOB procedure (laser-induced optical breakdown), and of course for tattooed scars from traumatic exogenous pigments (Fig. 10a–d).

Case 5 Acne Scars, Ice Pick Scars, and Dilated Pores

See Fig. 10a–d.

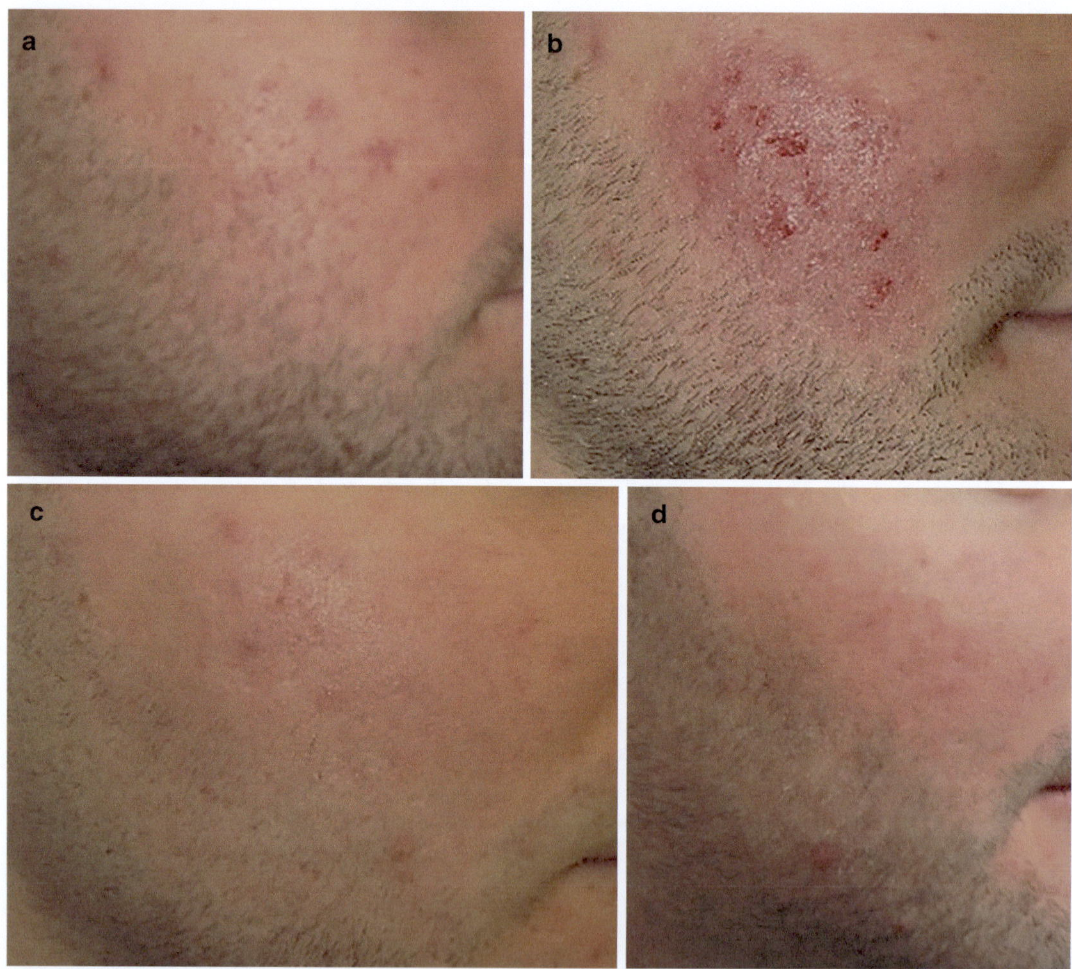

Fig. 10 (**a**) Acne scar and ice pick scar. (**b**) Petechial and erytheme jaust the use of the Q-switched laser 1064 nm in a stacking mode (8 J/cm^2; spots size 3 mm, 5 ns). (**c**) Result after three sessions 1 month apart. (**d**) Permanent result 4 years after. Courtesy of Hugues Cartier

Pulsed Polychromatic Light

Pulsed polychromatic light, flash lamp, or intense pulsed light (IPL) has the main characteristic of emitting photons of multiple wavelengths (Fig. 11). The spectral band is therefore wide, from 400 to 1200 nm, but the use of filters allows a contingent of photons to be filtered. The Intense Pulsed Light is indicated for acne, vascular, inflammatory, and pigmented scars [6] (Fig. 12a–d). It can be combined in the same session with photoacoustic or non-ablative lasers.

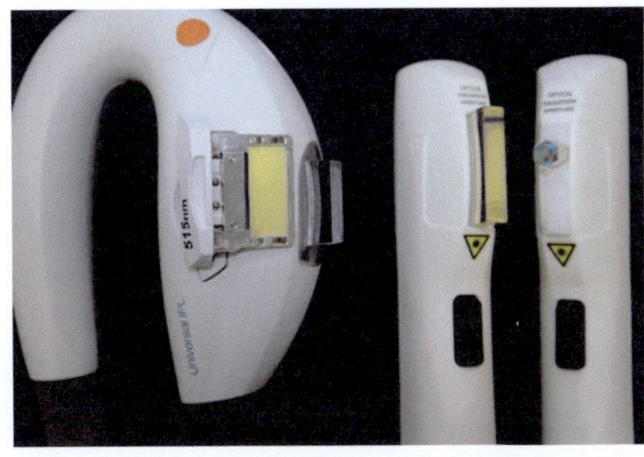

Fig. 11 Sample of IPL handpieces with the choice of the filtering system and the contact spot size. Courtesy of Hugues Cartier

Case 6 Acne Conglobata

See Fig. 12a–d.

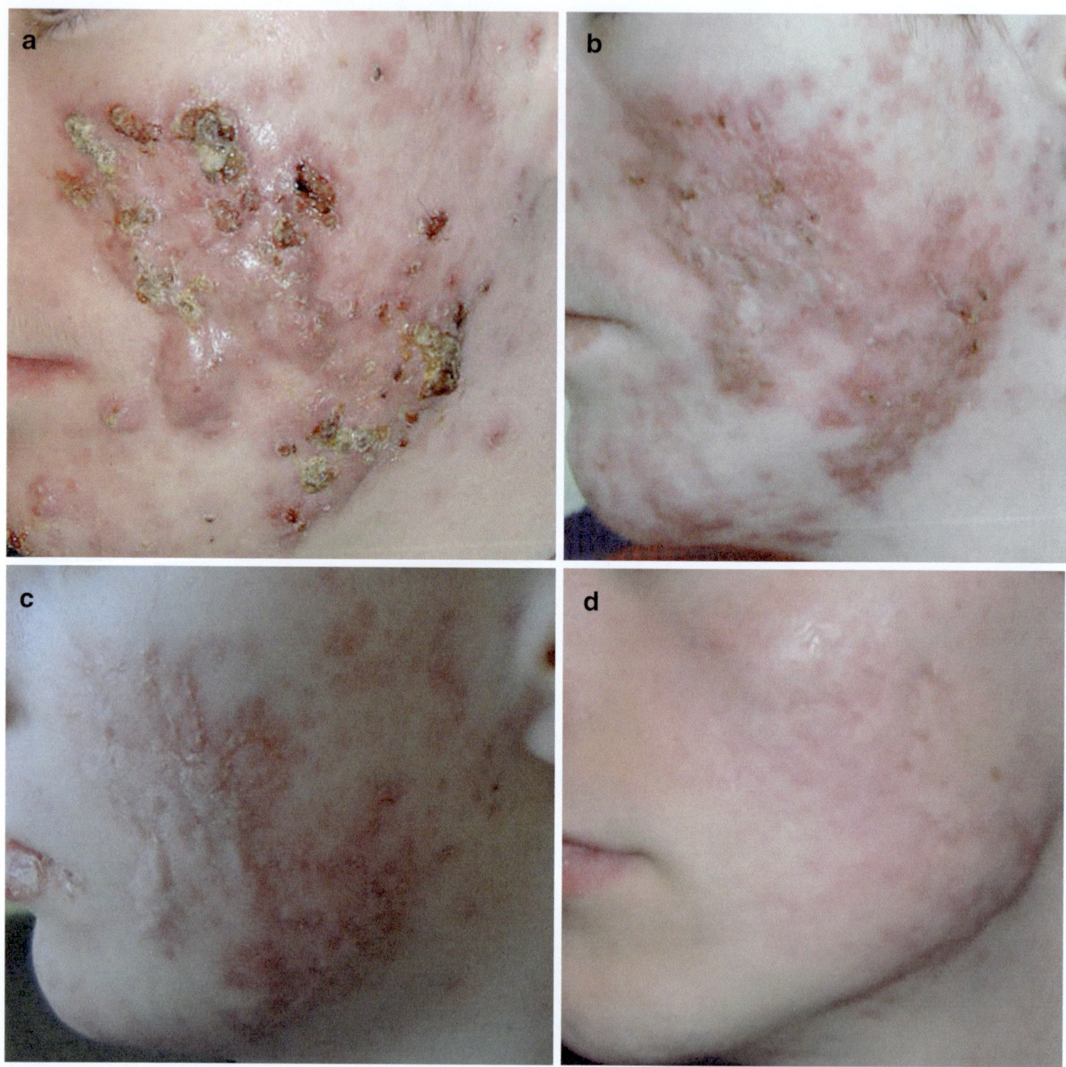

Fig. 12 **a**) Case 6 Fulminant acne treated by a combination of steroids, isotretinoin 5 then 10 mg/day + macrolides + metronidazole and emptying of abscess cysts. (**b**) Drying of cystic lesions but scarring may develop 2 months after. (**c**) After 4 months of the beginning of the treatment, 10 IPL sessions will be programmed over 15 months: 515 and 550 nm, 10 J/cm^2, double pulse 5 ms interpulse 10 ms. (**d**) Stabilised result at 30 months, the patient has received 9 months of isotretinoin at an average dose of 10 mg per day while being treated by IPL. Courtesy of Hugues Cartier

Light-Emitting Diodes (LEDs)

The use of LEDs can also respond to the management of a healing process [7]. It also responds to the choice of wavelength. In most publications, for inflammatory or recent scars, 630 nm is the first choice with infrared 850 nm. However, their benefit is the subject of debate. They have no deleterious effect except in the blue-violet (<450 nm) range. This spectral band can in fact prolong post-inflammatory pigmentation (Fig. 13a, b).

Case 7 Recent Traumatic Scar After Corrective Surgery

See Fig. 13a, b..

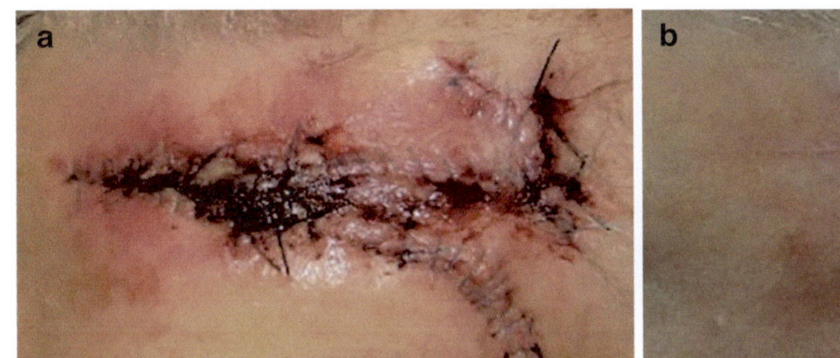
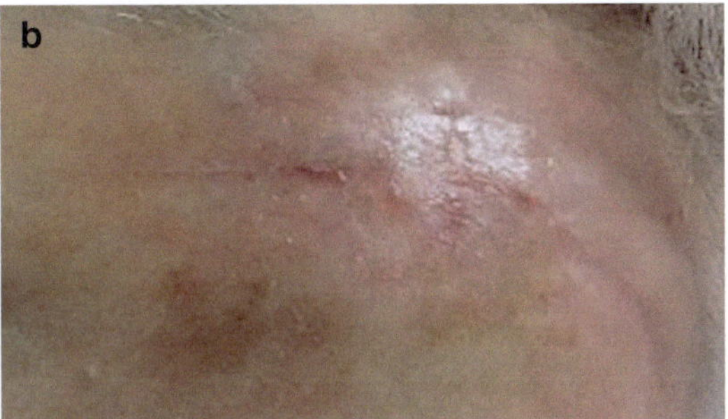

Fig. 13 (a) Fresh forehead traumatic scar. (b) Dramatical improvement after 3 months and 15 sessions of red 633 nm and infrared 850 nm LEDs: 20 J/cm², 15 min each. Courtesy of Hugues Cartier

Comments

The patient was hospitalized for a month, and we took advantage of this to offer her mixed LEDs every 2 days, always in combination with the classic postoperative healing procedure. We were surprised by the result and the textural quality of the scar. The choice of parameters and the number of sessions were empirical but there were no side effects.

Radiofrequency

Radiofrequency delivers only a thermal effect, unlike lasers.

Contact Radiofrequency

Contact radiofrequency by regular scanning allows mechanical remodeling while delivering heat, which we try to stabilize at around 50 °C thanks to thermal sensors. This is the same principle of infrared heat accumulation as the Nd-YAG 1064 laser.

Fractional Radiofrequency

This involves dozen electrodes applied in contact with the skin to cause surface thermocoagulation to regenerate it. It acts on less than 1 mm of skin thickness.

Radiofrequency with Micro-Needles (MRF)

This is like fractional ablative lasers. Physically, these are polarized needles that penetrate between 0.5 m and 4 mm deep to create thermal columns to fragment and remodel fibrosed or atrophic skin tissue (Fig. 14a–c).

There is a choice between insulated and unprotected needles. In the first case, only the tip will be able to deliver its full thermal energy. Depending on the thickness of the scar tissue, it will be necessary to make several passes to treat the entire scar volume. In the second case, the whole needle delivers this energy. This is also a source of discussion as to the possible choice. Note that needles can become damaged and blunt more quickly if the scars are very dense, unlike fractional ablative lasers.

Case 8 Fibrous Neck Acne Scar

See Fig. 14a–c.

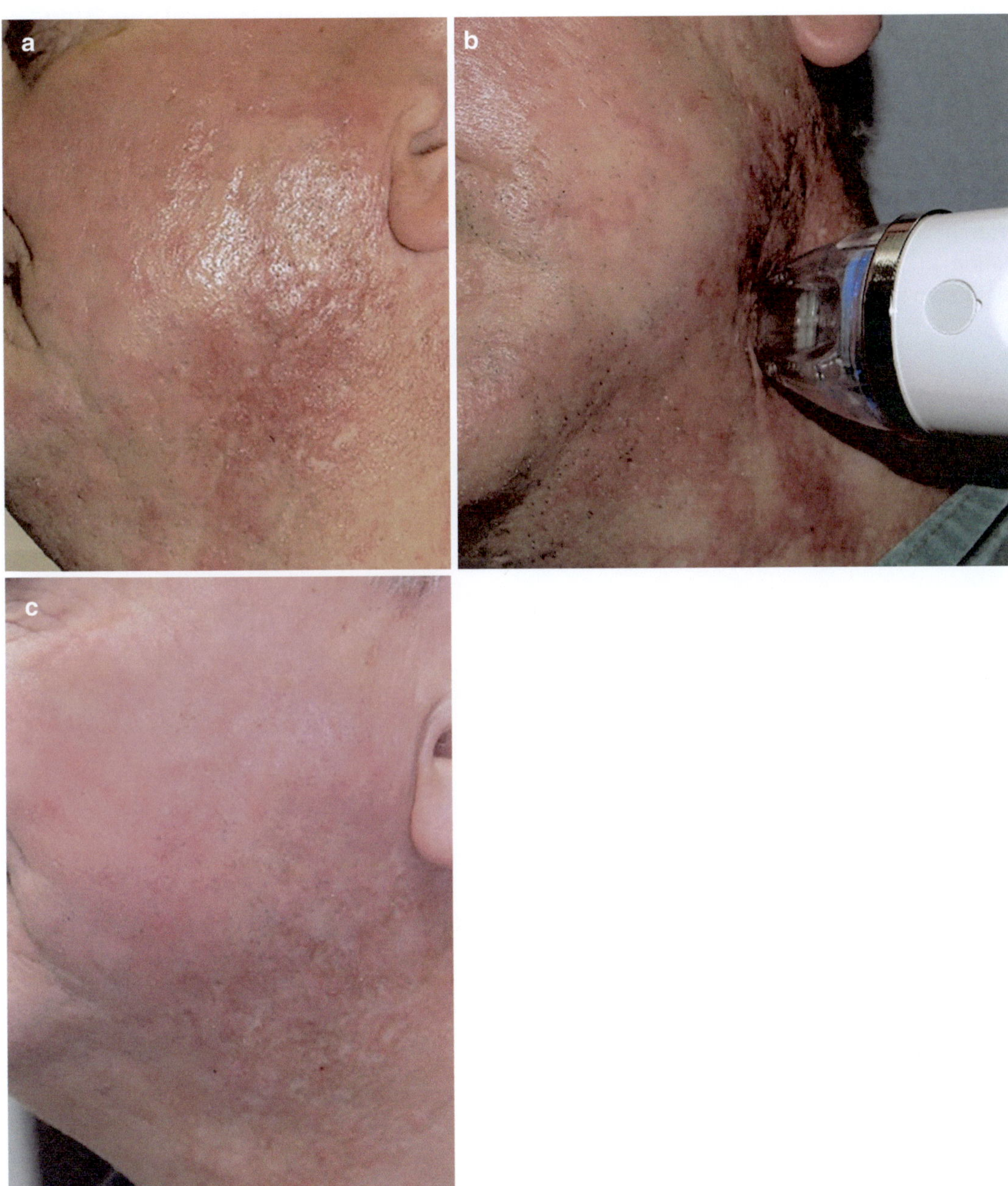

Fig. 14 (**a**) Fixed acne scar with fibrous tissue. (**b**) MRF (microneedle radiofrequency). Between 8 and 64 needles can penetrate simultaneously the skin depending on the device with a depth between 0.5 and 4 mm. (**c**) Improvement with a structure and texture modification after three sessions 2 months apart. Courtesy of Hugues Cartier

Other Waves

Shock Waves

Focused Ultrasound

These waves are focused according to the transducers used to create skin fusion points at more than 70 °C instantaneously: 1.5, 3.5, and 4.5 mm deep. High-intensity focused ultrasound (HIFU) is indicated for skin tightening and slackening. With the skin relaxation due to aging, the visualization of a scar is reaccentuated, and HIFU could help to reduce scar.

Mechanical Devices and Other Sources of Heat

Micro-Needling, Mechanical Subcision, and Scar Raising with Punch Biopsy

This is outside the scope of lasers and other waves, but mechanical techniques still can be used in the management of deep scarring, atrophic and mature scars (Fig. 15a–d).

They are not associated with a thermal effect and can be used without risk for scars on all phototypes [8].

Case 9 Acne Scar and Micro-Needling
See Fig. 15a–d.

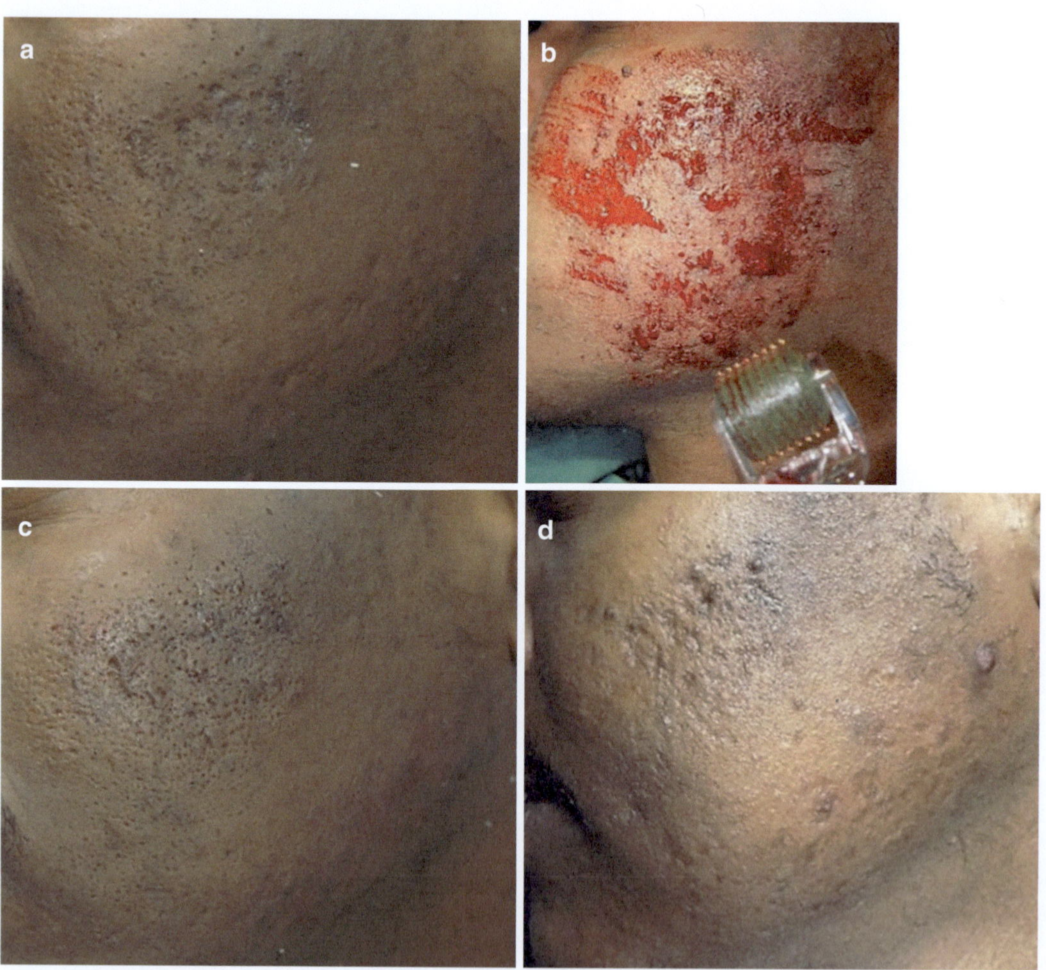

Fig. 15 (**a**) Atrophic acne scar, phototype VI. (**b**) Bleeding effect just after micro-needling. (**c**) Result after two sessions of micro-needling and fillers injection with hyaluronic acid. (**d**) Result 2 years after the last session with the re-appearance of scars. Courtesy of Hugues Cartier

Cryotherapy and Radiotherapy [9–10]

These two techniques are indicated for fixed keloid scars or after surgical removal of a keloid to avoid recurrence. Depending on the country, endocuritherapy is preferred by introducing an iridium thread into the keloid or now there is a focused cutaneous radiotherapy device that avoids the need for treatment in a leaded room in a radiotherapy center, which is normally the only one authorized to provide this type of radiation. The only system is SRT-100™ (Sensus Healthcare, Boca Raton, Florida) using a biologically effective dose (BED) of 30Gy with irradiation scheme of three 6Gy SRT treatments on Days 1, 2, and 3 following surgeries.

Cryosurgery without and with intralesional corticosteroids is effective and safe on young and small keloids not only as a destructive physical procedure but also by inducing biochemical and immunological scar rejuvenation.

Lasers in Surgical Scars

There is increasing evidence of the effectiveness of lasers, light-based devices, and others energy-based devices (EBD) in the postsurgical healing process. These different treatments occur at various times before or after surgery [11].

The Day Before Surgery with Non-ablative Fractional Laser

The concept of being able to treat a scar increasingly quickly stems from the work of Haedersdal et al. A single NAFL treatment at low to medium fluence performed 1 day prior, or in the early phases of wound healing, may have the potential to optimize scar formation in full wounds without side effects including dyschromia. It was a randomized, controlled, intra-individual trial with Erbium-glass 1540 nm NAFL versus no laser treatment on 16 subjects receiving 10 standardized full-thickness punch biopsy wounds. A single NAFL exposure has been assessed 1 day before the biopsy, immediately after, and 2 weeks after. Three fluence levels provided deep and superficial energy depositions (range 30–70 mJ/microbeam).

The results show that biopsy scars are invisible if the area is laser treated the day before the biopsy [12]. In clinical practice, treatment 24 h before the operation may be of interest [13].

Laser as an Early Procedure During Surgery

Automated Laser Diode 1210 nm [14]

The Laser-Assisted Skin Healing treatment induces a controlled heat stress that promotes tissue regeneration. This comparative trial is the first to evaluate the performance of a new automated 1210-nm laser system, compatible with all Fitzpatrick scale phototypes. The horizontal sutured incision of one breast was treated with the portable 1210-nm laser while in the operating theater. The other breast was used as the study control. Finally, at 24 weeks, the treated side had a 36% ($p < 0.038$) reduction in scar volume compared to the control group. At 52 weeks, there was a 29% ($p = 0.004$) reduction in volume, an 11% ($p = 0.017$) reduction in scar area, and a 17% ($p = 0.002$) improvement in the smoothness (roughness) of the scar compared to the control group. This procedure in facial skin surgery must benefit from more practical applications, but it is used for long scars of the body (Fig. 16a–d).

Result: Taking action at the end of the intervention is a promising way forward with limited risk. Courtesy of Francois Will

Case 10 Use of Diode 1210 nm for Scar

See Fig.(Fig. 16a–d).

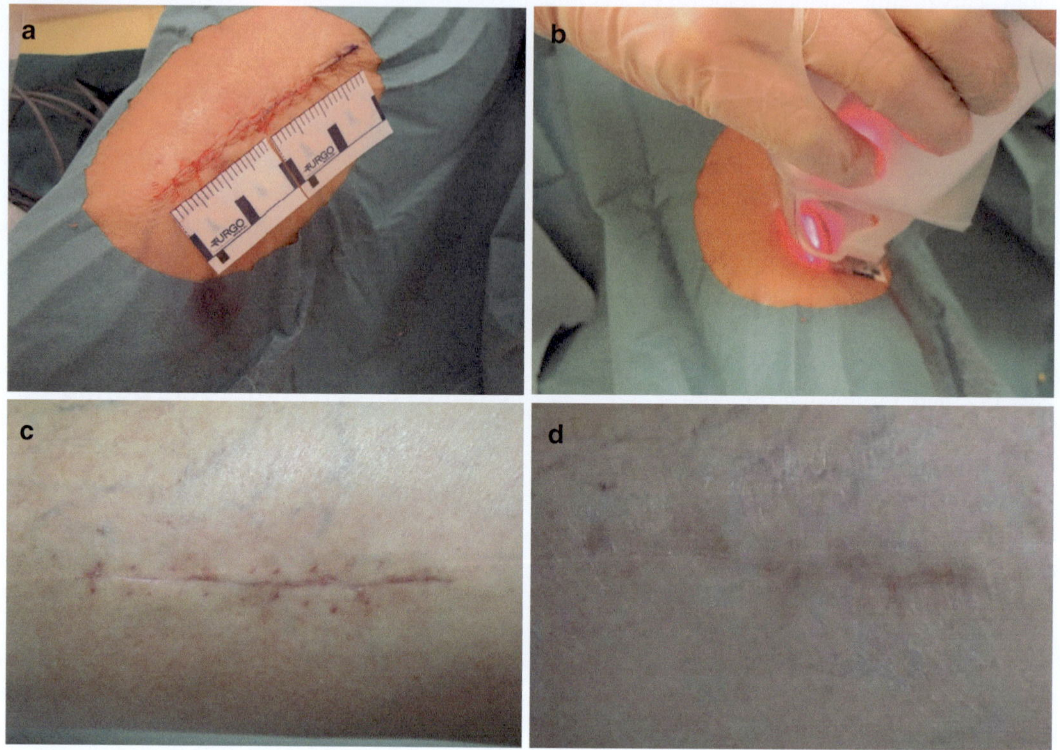

Fig. 16 (**a**) In an immediate postoperative surgical procedure: bar code for automatic settings. (**b**) Laser diode 1210 nm in action. (**c**) Laser diode 1210 nm: results after 1 month without inflammation. (**d**) Laser diode 1210 nm: results after 6 months. Courtesy of Francois Will

Laser as Soon as Possible After the Surgery, in the First 3 Months

Pulsed dye laser (PDL), ablative fractional laser (AFL), and non-ablative fractional laser (NAFL) are in the first line.

The PDL can be used as soon as the sutures are removed. This treatment performed in a period close to the inflammatory phase, and to the beginning of the proliferation phase, uses the vascular target due to vasodilatation and neo-angiogenesis to interfere with the complex phenomena of scarring.

A Vascular Laser Only

- Several studies have analyzed and compared the contribution of pulsed dye lasers (PDL), using different parameters and starting the treatment at different stages. Interesting results are presented with the use of PDL from suture removal, at low fluences: e.g., 10 mm 6 ms, 7 J/cm². This treatment, performed in a period close to the inflammatory phase and the beginning of the proliferation phase, uses the vascular target due to vasodilatation and neo-angiogenesis, to interfere with the complex healing phenomena [15] (Fig. 17a, b).
- The same is true with the KTP 532 laser on thyroidectomy scars. Each participant was treated using a 532-nm KTP laser (Gemini, Laserscope, San Jose, CA) two times at 2-week intervals. The laser treatment was done 2–3 weeks (average 15.5 days) after the total thyroidectomy surgery, which was around the time at which a surgical wound completes its epithelialization and the sutures have been removed. The laser treatment setting for each surgical scar was as follows: 10-mm spot size, 25-ms pulse duration, 8 J/cm² of fluence, 1.5 Hz, double pass. After two sessions of laser treatments using the 532-nm KTP laser, scars of the treated group showed cosmetically better outcomes than those in the untreated control group [16].

Case 11 Scar of the Nose After Derm Surgery for Basocellular Carcinoma
See Fig. (Fig. 17a, b).

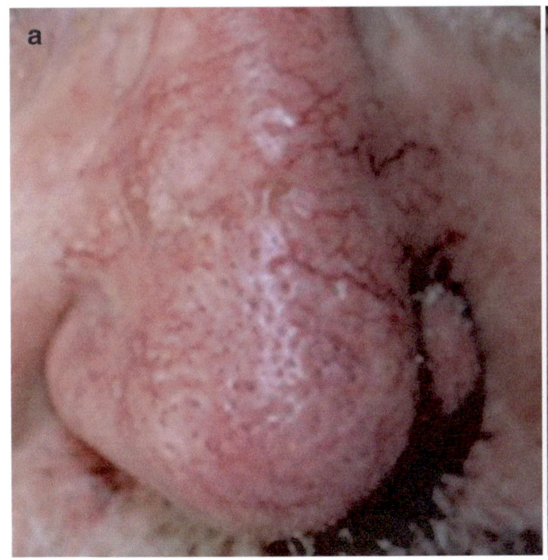
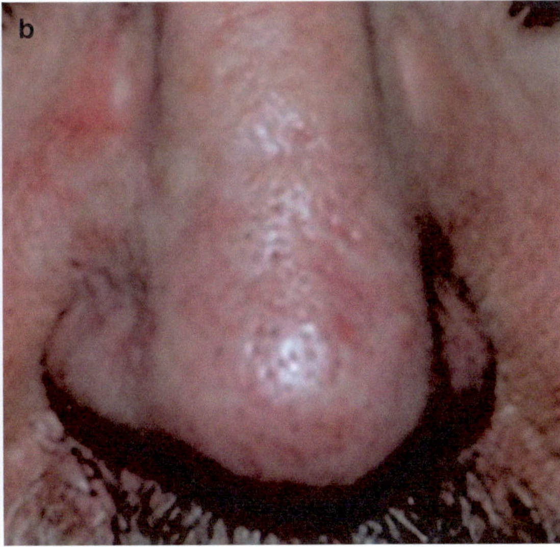

Fig. 17 (**a**) Nasoglabellar flap—vascular targets 1 month after surgery. (**b**) Result after 3 treatments at M1–M2–M3 with combined PDL/YAG Multiplex Cynosure setting 7 mm handpiece PDL 10 ms 9J short interval YAG 20 ms 45J. Courtesy of Francois Will

Non-ablative Fractional Laser

In this indication, the early use of a non-ablative fractional laser (NAFL) in the weeks following surgery has also shown favorable results in several studies for low densities even comparatively to Pulse Dye Laser [17].

In 2009, a Korean team treated linear thyroidectomy scars for 27 patients with a 1550 nm NAFL, starting in the second week, three times a month [18].

The same surgeon performed all the operations using the same surgical techniques. Each patient was treated four times at 1-month intervals using the same parameters (5×10-mm spot size, 10 mJ, 1500 spot/cm [2], static mode). Initiation of the first irradiation was made 2–3 weeks after the thyroidectomy.

The scar prevention effects were evaluated each month for 6 months after the thyroidectomy. The average Vancouver Scar Scale score (VSS) was lower in the laser treatment group. The global assessment also presented better cosmetic outcomes in the treatment group than in the controls. The NAFL can be safely applied in dark Asian skin without noticeable adverse effects.

Case 12 Traumatic Scar of the Glabella

See Fig. 18a–d.

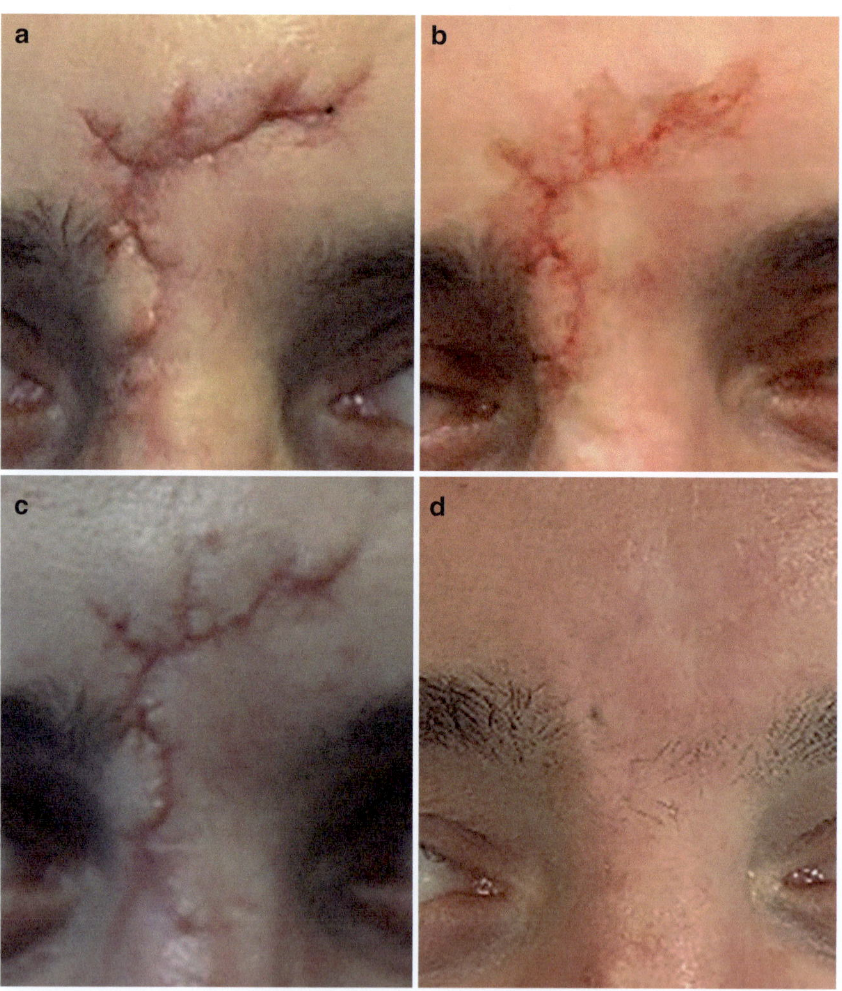

Fig. 18 (**a**) Post-traumatic scar and corrective surgery at 3 weeks with inhomogeneous contact between still swollen edges. (**b**) Erbium: YAG laser resurfacing + botulinum toxin injection to relax the glabellar muscles. (**c**) Pulsed dye laser 7 mm, 6 J/cm², 10 ms alternated every 2 months 3 times with non-ablative fractional laser 1550 nm 50 mJ, 3 ms followed by injection of a few drops of hyaluronic acid in the scar line (beware of major vascular risk area) while continuing with hyaluronic acid injections. (**d**) Result in line with expectations at 1 year with a discrete non-invasive scar line. Courtesy of Hugues Cartier

Comments

- *Alternative to the Erbium: YAG laser, the CO_2 laser also allows resurfacing but remains less precise for abrading borders.*
- *Alternative to pulsed dye laser, KTP laser 532 nm, 8 d/cm², 4 ms.*
- *Alternative to Erbium-glass laser 1550 nm, other wavelengths 1565, 1540 and Nd-YAP laser 1340 nm are also possible.*

Ablative or Non-ablative Fractional Laser, Which to Choose?

The great difficulty in most of these reported studies is to know the limits of one's own devices. One wonders on what criteria the authors base themselves to find the right settings for any device.

- Ibrahim et al. evaluated the use of CO_2 for postsurgical scars. A total of 27 Egyptian patients with recent postoperative scars were enrolled in this study. Three sessions of fractional CO_2 laser with a 1-month interval were started 4 weeks after surgery. Vancouver Scar Scale (VSS) was used as an assessment tool at 1 and 3 months after the final treatment. Patients reported their satisfaction using a subjective four-point scale. They demonstrated a statistically significant overall average improvement of the VSS (5.33 ± 1.33) before compared with (2.55 ± 1.06) 3 months after the last laser treatment ($P \leq 0.001$). The most significant improvements were found in pigmentation, height, and pliability [19].
- In a comparative study by Shin et al. [20], on the treatment of postoperative scars using non-ablative and ablative fractional lasers, the results may provide more clarity. They randomized 32 patients (mean age 42.1 years) of phototype III–V, with a thyroidectomy scar of 2–3 months. One-half of the scar was treated with non-ablative fractional laser and the other half with the ablative technique (Mosaic™ laser, Lutronic corporation). At the rate of two sessions 2 months apart, with similar parameters for the two modes: high energy 50–60 mJ and low density 5–8%. The

evaluation was done on photographic images, spectrophotometry, and durometer. Clinical improvement was not significantly different between the two systems; however, AFL was better at reducing scar hardness whereas NFL was superior for lightening color. But there is no miracle for vascular redness; the vascular laser seems to be the most interesting to use as soon as possible compared to any fractional lasers.

Vascular Laser with Fractional Laser: As Soon As Possible

- Kim and coll. report their results on the comparison of the pulsed dye laser (595 nm, 10 ms, 10 J/cm²), and the fractional CO_2 laser (AFL) (80 mJ/mtz, density 8% in two passes, spot 120 µm), in a prospective, comparative study on the same scar, for 14 patients with postsurgical scars of the face [12] and the abdomen. They observed comparable results between the two devices, with the LCP having a logically better action on pigmentation—vascularization—color and the CO_2 laser pliability—texture—height—thickness of the scar [21] (Fig. 18a–d).

Comments

- *Considering the vascular targets and the neocollagenesis in the healing process, we propose to our patients the combined treatment associating successively in the same session of LCP 595–10 mm 6 ms 7 J and AFL densities 5–10% for a power of 70–150 mJ. The results appear to us to be interesting, in accordance with the various publications, on postsurgical scars of the nose. This is an increasingly frequent situation after the removal of skin carcinoma in this area, in patients concerned about the visibility of their scar.*
- *We particularly insist on the prerequisite of a carcinologic surgery followed by a meticulous and optimal repair, the laser being an addi-*

tional technique that can only be used after a good repair surgery.

- *The treatment is started at the removal of the sutures, between D6 and D10, and repeated twice at 1-month intervals.*
- *This protocol brings quicker results in reducing the visibility of the scar and provides satisfaction to patients who wish to care for their scars after surgery.*

- *It can be debated that nose scars can improve spontaneously. Experience shows that we have no deleterious effect on the scarring process at the proposed parameters of our lasers (Fig. 19a–d).*

Case 13 Nose Surgical Scar for a Basocellular Carcinoma

See Fig. 19a–d.

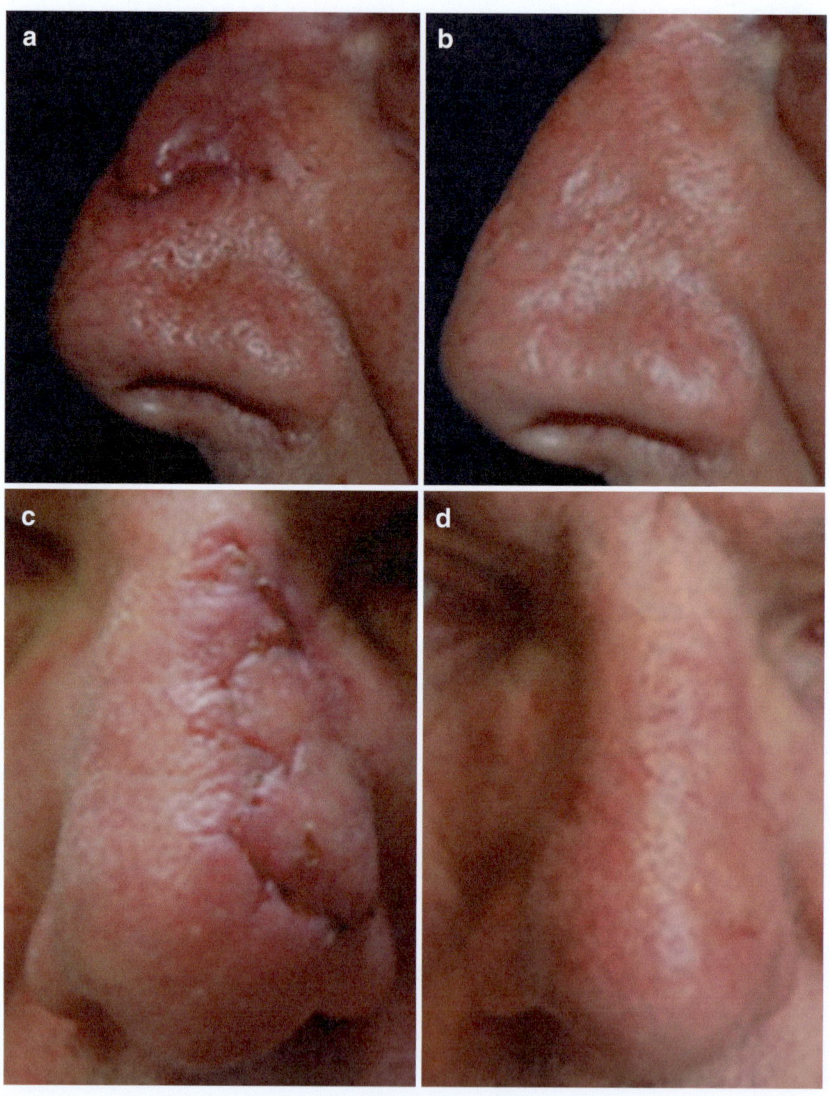

Fig. 19 (**a**) Surgical scar at Day 7 after flap of the nose. (**b**) Scars after 3 combined laser treatment PDL 10 mm–6 ms–7J and AFLCO$_2$ density 0.8–1 mm or (5%) fluence 70–120 mJ—start day 7 after surgery M1 and M2. (**c**) Surgical scar at Day 7 after flap of the nose. (**d**) Scars after 3 combined laser treatment PDL 10 mm–6 ms–7J and AFLCO$_2$ density 0.8–1 mm (or 5%) fluence 70–120 mJ—start day 7 after surgery M1 and M2. Courtesy of Francois Will

Key Point: Management of a Postsurgical Skin Scar

1. PRACTICAL, SIMPLE, and QUICK TREATMENT

   PDL (or KTP)/AFLCO$_2$ (or NAFL) laser combination—3 sessions: at D7 (removal of sutures)-M1–M2

2. MORE TECHNICAL IN THE OP ROOM

   A diode laser 1210 nm—especially plastic surgery

3. NEW MODALITIES SKIN TREATMENT BEFORE SURGERY

   Skin treatment to prepare the healing process before the operation: non-ablative fractional laser (NAFL)

Comments

– *There is no risk in offering laser sessions with low enough fluence parameters for a scar "under construction." In all the reviews, there is no mention that the laser has had a deleterious effect on the scarring process.*

– *The studies are difficult to compare, and it is not so easy to propose a codified protocol except for the thyroidectomy scar feature.*

– *Among the lasers and other energy-based devices (DBE), all can be of interest, and it is the laserist doctor who picks from their toolbox, while estimating the settings they find most useful.*

– *In this respect, the easiest laser to set up is the pulsed dye laser, as it is accepted that all that is needed is to provoke a sub-purple reaction. Whatever the situation, it forgives setting errors and systematically comes back as a reference on the day of the removal of the wires, or later for a scar that remains red or enlarges.*

– *The fractional non-ablative laser (Erbium-Glass 1540–1550–1565 and Nd-YAP 1340) is interesting when the scar hardens without being inflammatory. The depth of its radiation limits it to scars less than 2 mm thick to cover the entire scar volume, but it can be proposed for all phototypes.*

– *The CO$_2$ or fractional Er-YAG laser can be used as early as the removal of the sutures, on its own or in association with the pulsed dye. During the first 3 months, it can also be used if the edges of a scar are not well faced or if the scar is hypertrophied in order to facilitate the penetration of a topical corticoid or fluorouracil.*

– *IPL with short filters called vascular band, KTP 532 also in vascular mode, and LEDs to modulate the inflammatory process are proposed alternatives.*

– *Of course, all scars must be put to rest so that the inflammation does not persist and induce induration, hypertrophy, and enlargement. It is essential to fix it with a very thin hydrocolloid, silicone patches, a plaster, or compression garment according to the practitioner's choice.*

Finally, all these studies and comments tend to show that only the doctor can take the decision to offer a laser procedure. The problem being that most doctors do not practice laser treatment, it is more difficult to persuade them, in any case much more so than patients who are looking for recent technologies. It is obvious, but we all need a protocolization of the act to be reproducible and to offer the maximum to each patient. To date, the use of a systematic laser is neither possible nor necessary because in most cases, the scar will be fine, flexible, and in line with the expectations of the patient and the physician.

– *The semi-late treatment of a scar tissue in the making is variable and must be adapted to its type (atrophic, excessive, vascular, or fibrous, pigmented, or hypochromic...), its shape (surface, volume, thickness...), its location, and of course to the patient (history, age, ethnicity, phototype...).*

– *Lasers and other DBEs can be of appreciable help, but always combined with corticoids and physiotherapy: fixation-compression, massage-petrissage, or even a medical-spa treatment dedicated to the treatment of large areas, but to be discussed on a case-by-case basis. The choice of the device will depend on its penetration and on the target to be reached. The treatment is often long, 12–18 months. Is it worth it? Certainly, if the physician and the patient are determined and ... patient!*

Scars, What To Do After the 100 Days

However, it is questionable whether to propose a laser treatment at an early stage without knowing the scarring profile, even if we know its potential for risky situations; after the third month, we can more than suspect that the scar will not evolve as expected if it is already pathological or unsightly.

The analysis of the scar (color, height, suppleness, firmness, and the patient's phototype) remains the basis for considering a laser or EBD procedure regardless of the type of scar: inflammatory acne that leaves a depression, after effects of a burn or recent trauma, postsurgical scar. We must not neglect the patient's expectations and demands, for whom a mark, often on exposed areas, is the source of requests for treatment and medical and pharmaceutical nomadism. Also, while being reassuring on the often very favorable evolution, we must know how to propose risk-free treatments which may even bring benefits that we consider minimal, but which encourage compliance with the recommended measures.

If the Scar Tissue Is Still Red But Supple

Even if it tends to enlarge or thicken, only the constraint of a compression dressing is necessary. The use of dermocorticoids or patches is possible, as are pulsed dye lasers or vascular laser lamps, but no one knows whether they do not tend to encourage relaxation and therefore enlargement or perpetuated inflammation. Photo biomodulation by exposure to LEDs, particularly red (630 nm) and/or infrared, is a debated alternative that carries minor risk of aggravating the process.

If the Scar Thickens, Hardens, Itches, But Remains Red

There is a risk of hypertrophy, which may appear before the 100 days. For keloids, this is often the starting point for induration, but the genetic and topographical context must be put into perspective because the evolution is different from that of hypertrophic scars. The keloid must go beyond the scarring process, itches much more, and has no tendency to improve within 18 months in contrast to the hypertrophic scar.

In any case, we always recommend a pressure bandage with or without laser. We can add massaging—kneading and injectable corticoids in small quantities every 6–8 weeks or with the LADD procedure. Diprostene© is preferred to Kenacort-Kenalog©, which is more atrophying, for scar tissue that is not very thick and not yet indurated.

If the Scar Is Just Red or Pink, It Is Never Too Late for Vascular Lasers

- Pulsed dye laser in sub-purple photothermolysis mode preferably.
- Nd: YAG laser scanning has very low fluence (5 J/cm^2) and short times (0.5 ms) but it takes several hundred shots to heat beyond the sac-

rosanct 52 °C for a certain ill-defined time, and many sessions in the series that have been published for Nd:YAG.
- The sub-purpuric mode of the latest generations of KTP laser or intense pulsed light with vascular filters and pulse durations of less than 3 ms is an alternative to pulsed dye laser.

If the Scar Thickens, Hardens, White in Color

- It is more likely to be a fibrosis-type scar. It is therefore necessary to break the scar tissue either with a non-ablative or more aggressive ablative fractional laser.

Case 14 Nose Surgical Scar
See Fig. 20a, b.

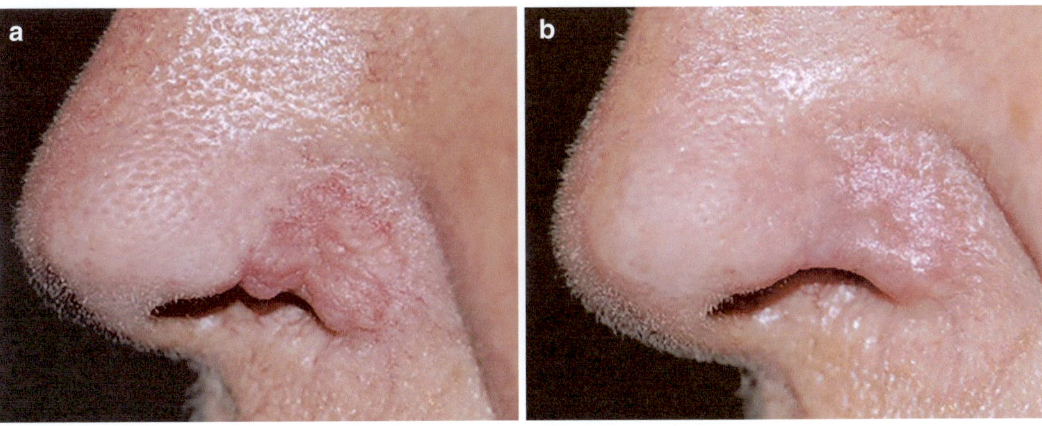

Fig. 20 (**a**) Just before Erbium: YAG resurfacing-sculpting of a total skin graft in a partially necrotic wallet. (**b**) Result in a single session. Courtesy of Thierry Fusade

– Microneedle radiofrequency is an alternative to soften the indurations laser. The use of corticoids is always interesting for their atrophying and softening effect but be careful with the quantity and concentration (to be diluted especially for the face or for children). It is possible to induce too much atrophy, giving the scar a stretch mark appearance with fine telangiectasias on either side, and their hypochromic effect.

If the Scar Falls Apart and Sags, Like a River Bed Without Water

– The connective tissue can be strengthened by recommending fractional ablative or non-ablative lasers (Fig. 20a, b) and the injection of hyaluronic acid to strengthen the scar wall (Fig. 21a–c). Some have tried tissue inducers such as highly diluted polylactic acid or calcium hydroxyapatite or platelet-rich plasma after microporation with inconsistent results. The injection of hyaluronic acid can be repeated every 6 weeks but without reusing the laser at the same time so as not to damage the hyaluronic acid structure. At least 3 months should be allowed for the hyaluronic acid to play its role as a tissue inducer if one wishes to combine the two.

Case 15 Facial Laceration Scars
See Fig. 21a–c.

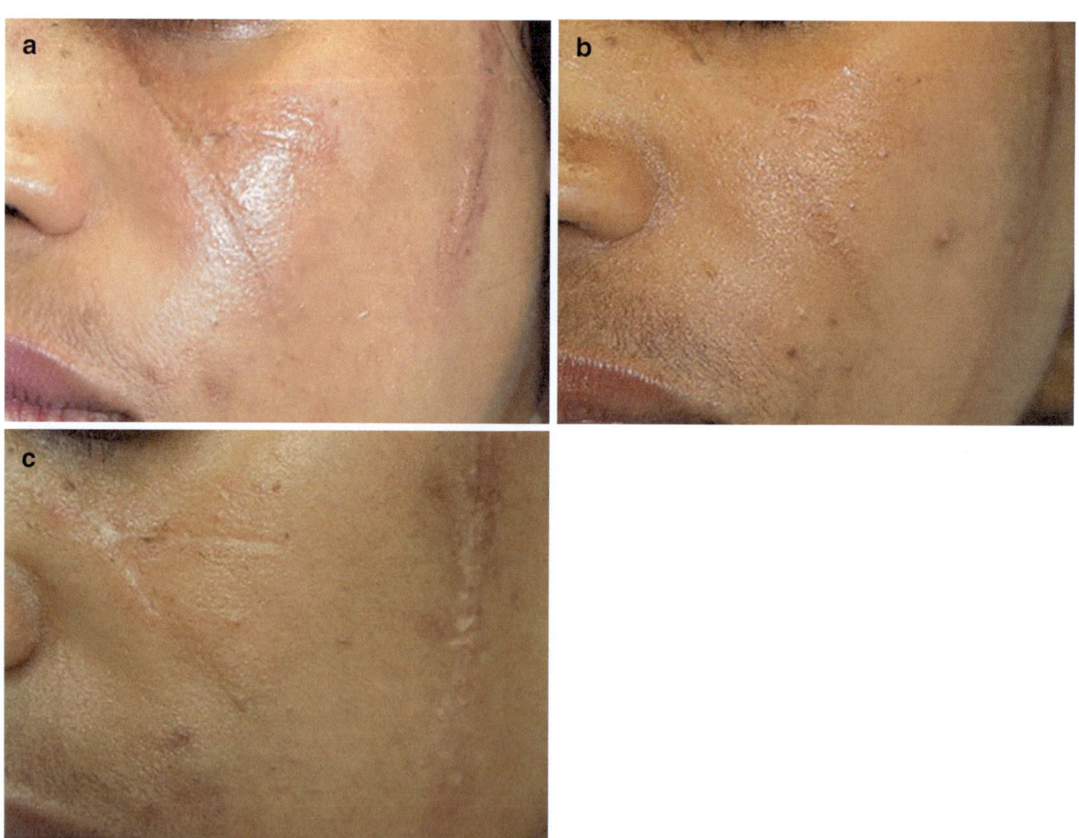

Fig. 21 (**a**) Traumatic atrophic scar (laceration). (**b**) Three sessions of non-ablative fractional laser 1550 nm, 40 mJ, 2.7 ms and filler injection with hyaluronic acid to elevate the scar fold. Injections were done just after each session, 2 months apart. (**c**) The result is incomplete with a scar that reappears on its upper half. And it is possible to reinject hyaluronic acid. The alternative would be the Er: YAG laser, which gives less depigmentation than CO_2. Courtesy of Hugues Cartier

Comments

We recommend the use of AFL or NAFL by adapting the parameters to the topography and skin texture of the scars, combining or not the PDL laser in the same session if an inflammatory aspect persists. The thicker the scars, with less and less flexibility, the more AFL is indicated.

- *For young atrophic scar, PDl or KTP or IPL first and as a second option NAFL and then AFL*
- *For established atrophic scars, NAFL then AFL or MRF and if necessary combined with soft tissue fillers and collagen inductors*

Inflammatory, Hypertrophic Scars and Keloids [22]

Inflammatory scars are defined by a redness that persists beyond the normal range. It is extremely variable from one subject to another because a scar can evolve over 1 year or more. It will remain so if its natural inflammation is prolonged. The hypertrophic scar is the volumetric translation of an inflammatory scar that expands to create indurated cords but without extending beyond the scar. Most of them fade spontaneously in 18 months, helped using corticoids, plasters that limit its movement and a gentle massage, to be decided on a case-by-case basis. If the healing process extends beyond the scar, it can be considered keloidal evolution like the classic butterfly scar. Both are inflammations but laser management is much more complicated, and we find in many publications a confusion between the two [23].

What To Do with a Hypertrophic Scar That Has Already Formed?

- The scar must be compressed with all the technical devices available: hydrocolloid, custom-made elastic fabric, and silicone patches almost permanently for at least 3 months when it is possible.

- The patient is advised to massage and knead the scar twice a week, either manually or mechanically, while continuing the permanent compression fixation.

In general, the combination of compression and massaging allows the scar to improve within 6 weeks to 3 months.

Nevertheless, it depends on the topography of the scar and whether it is under permanent tension. In this case, we do not recommend any massaging or compression to avoid overstressing the scar inflammation which will thicken even more if elongation movements are provoked. It is a case-by-case decision, and the use of lasers is subject to the condition of a real interest and not to perpetuate the inflammation.

- Our first line of treatment is based on the use of corticoids topically (cream or patch), but we keep the use of Pulsed Dye Laser (PDL) to reduce vascular and inflammation compromising in inflammatory phase.

We propose to our patients a treatment combined in the same session PDL (7 or 10 mm—3 or 6 ms—6–10 J/cm^2) followed by an intralesional injection of acetate of triamcinolone (TAC), 3 sessions spaced out of 1 month to weeks. Or a combination in some cases: removal with CO_2 laser followed by the prevention of the recurrences by sessions of AFL CO_2 followed at once by the topical application of TAP, "laser-assisted drug delivery" (LADD).

Inject corticoids into the scar either conventionally with a needle or by the LADD procedure with a fractional ablative laser to facilitate the penetration of drugs deeply into the skin (laser-assisted drug delivery), or using a roller with spikes or radiofrequency with penetrating needles is possible to create also small dermal holes. The interest of electric currents is to break the inflammatory bridges before they fibrose. The goal of using corticoids is to gain time because a hypertrophic scar typically does not improve over 18 months. However, a thick surgical scar will evolve by widening and by intervening as quickly as possible, what is gained in thickness will eventually be gained in less width.

– Vascular lasers can also be of interest. A recent study compared the effectiveness of pulsed dye laser vs pulsed dye laser combined with ultrapulse fractional CO_2 laser in the treatment of immature red hypertrophic scars [24] (Figs. 22 and 23a, b).

"Fifty-six patients (56 sites) were randomly divided into a treatment group and control group. The control group was treated with the 595 nm PDL at a fluence of 7–15 J/cm^2 and pulse widths of 1.5–3 ms, 7 mm spot size. The treatment group was treated with a fractional CO_2 laser (UltraPulse CO_2: Deep FX, Energy: 30–50 mJ, Frequency: 300 Hz, Density 5%, Scan Shape, and Spot Size were decided by shape and area of scar) after utilizing the 595 nm adjustable pulse width PDL (Fluence: 7–15 J/cm^2, Pulse: 1.5–3 ms, Spot size: 7 mm). MEBT/MEBO, previously described as a post-treatment wound ointment, was used after laser treatment. The scars of the treatment group and the control group were evaluated for changes in pigment, height, vascularity, and pliability using the Vancouver Scar Scale (VSS) after two laser treatments."

Finally, the total VSS score, as well as the score for melanin, height, vascularity, and pliability in both groups, showed an obvious decrease following the treatments. There were statistically significant differences between before treatment and after treatment ($P < 0.05$); however, the total score of the VSS, and score of the melanin, height, vascularity, and pliability in the control group decreased more than that of treatment group, and there was a statistically significant difference ($P < 0.05$).

The 595 nm adjustable pulse width PDL combined with the fractional CO_2 laser appears to have a beneficial clinical effect on fresh red hypertrophic scars, with no severe adverse reactions seen.

Vascular IPL or KTP 532 nm therapy also offers a safe and effective means of hypertrophic scar treatment [25, 26]. The settings vary depending on the device.

Case 16 Hypertrophic Scar After Wrinkles Resurfacing on the Upper Lip

See Fig. 23a, b.

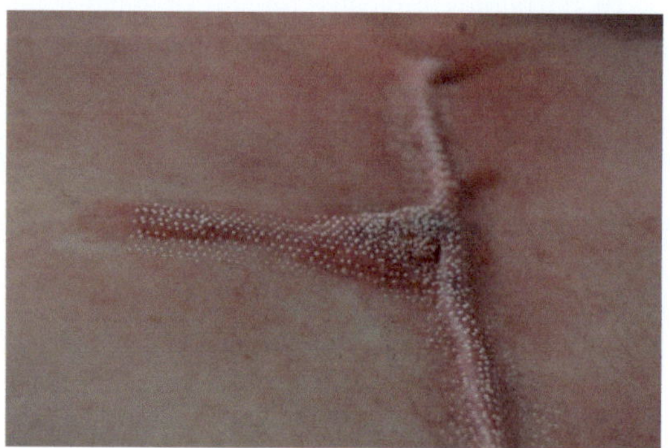

Fig. 22 Immature hypertrophic scar: combined treatment with PDL and Laser (AFLCO$_2$) Assisted Drug Delivery (LADD). Courtesy of Thierry Fusade

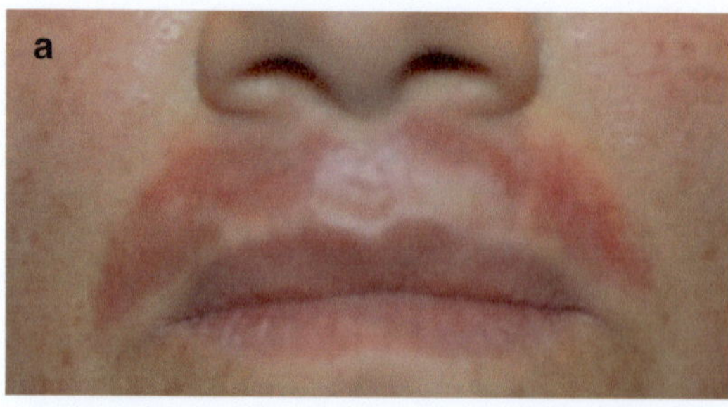
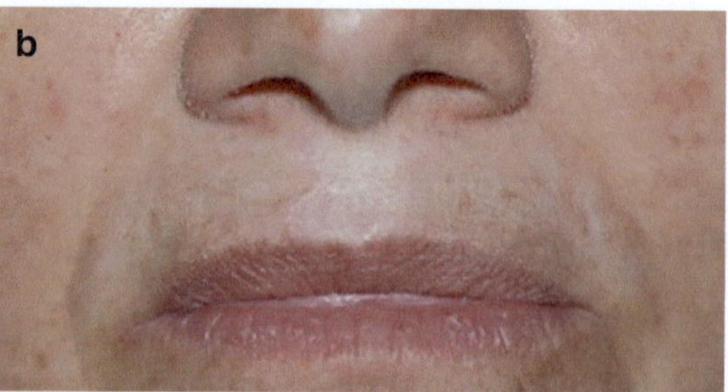

Fig. 23 (a) Mixed hypertrophic and keloid scar after an upper lip resurfacing with Er: YAG laser. (b) Result after 3 sessions of pulsed dye laser (595 nm, 6 J/cm^2, 1.5 ms, spot size 7 mm) and intralesional injection of diluted injectable corticosteroids, follow-up 18 months. Courtesy of Thierry Fusade

Keloids

This subject alone could be an entire chapter. The genetic and topographical context makes its management complex with medical and surgical advice. Either the scar is surgically removed, generally intralesionally, or by reducing tension forces with flaps, and the treatment is started from scratch with rigorous follow-up, which requires compression and corticosteroid injections for several months (Fig. 24).

Typically, a needle can be used to inject the scar. However, depending on the scar's thickness or the difficulty of injecting into it, techniques can be used to facilitate the delivery of corticosteroids. The LADD procedure involves using a fractional ablative laser, MRF, or simple mechanical micro-needling that creates deep wells in the skin (laser-assisted drug delivery). The dedicated devices like the mechanical Dermojet© or the pneumatic needle-less liquid jet technology injection as Enerjet© are options to deliver drugs into the skin. The jet disperses therapeutic substance in the dermis with less pain (velocity 150 ms) vertically (controlled depth penetration up to 6 mm) and laterally (10 mm). This technique is used for hypertrophic keloids with injection of drugs as 5FU and corticoids (Figs. 5a, b and 26a–c).

For atrophic scars, an effect of de-anchoring the scar base can be achieved by injecting substances like hyaluronic acid, which elevates and provides support for the scar which has been raised.

- Pulsed Dye Laser is probably the easiest to use (Fig. 25a, b). The settings are variable, with an emission time of 0.45–40 ms and an energy of 6–10 J/cm^2. Manuskiatti et al. compare these two extreme emission times and conclude that the volume of keloidal or hypertrophic median sternotomy scar segments treated with 0.45 and 40 ms pulses decreases significantly after two treatments. Segments treated with 0.45-ms pulse widths showed significantly greater improvement than those treated with 40-ms pulses after three treatments. The elasticity of the 0.45-ms segments was notably higher than that of the 40-ms segments after two treatments. The pulse width had no significant effect on the improvement of scar erythema. Additionally, PDL at 595 nm was safe even in dark-skinned patients [27].

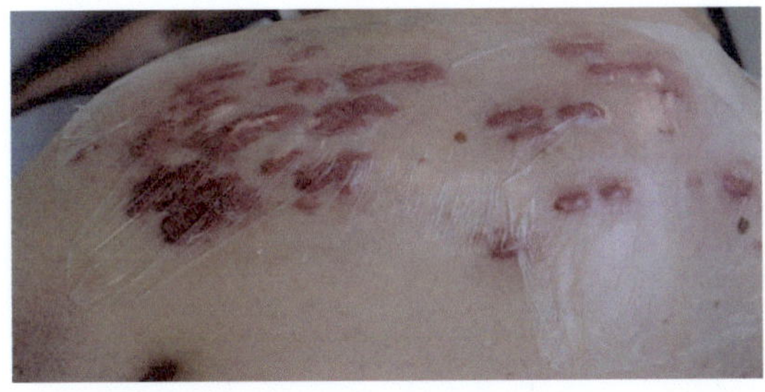

Fig. 24 Keloids: combined PDL and LADD treatment with triamcinolone acetate under occlusive tape. Courtesy of Thierry Fusade

Case 17 Chest Keloids
See Fig. 25a, b.

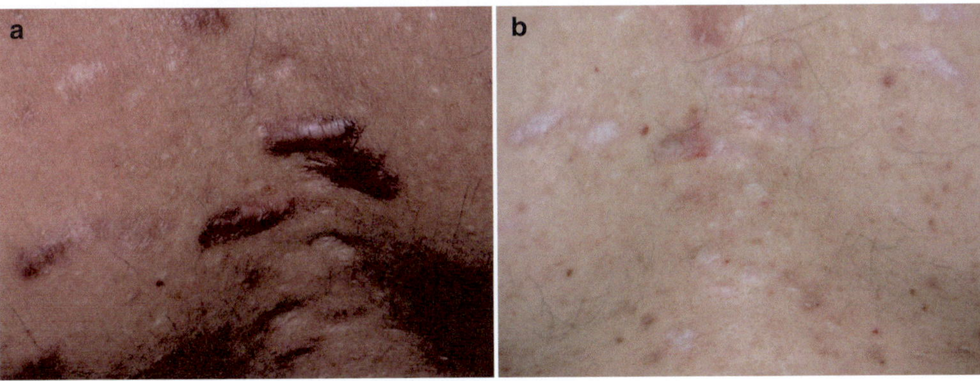

Fig. 25 (**a**) Just after PDL on keloids setting 595 nm, handpiece 10 mm 6 ms 7 J/cm^2. (**b**) No recurrence of keloids 6 years after 3 sessions of combination PDL and TAC injection inside in same sessions. Courtesy of Thierry Fusade

Comments

For a limited and young keloid, use in a combined treatment with pulsed dye laser and corticosteroids is indicated. The use of pulsed intense lights was also documented in these indications. A flash of external radiotherapy or endocurie therapy in the immediate postoperative period can also be very effective but few French teams offer them for fear of the risk of radiodermatitis and its long-term consequences. Focused radiotherapy is now available, and some dermatological centers are authorized to use it.

Case 18 Classic Abdominal Keloid After Surgery

See Fig. 26a–e.

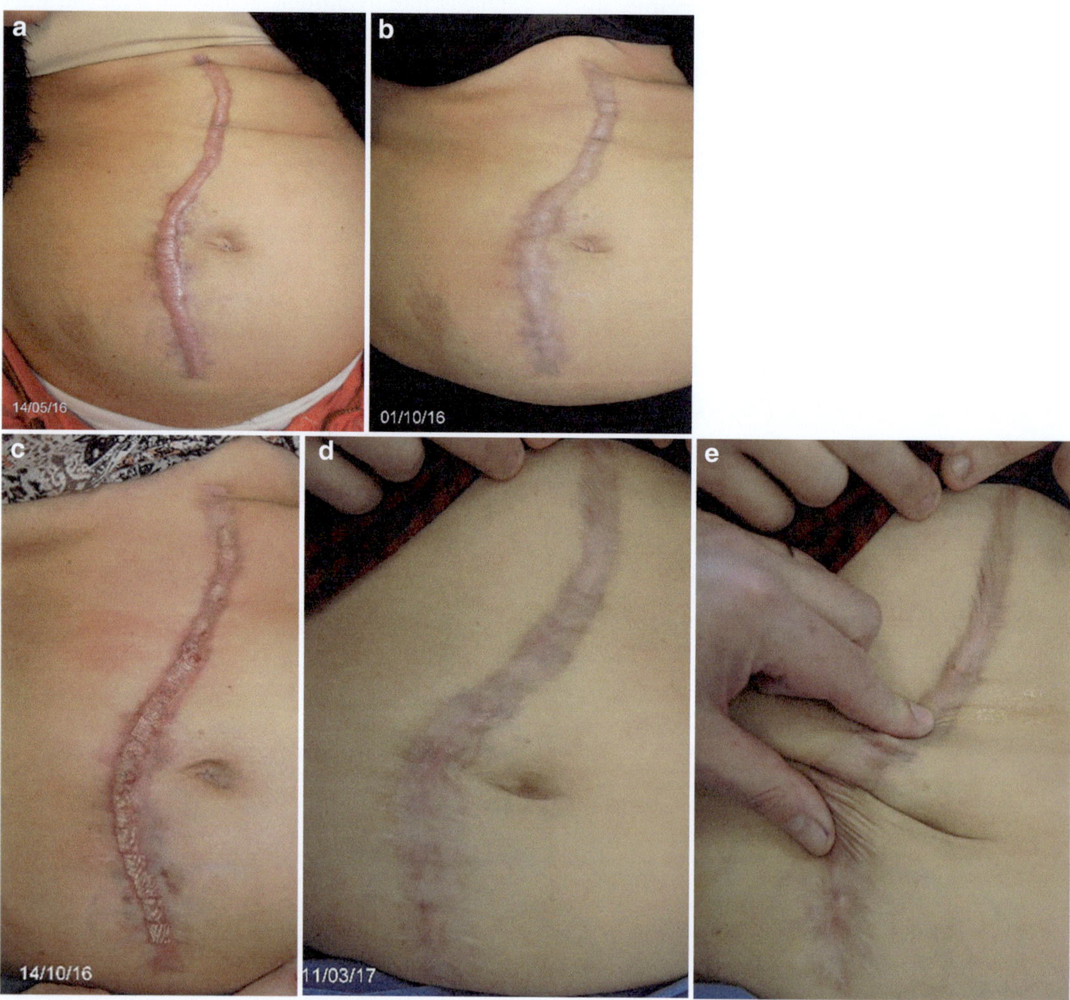

Fig. 26 (a) Classic keloid after abdominal suture in a patient with a genetic predisposition to keloids. (b) Result after 4 sessions of ablative fractional Laser in combination with steroid injection and application under tape every 6 weeks (LADD procedure). (c) Just after ablative CO_2 fractional laser. (d) Result after 6 sessions of LADD (laser-assisted drugs delivery) and 15 months follow-up. (e) The LADD procedure has reduced the thickness and pruritus and given the patient comfort with a more flexible scar. Courtesy of Hugues Cartier

Comments

If the keloid is fixed, less inflammatory, and fibrous, the use of fractionated ablative lasers or conventional methods to flatten or surgically cut the keloid is possible but the associated use of corticosteroids will be essential anyway. Some colleagues combine the injection of corticosteroids (10–40 mg/cc TAC/triamcinolone) and 5 Fluorouracil (50 mg/cc) with a dedicated needle or device to facilitate injection. Other lasers are useless as their thermal and penetration properties are limited and may even sustain inflammation. In another context, wound healing often responds to surgical intervention to reduce traction forces. The high-penetration fractional CO_2 laser is a way to gain a few degrees of flexibility. The principle is based on dilaceration of the scar tissue to make it more flexible, but it will not have the elasticity of normal skin. Some colleagues recommend the combined use of the fractional CO_2 laser and the pulsed dye laser after surgery for long-lasting results such as ear keloids after resection [28] (Figs. 27a–c, 28a, b, 29a, b).

Case 19 Lobe Keloid in Phototype V, African Type

See Fig. 27a–c.

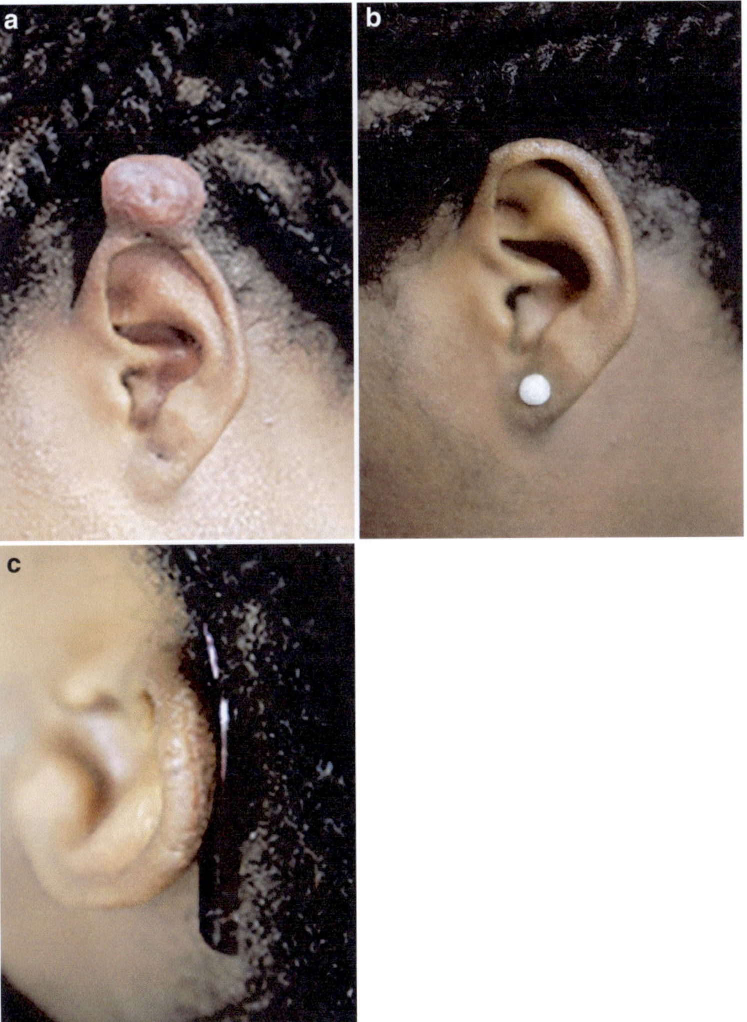

Fig. 27 (a) Auricular's keloid, genetic predisposition for skin phototype V or VI. (b) Debulking of keloids after a combination of AFL on the basement of the scar, corticoids, and maintenance by PDL to avoid recurrence. (c) Result at 9 months without recurrence. Courtesy of Hugues Cartier

Comments

For thick or more mature limited keloids: excision-basement treatment with CO_2 laser and then prevention of the recurrences by sessions of AFL CO_2/PDL followed at once by the topical application of TAC is also another possibility.

Case 20 Brest Keloid After Mastopexy

See Fig. 28a, b.

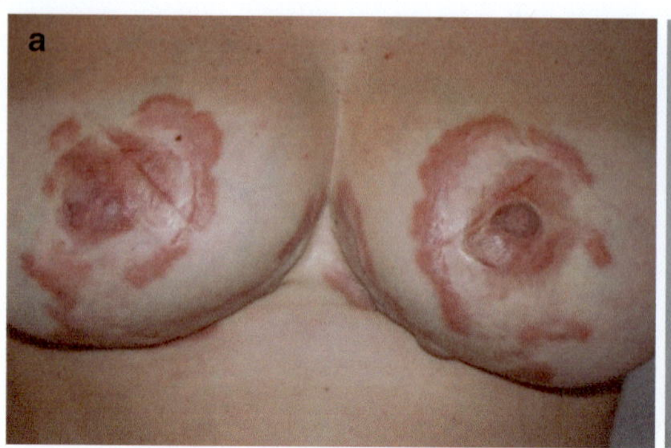
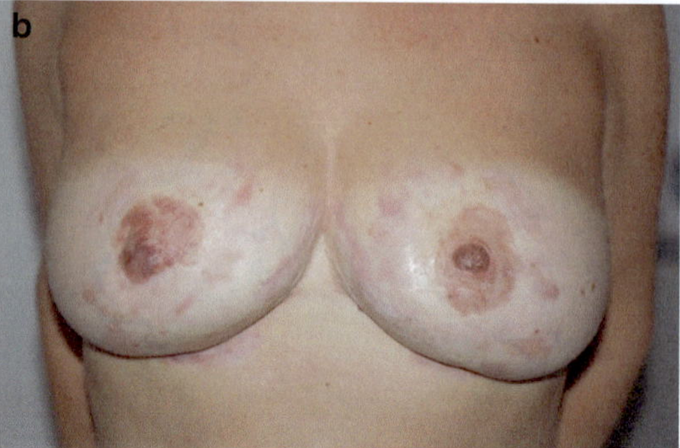

Fig. 28 (**a**) Treatment combining compression, intra-lesional corticoids, and pulsed dye laser 6.5 days/3 ms then 6 days/1.5 ms pam 7. (**b**) Result after 5 sessions and 15 months of follow-up. Courtesy of Thierry Fusade

Case 21 Keloid and Hypertrophic Scar of the Wrist

See Fig. 29a, b.

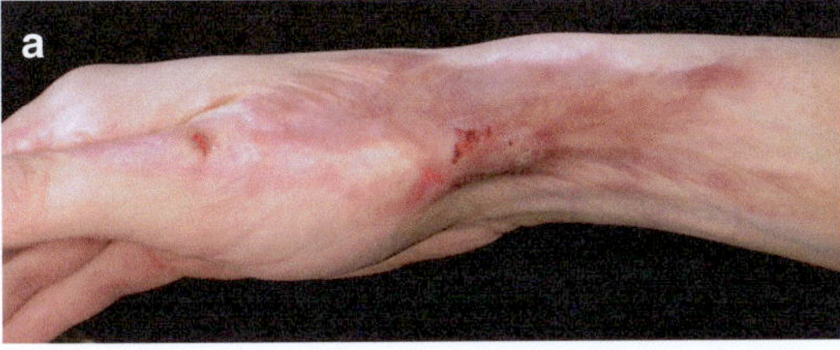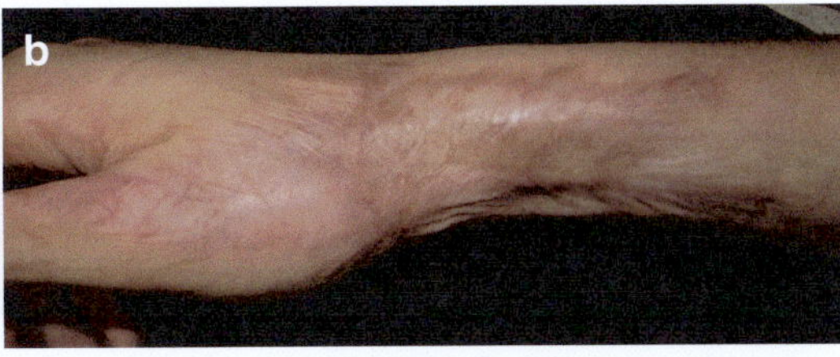

Fig. 29 (**a**) Fixed old scar of the wrist. (**b**) Result at 15 months after a combination of fractional CO$_2$ laser (spot size 120 microns, 1 ms time emission, density 5%, 90–130 mJ) with in same time 5 corticosteroid procedures every 2 months to ameliorate thickness, roughness, pliability. Courtesy of Hugues Cartier

Comments

- *The role of the CO_2 laser is to fragment the scar fibrosis. Corticosteroids reduce any inflammatory process resulting from the thermal shock of the laser and cause atrophoderma of the fixed scar tissue generating the mobilization of the wrist movement.*
- *The alternative of micro-needling with radio-frequency or fractional Er: YAG is, respectively, limited by the difficulty of penetrating strong fibrous scar tissue and less laser beam generation compared to a CO_2 laser.*

Vascular Scars

The vascular network that appears at the edge of the scar may be the consequence of repeated use of corticosteroids but may also appear spontaneously, neoangiogenesis being part of any scarring process. Neoangiogenesis is often seen after facelift or reconstructive surgery of the nose. These vessels are often fine and superficial and are easily treated with all vascular lasers (Fig. 30a, b).

Case 22 Telangiectatic Network on Both Sides of the Scar
See Fig. 30a, b.

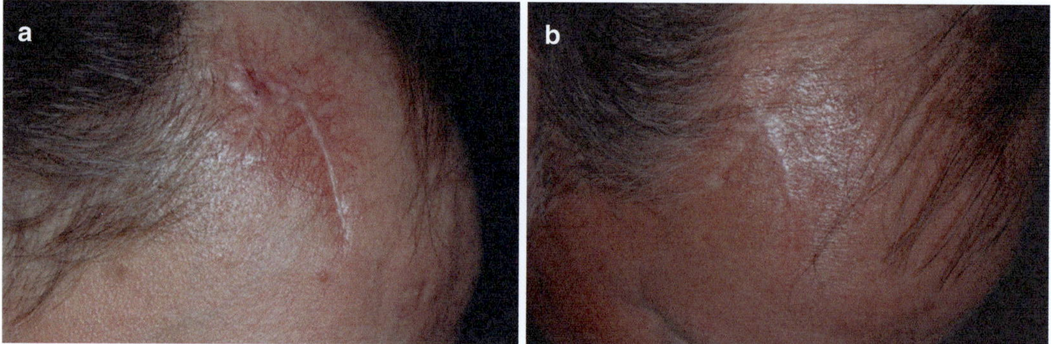

Fig. 30 (**a**) Development of telangiectasias on both sides of the frontal surgical scar. (**b**) Result after a single session of pulsed dye laser. Courtesy of Francois Will

Case 23 Chalazodermic Scar
See Fig. 31a, b.

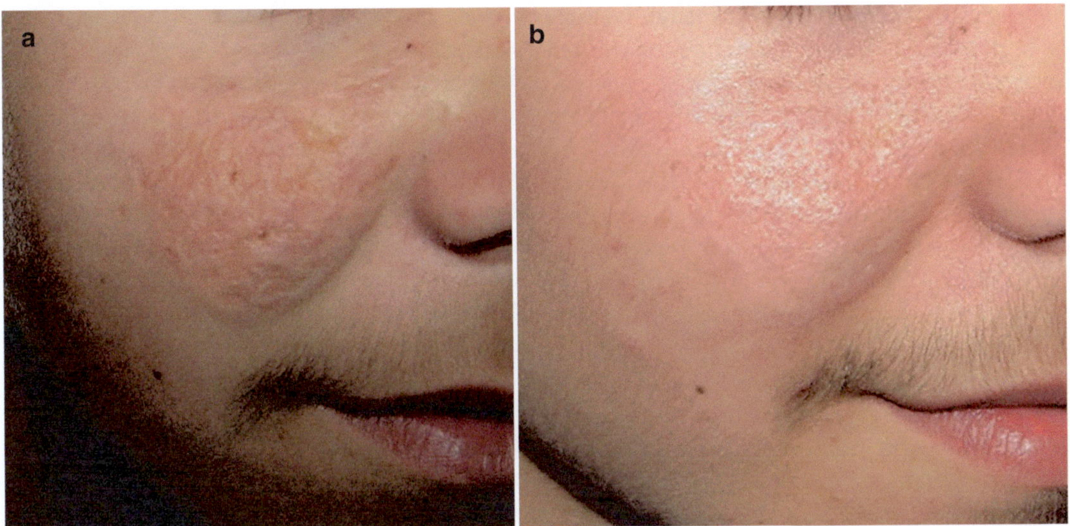

Fig. 31 (**a**) Old face hemangioma looks like as a chalazodermic scar. (**b**) Before and after a single session of classic resurfacing by CO_2 laser. Courtesy of Thierry Fusade

Hyperpigmented Scars [29]

The genesis of hyperpigmentation following a cutaneous trauma, whether spontaneous, postsurgical, or after an aesthetic procedure, more often laser or peel, seems to respond to the same physiology: post-inflammatory hyperpigmentation (PIH) and/or lack of sun protection.

In the case of prolonged inflammation, a mechanism of photo-protection with the production of melanin and then the export of melanosomes to neighboring keratinocytes is put in place. In the case of hyperpigmentation, the melanin can be found in the horny layer but also in the dermis where it is distributed in extracellular or intra-macrophagic (melanophagic) lumps: this is known as pigment incontinence. Pigment incontinence occurs very frequently in PIH because there is an alteration of the basement membrane. However, this varies according to the initial inflammatory process (e.g., lichen where it is major because the inflammatory infiltrate nibbles at the membrane).

From a therapeutic point of view, corticosteroids are still the basis of treatment as early as possible for subjects at risk. Their effectiveness is explained by their anti-prostaglandin action, which is involved in the physiological process.

If we can hope for a reduction of a simple post-inflammatory pigmentation spontaneously in 1 year, it is much more difficult to do so for a hyperpigmented scar.

As a preventive measure, as demonstrated by Passeron et al., it is obvious that the scarring area should be kept away from sunlight and even from ambient light. It is even more important to avoid placing patients under LEDs in the blue-violet spectrum during the healing phase, which would promote prolonged pigmentation just as much as UV light and for even longer.

To regulate fixed pigmentation, anti-tyrosinase depigmenting topicals are initially recommended, with hydroquinone at different concentrations in classic formulations such as Kligman's trio. If hydroquinone, which already has a pro-inflammatory power, is combined with active ingredients that accelerate cell turnover such as AHAs or topical retinoids, then care must be taken not to perpetuate the inflammation. It is therefore necessary to limit their use over time and adapt their concentration or add corticoids or alternate with other bleaching ingredients as kojic acid and azelaic acid with lower risk of definitive hypochromia.

Depigmenting peels are only the most aggressive version of the use of topicals; it should be kept in mind that they can themselves induce reactive pigmentation. Their use should be considered in the light of the pros and cons.

The use of tranexamic acid seems, according to publications, to be less useful in recent hyperpigmented scars. It is identical to post-inflammatory pigmentations according to the experience of some authors, unlike melasma for which it is increasingly prescribed. It will be necessary to investigate its topical use once the right formula has been found, as in this form it carries far fewer risks of side effects.

In the context of lasers, there are very few publications on the subject because it is necessary to empty the melanosomes without causing inflammation, which would induce an infernal cycle through a feed-back effect. This is also the reason why a test area and the very early use of corticoids are recommended after any kind of laser, including ablative ones, all the more so as the phototype is high.

- Few cases of laser-related PIH of the face were successfully treated by combined therapy with 578-/511-nm copper bromide laser and light-emitting diodes (LEDs) [30].

– The effect of the different Q-switched lasers on normal or hyperpigmented skin is comparable; only the depth of penetration varies according to the equipment used. Because of the principle of selective photothermolysis, the damage caused to the melanosomes is followed by cellular destruction of the melanocytes and keratinocytes loaded with pigments. Histological studies after triggered laser treatment on normal skin show a correlation between the extent of epidermal damage and the fluences delivered and the initial level of pigmentation. The anomalies usually encountered after exposure to triggered pigment lasers are ballooning of melanocytes and keratinocytes. These same studies have made it possible to determine a threshold fluence. Below this fluence, the destruction of melanosomes is not associated with a joint destruction of melanocytes and a reactive paradoxical hyperpigmentation may result. Interaction with factors inhibiting melanogenesis would cause an increase in tyrosinase activity resulting in an effect equivalent to that seen in post-inflammatory hyperpigmentation.

If, however, hyperpigmentation occurs, and one wishes to propose laser treatment

• Most authors on the subject recommend either low fluence with nano or picosecond triggered lasers, emitting either at 532 or 694–670 nm (rather in fractionated mode) or at 755 nm and with caution, the one that is most recommended remains 1064 nm, still like the one with melasma but with a superior benefit in terms of long-term result it seems (Fig. 32a–e). It is however difficult to give a threshold fluence. Based on data from Asian publications, they are low, often less than 1.5 J with a 1064 nm nanosecond laser.

– The other range of laser recommended is based on fractionated non-ablative lasers, also with low fluence, of the order of 15–35 mJ/MTZ for emission durations of less than 3 ms, but with caution and a test area.

– The outsider is the flash lamp or pulsed polychromatic light with a modulation of the spectral band, the number of pulses and interpulses, and a low fluence to avoid any rebound of the hyperpigmentation. The number of passes required for improvement can be in the order of 3–5.

– Fractional ablative and non-ablative lasers also improve the hyperchromy of burn scars by homogenizing them. Combinations are also possible, such as a combination of non-ablative fractional laser and pulsed light, pigment laser, or pulsed light and peeling.

– Moreover, treatment of laser-induced PIH remains a challenge. To prevent PIH, especially for skin of color, with AFL prefers a low density of 1–5% MTZ while keeping the energy high and the pulse duration time short, less than 1 ms. Do not forget to use topical corticosteroids, if necessary, immediately after the session and for a few days. There is no longer any risk of causing an infection. The use of topical or oral tranexamic acid is not relevant.

– In conclusion, hyperpigmented scars and post-inflammatory pigmentation are treated in the same way, but with more hope for the latter: sun protection is always essential, and dermo-corticoids should be used at an early stage for subjects at risk or with a high phototype. The later we intervene, the more complex the treatment becomes.

Case 24 Hyperpigmented Scars of the Nose
See Fig. 32a–e.

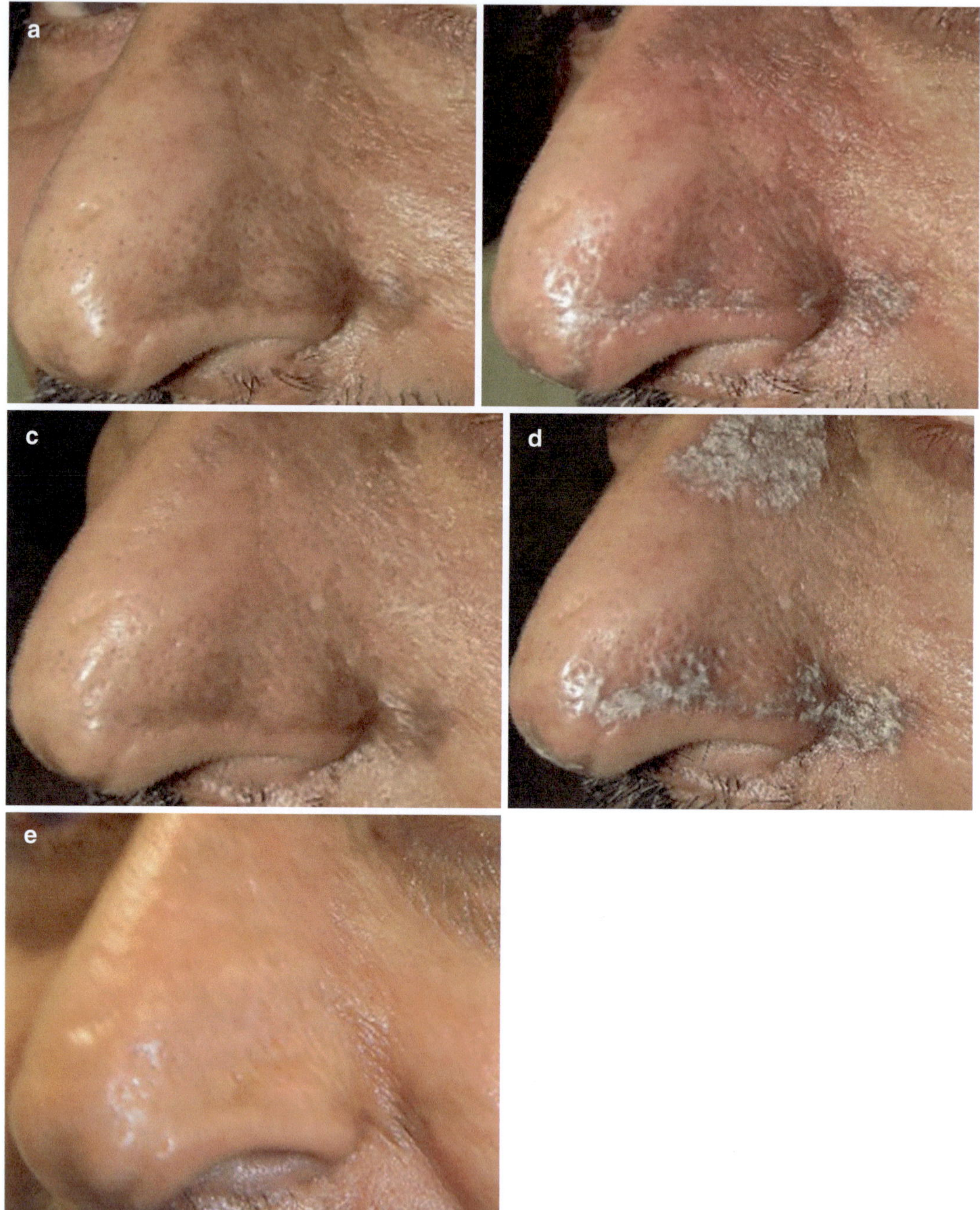

Fig. 32 (**a**) Old and fided hyperpigmented traumatic scar of the nose. (**b**) Just after the first session of Q-switched laser 532: 0.8 J/cm², 5 ns. (**c**) Disappointing results after the first session of Q-switched 532 laser. (**d**) Just after with higher energy 3 J/cm² than the previous settings, 5 ns, spot 4 mm plus betamethasone cream twice a day 10 days. (**e**) Dramatical improvement after 3 sessions after Q-switched 532 nm laser. Courtesy of Hugues Cartier

Hypopigmented Scars

After a suture or a deep burn, it is usual to observe a definitive achromy due to the lack of hair follicles present in the depths, reservoirs of melanocyte stem cells, which allow pigmentary resurgence. But if there are still some stem cells capable of differentiating into melanocytes, they retain the ability to form melanin when they migrate to the hair bulbs or to the epidermis, which still allows repigmentation. Although there are no more melanocytes in black skin than in white skin, the melanosomes are larger and more numerous, and more mature, i.e., more "reactive" (Fig. 33a–c).

Case 25 Forehead Traumatic Scar
See Fig. 33a–c.

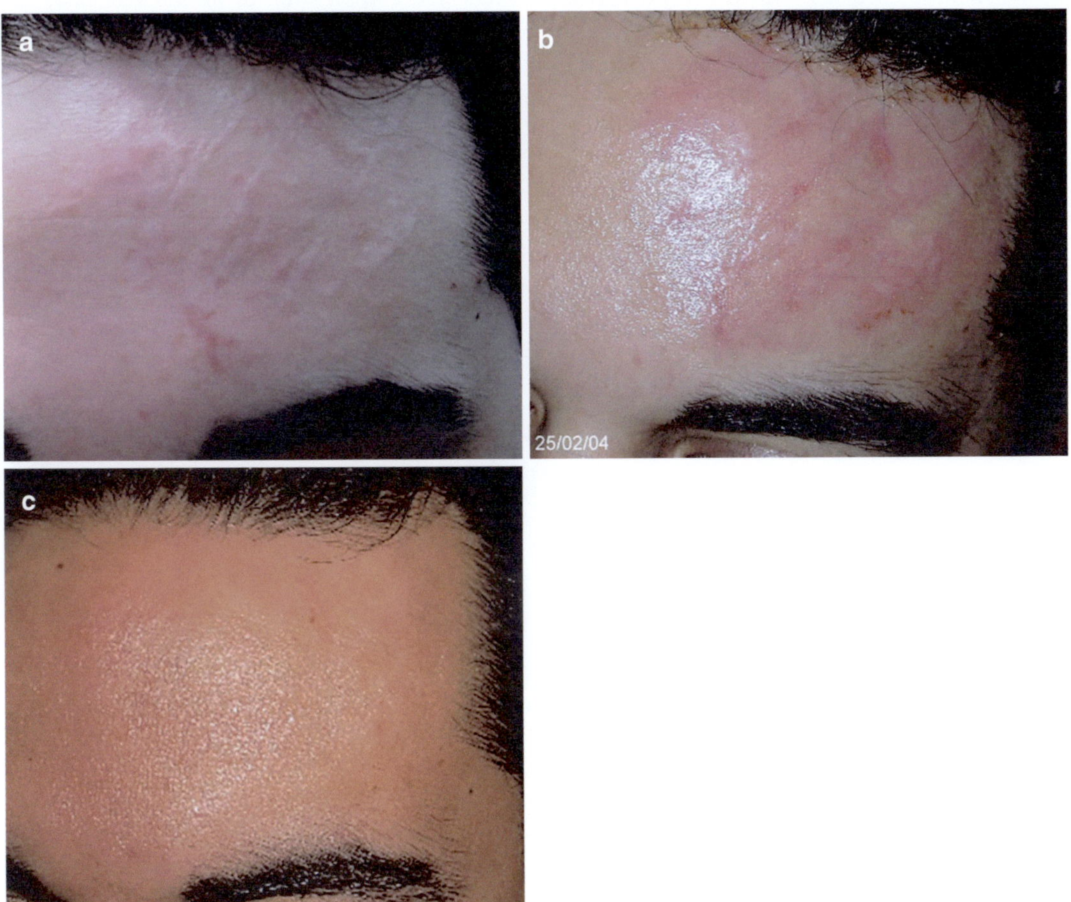

Fig. 33 (**a**) Hypochromic forehead scar. (**b**) Three weeks after Erbium: YAG dermabrasion. (**c**) Results 5 years after a single session with almost complete recovery of the hypochromy. Courtesy of Hugues Cartier

Thus, when faced with a so-called mature scar made up of fixed tissue, as the achromy appears well after 3 months, it is extremely difficult to recolor naturally.

There are nevertheless several strategies if we think that there may be a few melanocytes or stem cells left in "disarray" capable of differentiating into melanocytes, particularly in burn scars, and we can try to stimulate them.

- Moderate sun exposure (like vitiligo, these areas are more "sensitive" to UV rays) and the use of localized phototherapy by laser or 310 nm excimer lamp can be effective, but patience is required and at least 6 months are necessary before any results are obtained, which must be maintained at least at the beginning.

Techniques are often combined for better results

- Ablative lasers, particularly fractionated or micro-needling, have their place. It has been shown that these ablative techniques can stimulate cell differentiation pathways and lead to the reappearance of hair and/or sweat appendages in old scars.

After failure of these techniques or if it is thought that there are no cells that can be stimulated, always in association with phototherapy or natural heliotherapy, attempts at melanocyte self-grafting should be made. The laser group of the French dermatology society had conducted a prospective study proposing, in hypopigmented scars, the combination of an ablative laser and autografting by spraying a melanocyte suspension obtained with the Viticell© kit from Genevrier. The results were very inconsistent because the grafting of these particularly fragile cells was not obvious on scar tissue and fibrous, not very conducive to cell migration unlike vitiligo where this technique is effective (Fig. 34a–g).

Medical dermopigmentation is a risk-free indication that satisfies numerous patients, particularly in the reconstruction and pigmentation of the areola.

Case 26 Hypochromic Scar, Fibrous Tissue Forearm

See Fig. 34a–g.

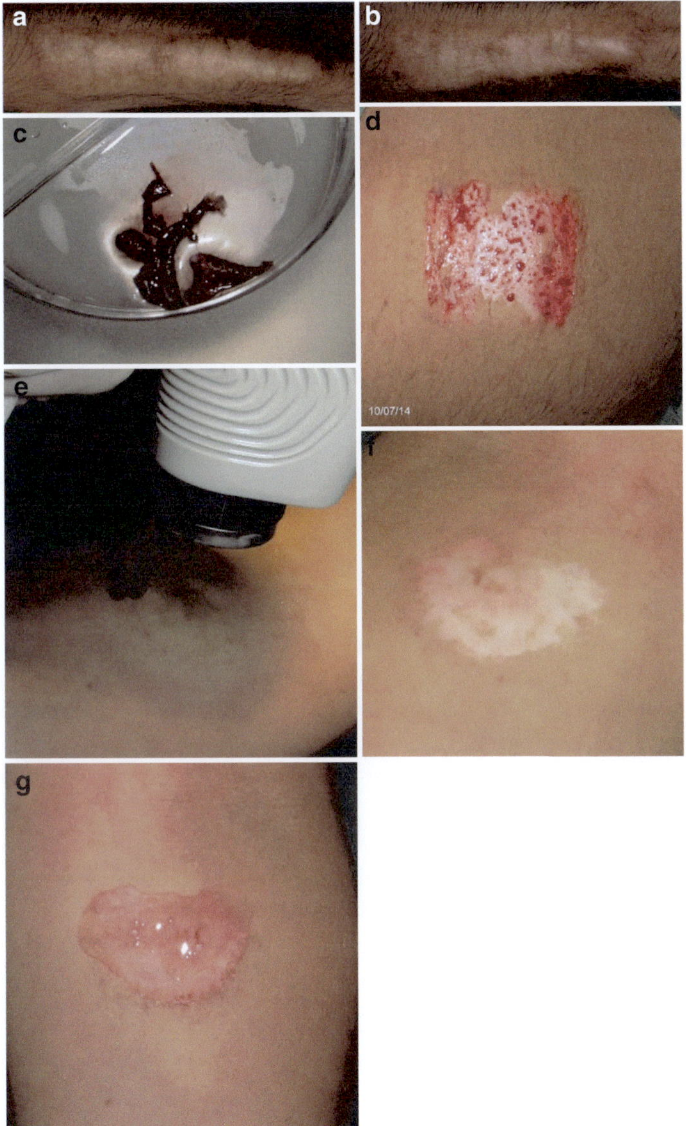

Fig. 34 (**a**) Melanocytic grafts after scarring of the forearm. (**b**) Result 7 months after the transplant, slight reduction in pigmented areas. (**c**) Skin grafting before chemical separation to recover suspended melanocytes by the Viticell© process. (**d**) The grafted area is first prepared by gentle abrasion with a CO_2 or Erbium: YAG ablative laser. (**e**) The grafted area is first prepared by superficial abrasion with a CO_2 or an Erbium: YAG laser. (**f**) The objective is simply to prepare the area to be grafted by removing the epidermal layer and the superficial dermis. If the abrasion is too deep, the melanocytes will not be viable. (**g**) Deposition of the melanocyte suspension on the area to be grafted, which has been previously abraded. This deposit will be maintained in place by an occlusive dressing for 5 days. (**a**)

Melanocytic grafts after scarring of the forearm. (**b**) Result 7 months after the transplant, slight reduction in pigmented areas. (**c**) Skin grafting before chemical separation to recover suspended melanocytes by the Viticell© process. (**d**) The grafted area is first prepared by gentle abrasion with a CO_2 or Erbium: YAG ablative laser. (**e**) The grafted area is first prepared by superficial abrasion with a CO_2 or an Erbium: YAG laser. (**f**) The objective is simply to prepare the area to be grafted by removing the epidermal layer and the superficial dermis. If the abrasion is too deep, the melanocytes will not be viable. (**g**) Deposition of the melanocyte suspension on the area to be grafted, which has been previously abraded. This deposit will be maintained in place by an occlusive dressing for 5 days

Comments

- *For acne scars and small hypopigmented scars, some of us recommend NAFL, AFL, or MRF, topical application of bimatoprost plus topical application of 0.25% retinoids to stimulate dormant stem cells or melanocytes to "wake them up."*
- *In our experience, the melanocyte grafting procedure works better for vitiligo than for scars with a fibrous tissue that is probably not hospitable to fragile melanocytes.*

Mature, Fixed Scars with Relief Alterations

Thick Scars

Provided that there are no signs of hypertrophic scarring or keloids, all raised scars can be treated with a pulse laser.

Before considering a dermabrasion, scars subjected to repeated tensional efforts should be screened, especially in the nasolabial fold or the upper white lip. In these two situations, the great mobility induced by the opening of the mouth does not allow a satisfactory leveling, the permanent tensional efforts (elocution, mastication) inducing a new inflammatory hypertrophic process by a mechanical stretching effect.

For other scars, the abrasion will be progressive, so controlling the depth of treatment and remaining particularly cautious on scarred areas without annexes (deep burns) is important. It should always be kept in mind that a second treatment is always preferable to a too deep abrasion.

Atrophic Scars

Depressed scars must first be surgically revised when possible: the principle is to resect all or parts of the most damaged areas. This surgery is only possible if the scar orientation is good and if the tension on the edges is sufficiently limited not to cause secondary enlargement. Certain large scars can sometimes benefit from lifting, such as chicken pox or wide scars. Otherwise, laser dermabrasion will focus on the scar margins, softening steep slopes to make the depression less visible by blurring shadows in natural light (Fig. 35a–i).

Chalazodermic Scars

A typical example of a chalazodermic scar is the aftermath of a blowing hemangioma. The skin appears very thin, the dermis no longer ensuring its support function and leaving the underlying hypodermis to appear like a hernia or, on the contrary, drawing a depression linked to this thinning. This type of scar is one of the best indications for fractional lasers; however, in certain situations partial results may indicate the use of a pulsed CO_2 laser (Fig. 31a, b).

Case 27 Atrophic and Dehiscent Scar After Corrective Surgery

See Fig. 35a–i.

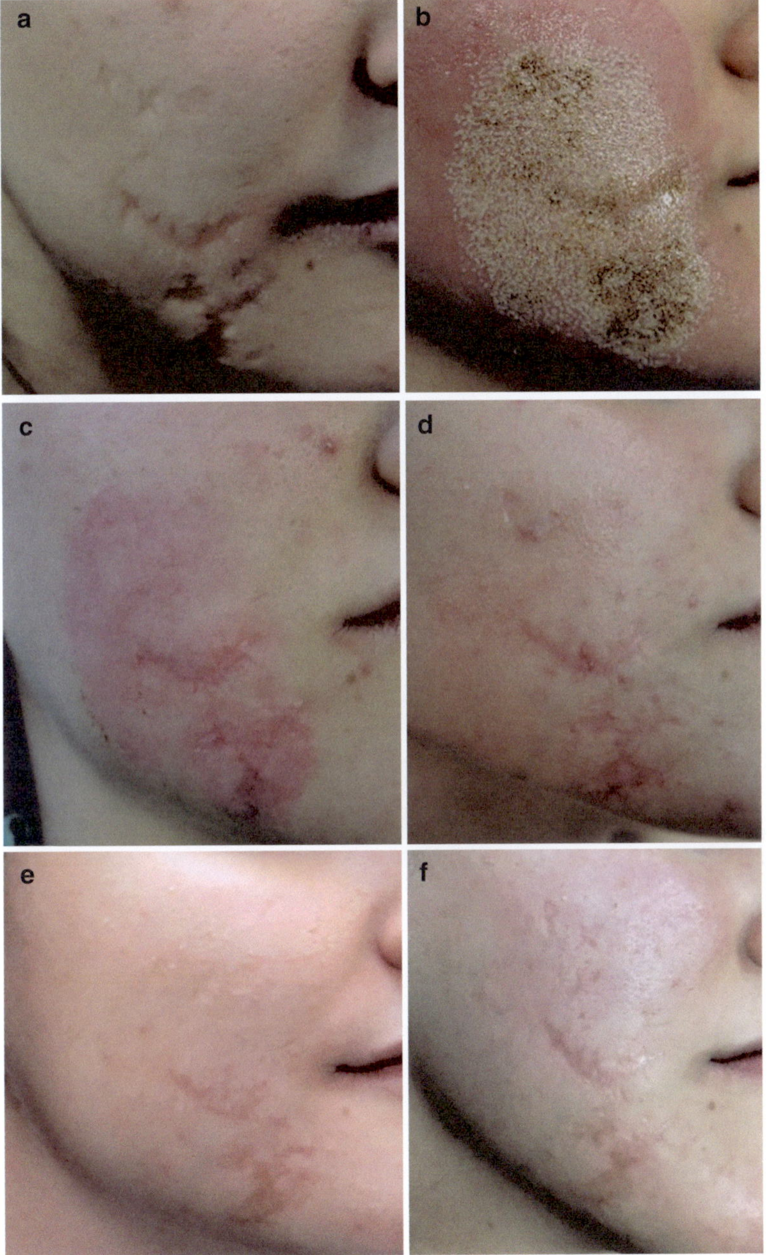

Fig. 35 (a) Old and mature facial post-traumatic scar (dog bite).(b) Resurfacing of the scar base and its edges and then passing more widely beyond the scar in fractional mode to avoid edge effects. (c) Seven days after the laser procedure and injection of hyaluronic acid below and inside the scar. (d) Result at 1 month after the combination laser and fillers injection. (e) Result at for 4 months after the combination laser and fillers injection. (f) Stability of the scar over 3 years without any other modality since. (g) Chalazodermic scar in smiling. (h) Structural modification, pliability-elasticity-roughness at 4 months. (i) Maintenance of this structural and textural change at 3 years after a mix of ablative laser and AH fillers. Courtesy of Hugues Cartier

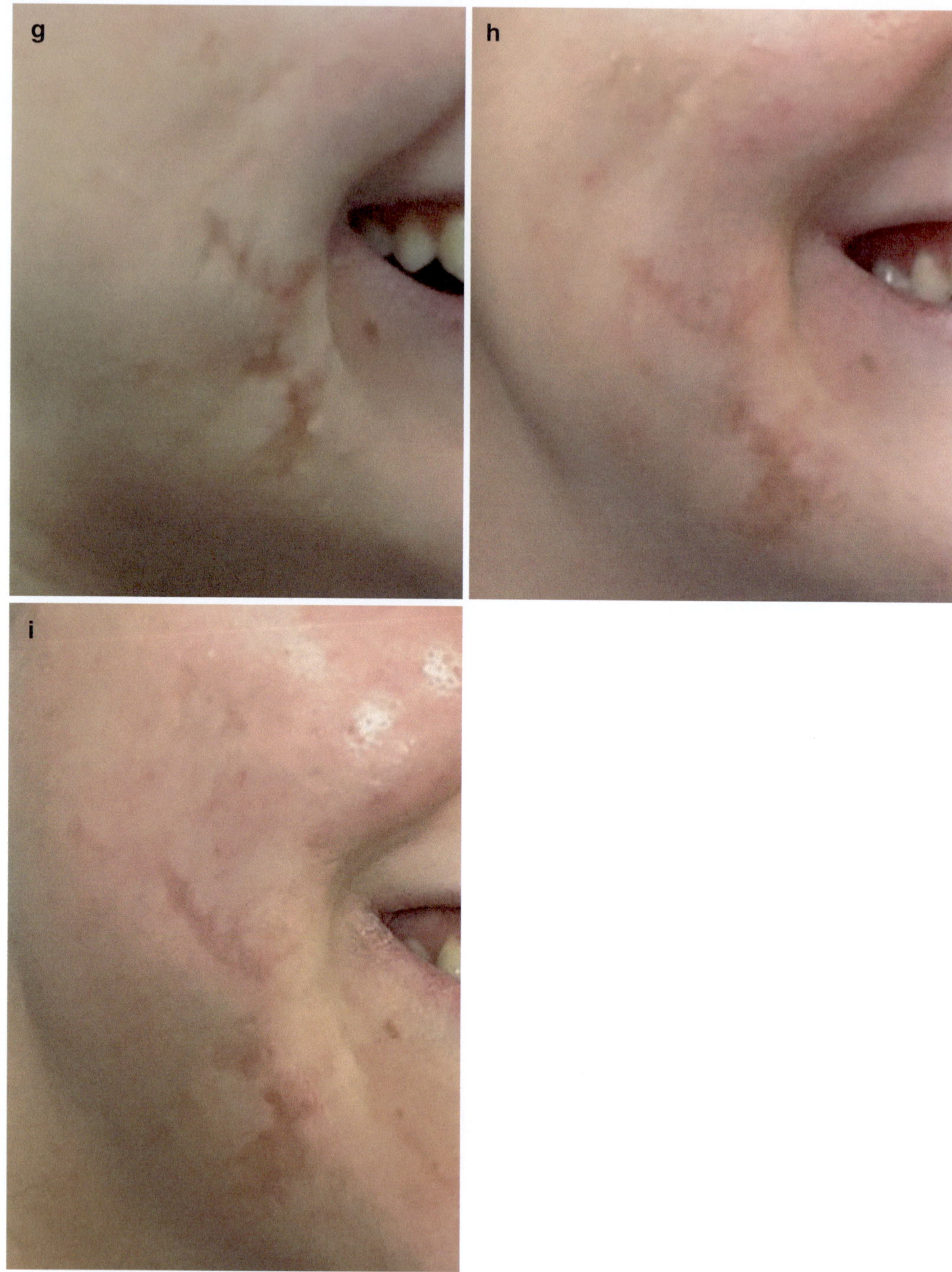

Fig. 35 (continued)

Acne Scar

Acne scars occur consequent to abnormal wound healing following sebaceous follicular inflammation in acne.

Various types of acne scars are ice pick, rolling, pox scar, hypertrophic, and keloidal. Different modalities of treatment include subcision, dermaroller, radio frequency therapy, punch excision, chemical peeling, and lasers.

After ensuring that there are no progressive acne lesions during the interview, it is the analysis of the scars during the preliminary consultation that will enable the therapeutic attitude to be specified. We will thus separate spontaneously regressive sequelae and permanent sequelae and determine the nature of the latter [31].

Active Acne with Inflammation, Why Wait?

Acne, also known as acne vulgaris within the medical community, is a chronic inflammatory skin condition. Acne can grow everywhere, but the more common spots for breakouts are the face (particularly the cheeks and forehead), back, chest, and shoulders. It can be improved with over-the-counter treatments, but more severe forms of the condition would require medical intervention. There are several types of acne, from blackheads to conglobata. But although we have a medical arsenal to treat this acne, the use of lasers and BEDs can be helpful. Indeed, the risk of scarring must be considered, and its early management is debated [32].

For inflammatory acne, we can propose photo-biomodulation with LEDs alone or optimize it with dynamic phototherapy. Without going back over the photo-chemical mechanism, the results are quite interesting (Fig. 36a–c). Encapsulated gold particles activated by Nd-YAG laser shots are also another therapeutic option (Sebacia ©) while waiting for the new wavelengths dedicated to acne which are currently being researched. To target *P. acnes* and its secretion, it is necessary to damage the sebaceous glands to stop or minimize sebum production. Optically, at 1726 nm, fat and sebum absorb twice as much as compared to H_2O.

Pulsed dye laser, Nd-YAG 1064 nm, and non-fractional and non-ablative such as Nd-YAP 1340 nm are other options to eliminate active acne, but they are often a temporary effect. For mature women, laser therapy may nevertheless be an alternative to conventional drugs and topical ointments in treatment impasse [33] (Fig. 37a–d).

**Case 28 Active Acne with High Risk of Scars
Treated by Photo-Dynamic Therapy**
See Fig. 36a–c.

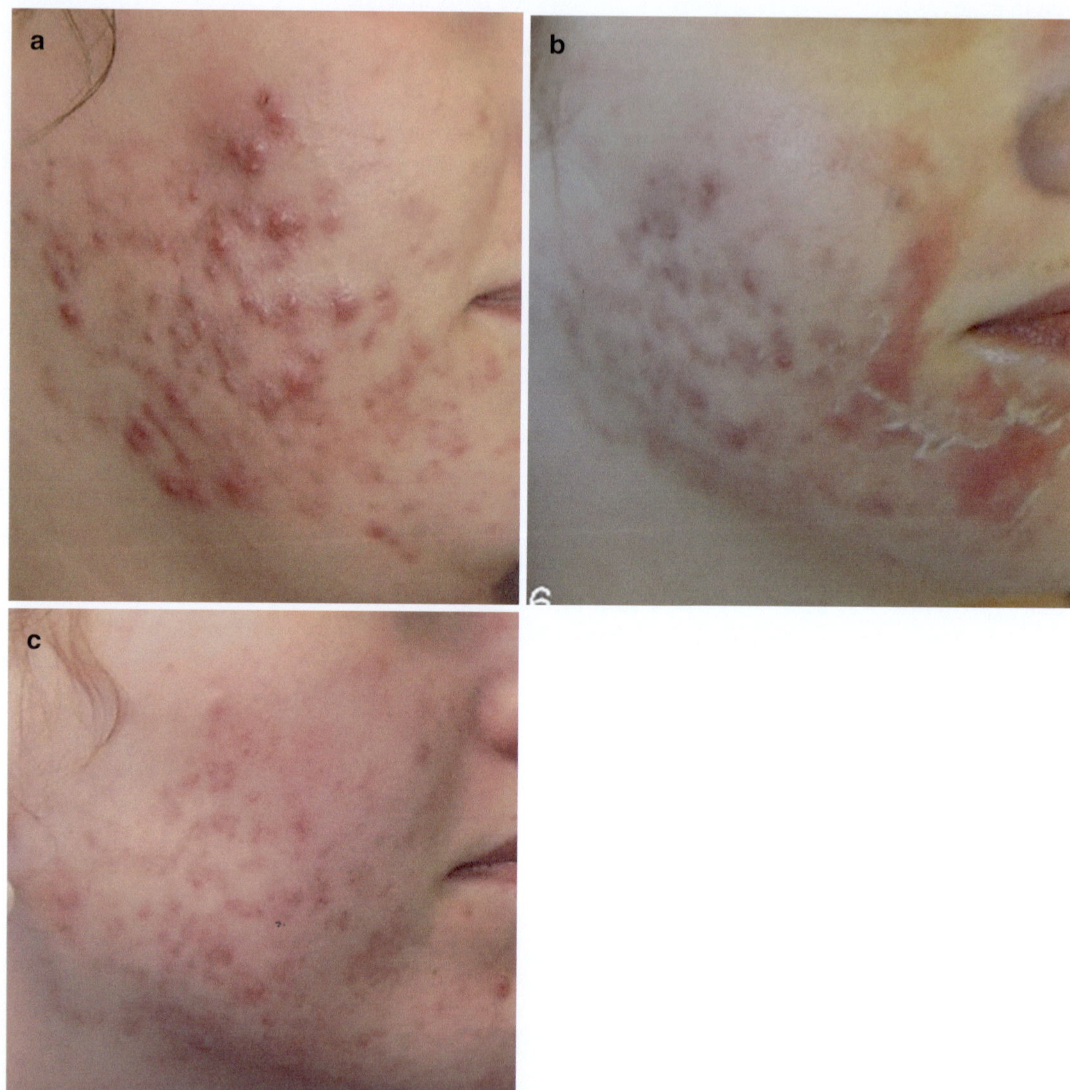

Fig. 36 (**a**) Active acne in a patient who refuses all systemic treatment for a desire to become pregnant. (**b**) Inflammatory reaction with moderate desquamation after a session of dynamic phototherapy with 5-ALA cream 20%. (**c**) Complete reduction of active acne after 3 sessions of PDT and persistence of acne scars to be treated later. Courtesy of Hugues Cartier

Case 29 Active Acne Scars with Inflammation and High Risk of Atrophic and Ice Pick Scars

See Fig. 37a–d.

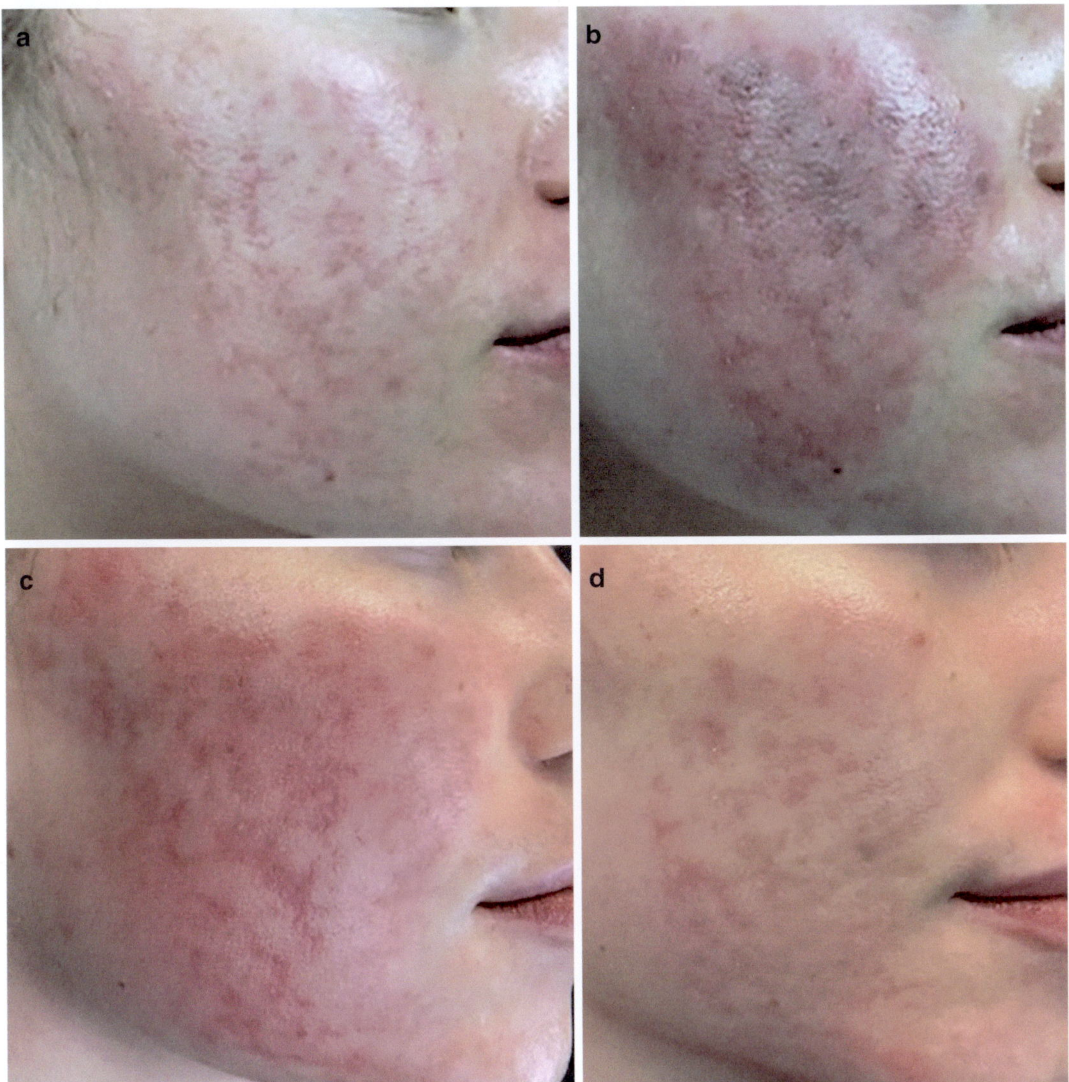

Fig. 37 **a**) Inflammate acne scars. (**b**) Pulse dye laser to reduce inflammation settings 6 ms, 10 J/cm², 10 mm spot size. (**c**) Nd: YAP 1340 nm to reduce scars in progress, setting: 100 MTZ/cm², 110 mJ/MTZ, 5 ms. (**d**) Stabilization of acne scar in progress by an alternating treatment between PDL and Nd: YAP, 4 sessions in 5 months. Courtesy of Hugues Cartier

Comments

While treatment of active acne with lasers has been successful, many studies are limited by the lack of control populations and comparison to standard therapies for active acne. Laser therapies are increasingly becoming part of or an adjunct to the medical treatment of active acne and are a useful treatment modality.

For Fixed Acne Scars

Changes in the skin's micro-relief for acne scars.

These are the most frequent scarring manifestation: the skin grain becomes coarser, irregular, and takes on a dull appearance. These irregularities are made up of dilated pores induced by the progressive dilation of the sebaceous ostia by hyper-seborrhea.

Alterations to the Skin's Micro-Relief

Fractional lasers are of great interest here. Their use in ablative, non-ablative, or mixed mode makes it possible to obtain in three to four sessions spaced at least 2 months apart (to benefit from the early remodeling phase of the previous session) a regularization of the skin surface allowing a visible softening of the skin texture (Fig. 38a–d).

– Fractional lasers remain the first-line treatment for ostial dilatation. They reduce the diameter of the pores by contraction and dermal densification and regularize surface irregularities by their tensor effect.

Case 30 Acne Scars with Ice Pick and Enlarged Pores

See Fig. 38a–d.

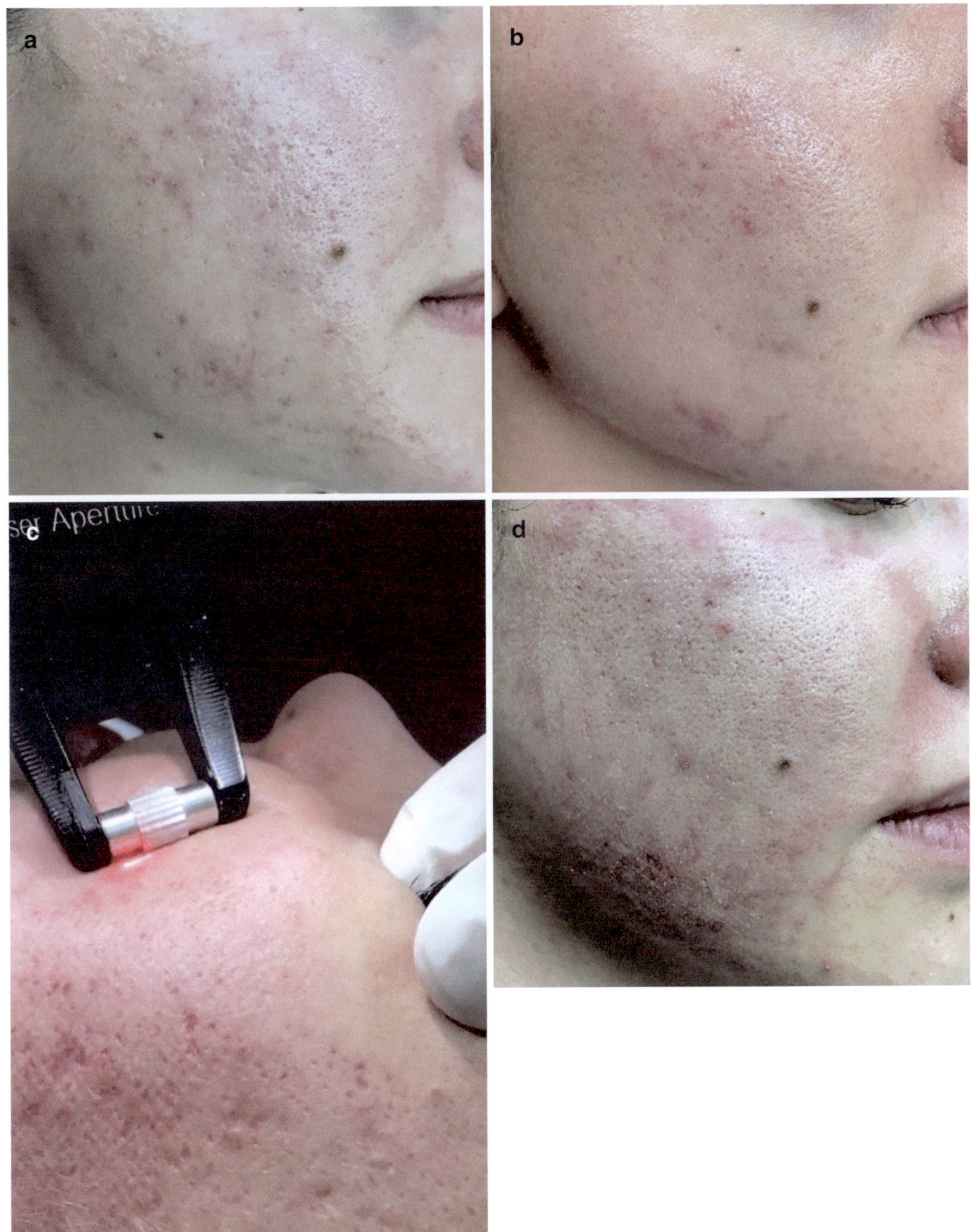

Fig. 38 a) Dilated pores, atrophic and ice pick acne scars. (**b**) Result after four sessions at 6 weeks apart. (**c**) NAFL 1550 nm laser treatment: 50 mJ, 3 ms. (**d**) NAFL linear beam mode: 50 mJ, 3 ms, 25% density, 3 passes. Courtesy of Hugues Cartier

Comments

The use of non-ablative fractional lasers including phototypes IV, V, and VI is possible with a much lower risk of triggering post-inflammatory pigmentation than with fractional ablative lasers. Wherever possible, they should be recommended as a first option.

— Depressed scars require a more complex two-stage sequence. Scar raising is the first essential step prior to laser abrasion when the depressions are deep; it is performed under local anesthesia. The isolated fragment is placed slightly above the surface of the adjacent skin using a punch with a diameter greater than the scar to be raised. Subcision and dermal graft can be combined. Coagulation will maintain the lift in its new position. Fatty plasters are changed daily for the first 4 days following the operation, after which the lifts are left in the open air. In the time interval between this procedure and the laser abrasion, the appearance is reminiscent of a papular acne flare-up. Laser abrasion is performed at least 1 month after the first procedure (Fig. 39a–d).

Anatomical unit performs laser dermabrasion, depending on the skin's laxity and therefore often depending on the age of the patients concerned. In young patients, abrasion with a low thermal effect is done with the Erbium: YAG laser. The demand for scar correction in older people requires the use of the CO_2 laser which leads to a real re-draping by dermal contraction in addition to leveling. Postoperative erythema is prolonged (2–3 months versus 4–6 months) [34, 35].

Case 31 Ablative and Resurfacing Procedure with CO₂ Laser

See Fig. 39a–d.

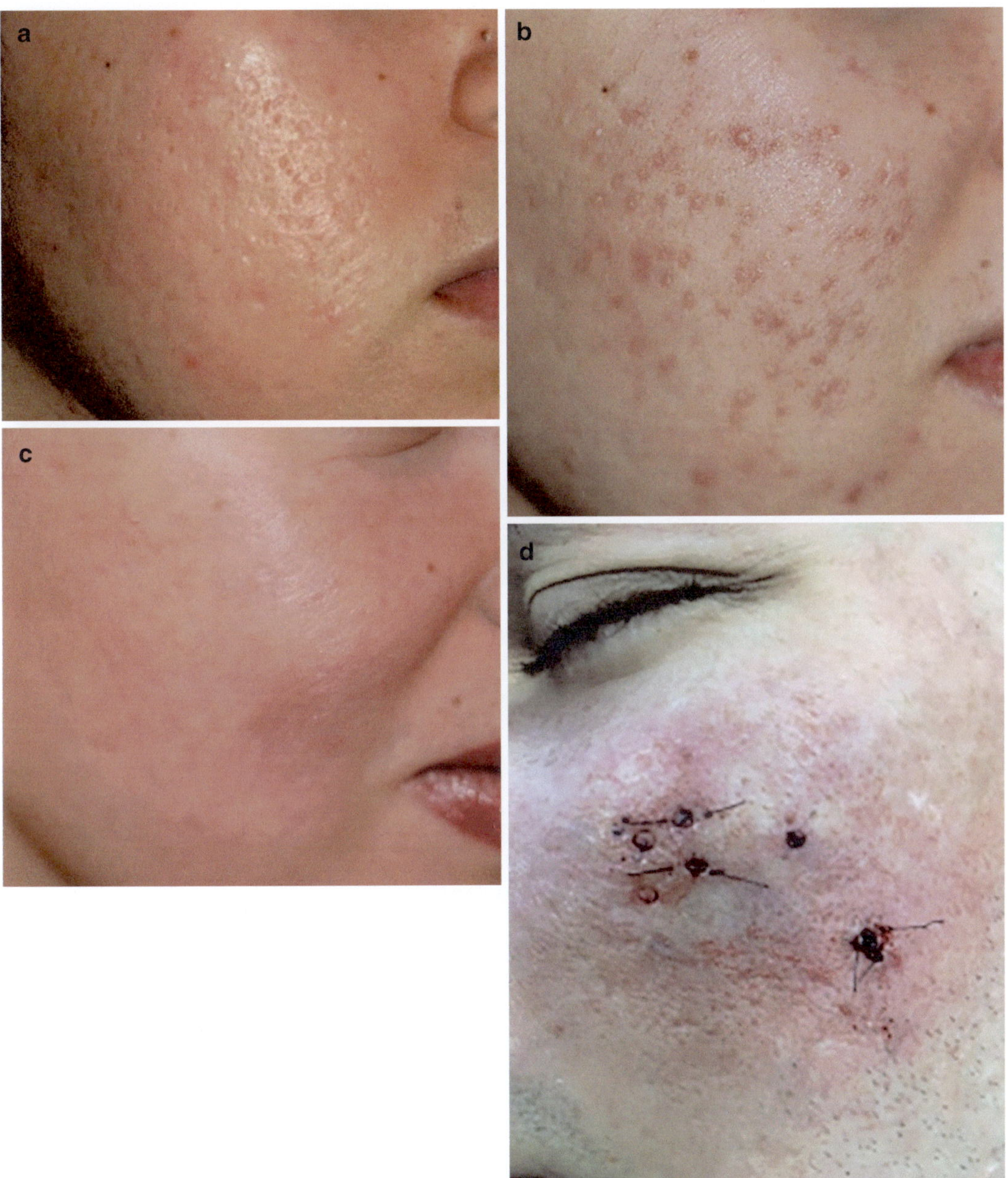

Fig. 39 (**a**) Mixed acne scars: pox scars, chicken pox scars, atrophic and ice pick scars. (**b**) Healing time after acne scar raising and before resurfacing of the area by CO₂ laser. (**c**) Final result after one session of ablative CO₂ laser. Courtesy of Thierry Fusade. (**d**) Acne scar raising with punch biopsy adapted to the size of the scar. Courtesy of Hugues Cartier

Case 32 Ice Pick Scars of the Nose
See Fig. 40a–d.

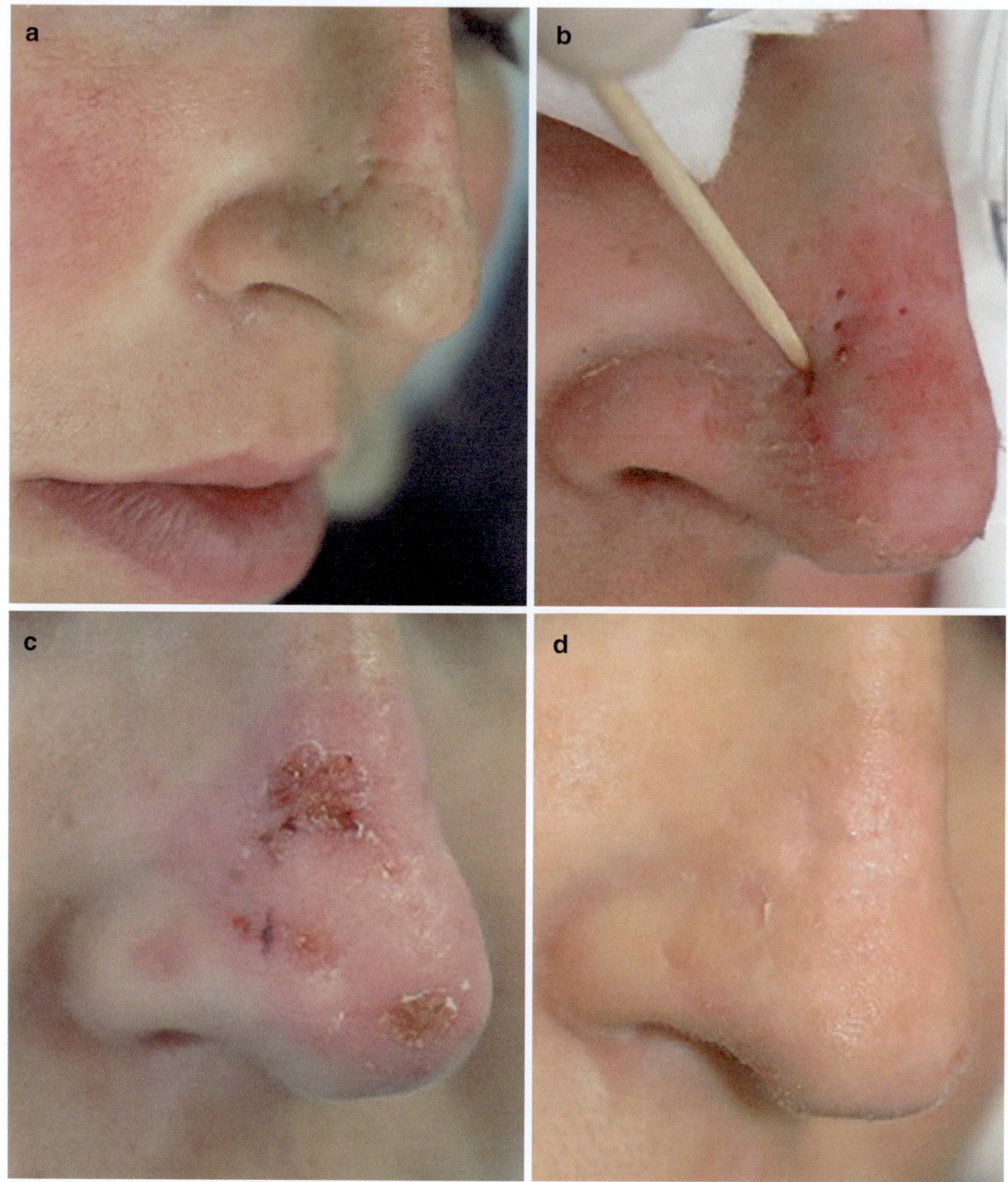

Fig. 40 (**a**) Ice pick scar or dilated pore treated by the phenol cross technique in one session. (**b**) The solution is slid on with a sharpened wooden stick. (**c**) Healing time with crusty dermal (**d**) Scar tissue elevation can be obtained by injecting a small amount of hyaluronic acid. Courtesy of Hugues Cartier

Comments

- *Ice pick scars will benefit firstly from surgical removal with punch and secondary suture when possible. The chemical technique TCA or Phenol Cross is an alternative but sometimes it can open up ice pick scars even more (Fig. 40a–d). In some cases, the use of the TCA/Phenol cross may open up the enlarged pores further. It is preferable to remove surgically and then smooth the scar surface with a CO_2 or Erbium: YAG ablative laser.*
- *In the situation where depressed scars are predominant and the after effects appear too burdensome for patients to manage, ablative fractional lasers can also be used.*
- *With AFL, the depth of treatment must be favored over density and thermal diffusion appears to be a determining factor. Thus, whatever the type of fractional laser used, the power, energy, and/or time of the unit pulses (dwelling) will be chosen to be high, while the density of the thermal cones (MTZ) or ablation will be medium or low. The session can be repeated.*
- *With the same parameters, the greatest improvements are obtained during the first sessions.*
- *Dermal grafting, injection of polylactic acid, calcium hydroxyapatite, and hyaluronic acid are now very common for scar lifting, reduction of pox scar, depression, or rolling scars, alone and especially in combination with laser remodeling, especially AFL and NAFL or MRF.*
- *To trim the shoulders of depressed, chickenpox scar, pox scar, or rolling scars and to reduce the difference in height at the surface of the skin, you can use a drilling method with a donut-shaped design of the laser scanner or use a handpiece with a spot size of less than 1 mm in pulse or continuous mode to reduce the border edge (Fig. 41a–j, 42a–e, and 43a,b).*

Case 33 Ablative Fractional Laser for Atrophic Acne Scars To

See Fig. 41a–j.

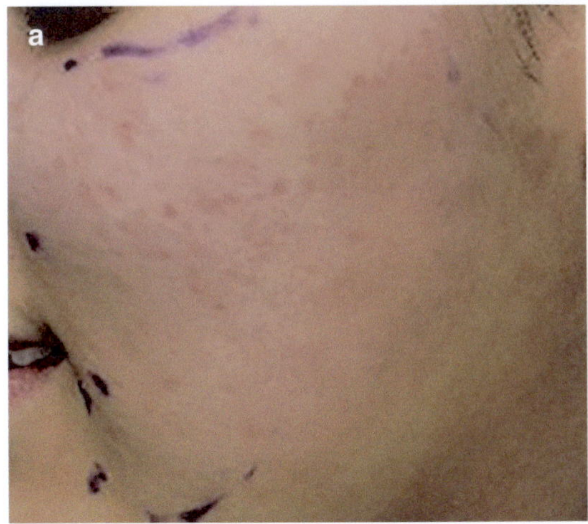
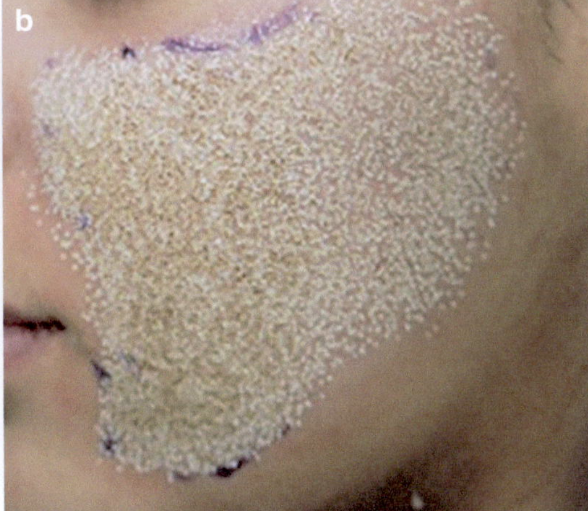
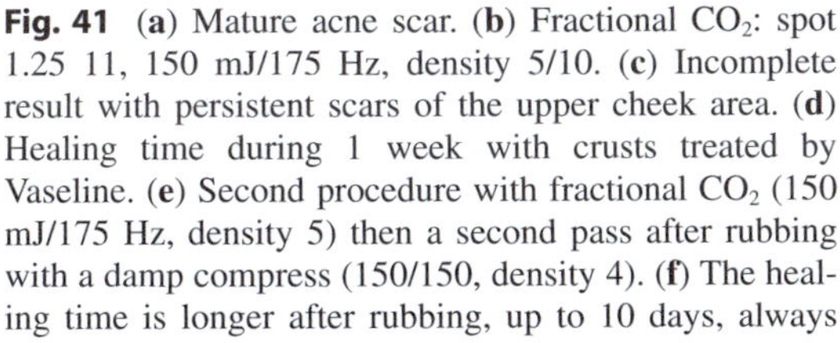

Fig. 41 (a) Mature acne scar. (b) Fractional CO_2: spot 1.25 11, 150 mJ/175 Hz, density 5/10. (c) Incomplete result with persistent scars of the upper cheek area. (d) Healing time during 1 week with crusts treated by Vaseline. (e) Second procedure with fractional CO_2 (150 mJ/175 Hz, density 5) then a second pass after rubbing with a damp compress (150/150, density 4). (f) The healing time is longer after rubbing, up to 10 days, always with Vaseline as a protective ointment. (g) Inflammation and redness treated by a short pulse of bethametasone cream during 5 days to avoid a higher risk of post-inflammation-hyperpigmentation (PIH). (h) Slight PIH, to be managed with time and sunscreen. (i) Result after two ablative procedures 8 months after. (j) Final result after two ablative procedures 6 years after. Courtesy of Hugues Cartier

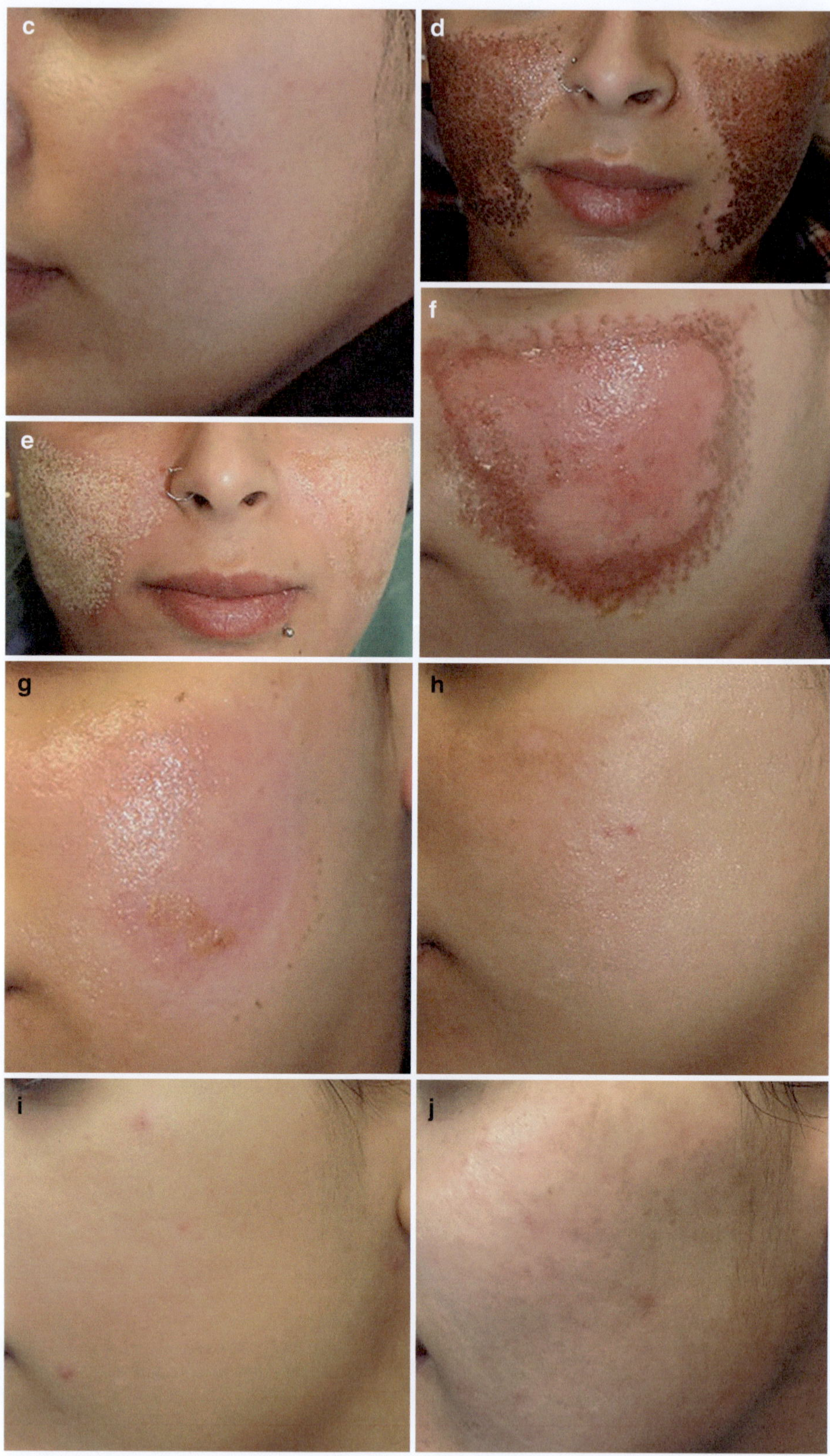

Fig. 41 (continued)

Case 34 Complex Acne Scars and Combined Procedure Er: YAG Plus CO$_2$

See Fig. 42a–e.

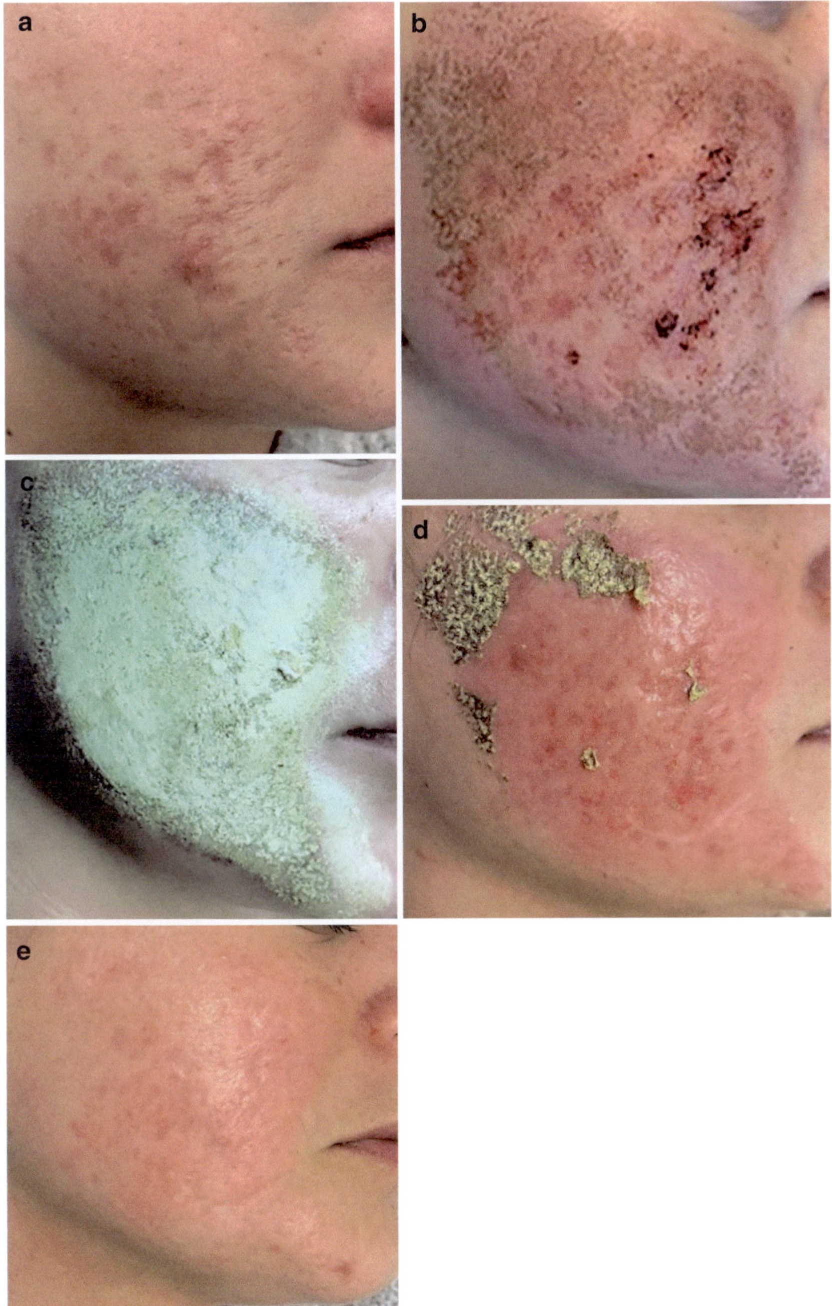

Fig. 42 (a) Acne scars: pox scar, rolling, pathomimics, failure TCA cross-session. (b) Just after ablative laser: first pass with Er: YAG (10 J/cm^2, 1500 µs) and then second pass with fractional (CO$_2$ 150 mJ, 150 Hz, 1.25 mm spot size, density 6). (c) Wound healing with application of mimosa powder, usually used after a phenol peel to avoid scratching by the patient. (d) Detachment of the mimosa crust on the eighth day. (e) Dramatical improvment 3 months after one session of Er: YAG + CO$_2$. Courtesy of Hugues Cartier

Comments

– *Rolling scars caused by underlying fat melting are too deep to be improved by laser. It is illusory to expect treatments with fractional pulsed lasers or laser resurfacing on this type of lesion to have a tensor effect that lasts more than a few months. Their correction is obtained by filling with an injection of hyaluronic acid. The choice of cross-linking depends on the depth of the lesions to be treated. Lipo-structure is only exceptionally proposed for the most severe lesions. Slow resorption occurs in sites that are not much mobilized by facial expressions, and the results often persist for 18–24 months (Fig. 43a, b).*

Case 35 Rolling and Atrophic Scars and Hyaluronic Acid

See Fig. 43a, b.

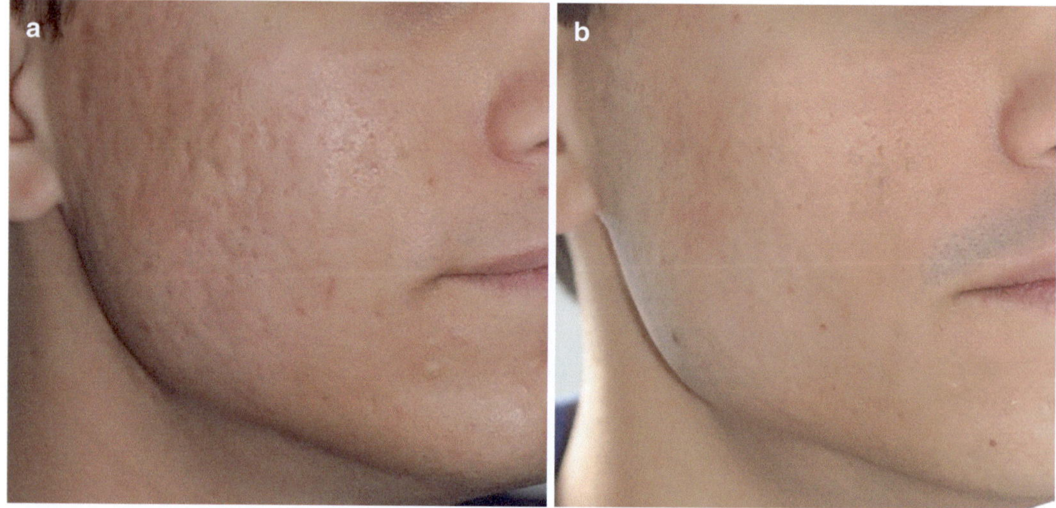

Fig. 43 (**a**) Mature acne scar. (**b**) Expected result at 9 months after 2 sessions, 1 month apart, of hyaluronic acid injection below and inside scars (medium G′) without any laser or EBD. Courtesy of Thierry Fusade

Comments

- *Ice pick scars need to be raised at first.*
- *Rolling scar can be reduced by injecting fillers alone. Hyaluronic acid raises scar tissue and stimulates neocollagenesis.*
- *The durability of HA is variable but in fibrous tissue, it can be stable for years. Other injectables as inductors can be used as PLLA (polylactic acid) or CaHA (hydroxyapatite of calcium) (Figs. 44a–h).*
- *Complex bridge scars and fixed retractile depressions benefit from surgical removal. The subcision is proposed for a long time to break the fibrous bridges, but it can sometimes be disappointing because the scar may reform a fibrous flange after a few weeks unless a resorbable material (Hyaluronic Acid) is used. At the time of surgical revision, to avoid secondary scar enlargement, particular attention must be paid to the suture in 2 or 3 planes with perfect confrontation of the deep plane.*
- *For residual erythema and post-inflammatory hyperpigmentation on dark skins, we are usually content to wait for regression, as these marks are always involutivity within few months. However, we can also suggest laser treatment as Nd:YAG long pulse in fast motion mode, non-ablative fractional and vascular laser as pulsed dye laser.*

Case 36 Mixed and Complex Acne Scars

See Fig. 44a–h.

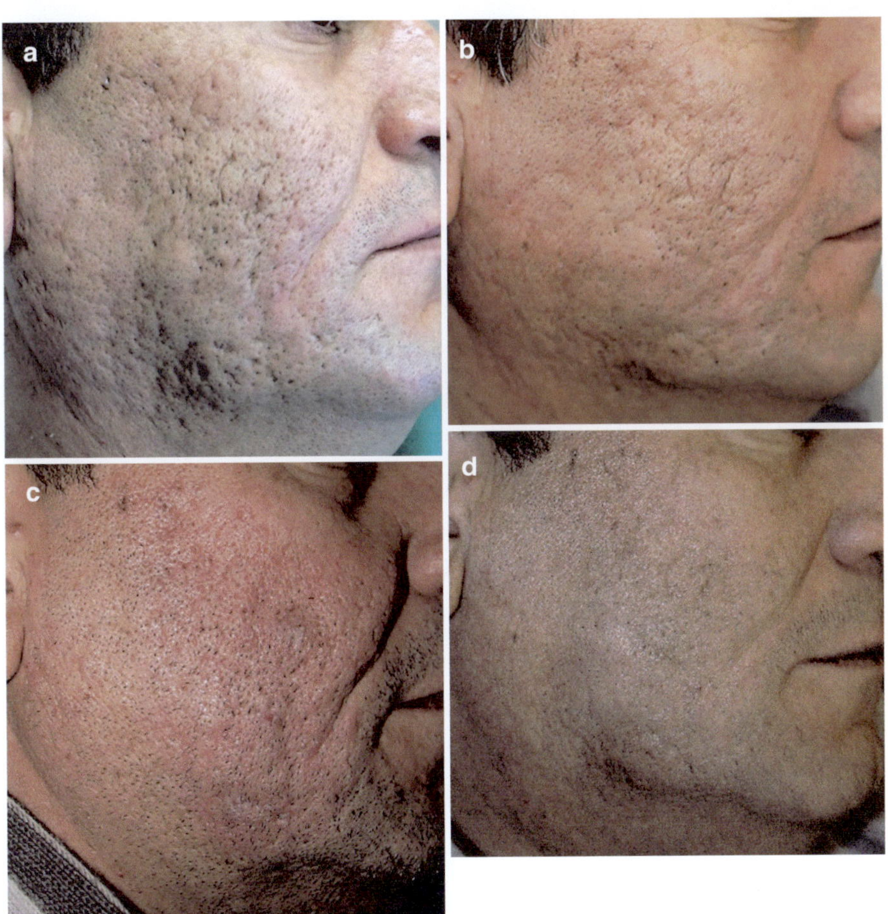

Fig. 44 (**a**) Acne scar with deep ice pick, atrophic and chicken pox scars. (**b**) One year of combined treatment. (**c**) After a second year of a combined treatment. (**d**) Final result after 2 sessions of MRF, 1 Er:YAG, 5 sessions of fractional CO_2, 2 sessions of PLLA. (**e**) Abrasion with Er:YAG + fractional CO_2. (**f**) Abrasion with CO_2 then fractionated CO_2 in second and third passes. (**g**) MRF (microneedle radiofrequency) combined with subcision and diluted subdermal poly-lactic acid injection. (**h**) Fractional CO_2 laser. Courtesy of Hugues Cartier

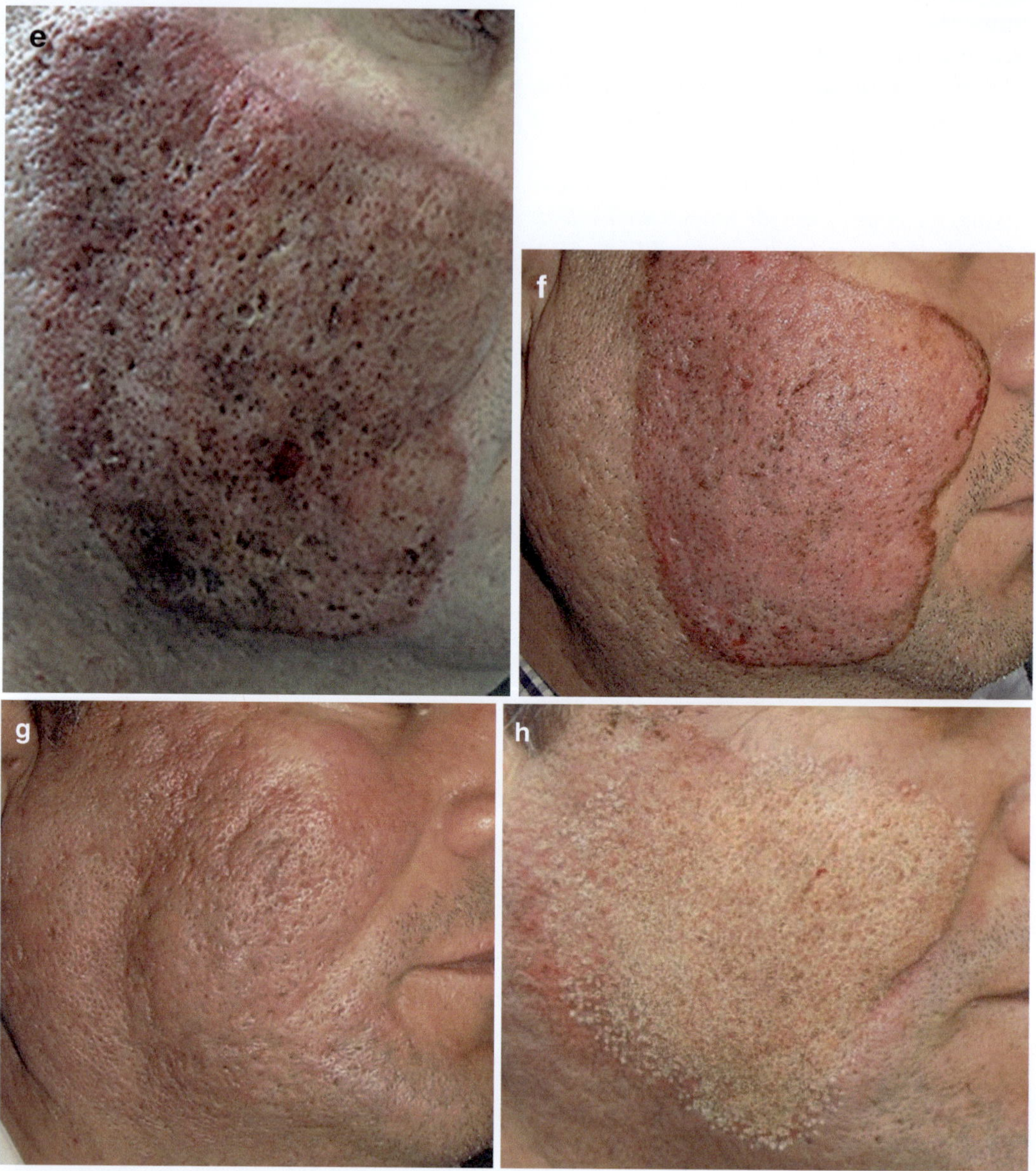

Fig. 44 (continued)

Comments

When acne scars are fixed, several solutions are possible. We distinguish between fractional abrasive or classical resurfacing techniques and fractional non-ablative lasers. The type of scar, the risk of PIH on darker phototypes, and the speed of the procedure are all factors that must be considered in order to achieve the desired results.

Ablative lasers are certainly effective, but one must accept the constraints of the postoperative period with oozing, crusty phase, and long-lasting erythema. Anything that is not ablative will take more time, and especially more sessions, to see the effects but with minimal after effects such as edema and very transient redness.

Overall, it should be remembered that the multiplicity of treatments does not realistically allow patients to be offered at all the stages. It is here that the importance of a good dialogue aimed at identifying individual motivations enables the scar priorities of each patient to be determined and therefore for the greatest therapeutic effectiveness to be proposed.

What to Do for Burn Scars?

Of course, all laser indications must be adapted according to the type and age of the scars. As with surgery, it appears necessary to intervene during the healing phase.

Vascular lasers such as the PDL are the keystone of this first photonic treatment. As the skin tightens, contracts, or aberrant scars appear, NAFLs and AFLs should be used.

The use of corticosteroids is also essential and is necessary to reduce an inflammatory process that is getting out of control. The use of the cohort of other drugs is also compatible for all scars to avoid retraction, hypertrophy, etc. or, botulinum toxin, 5FU, or platelet-rich plasma for example.

For mature and old scars, AFL CO_2 or Erbium: YAG are the first line of classic resurfacing (impulsion mode or fractional mode to a depth of 3.5 mm (maximum of 10% density, spot size less 150 μm, as much as possible in hyperpulse mode less 1 ms time delay to avoid overscars)) (Figs. 45a, b and 46a, b).

Case 37 Skin Burn of the Forehead
See Fig. 45a, b.

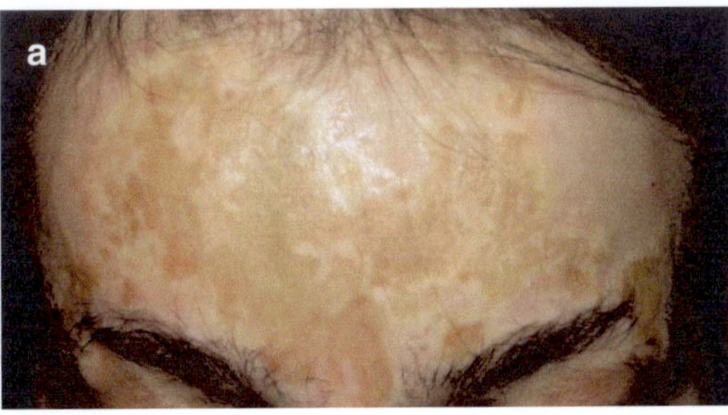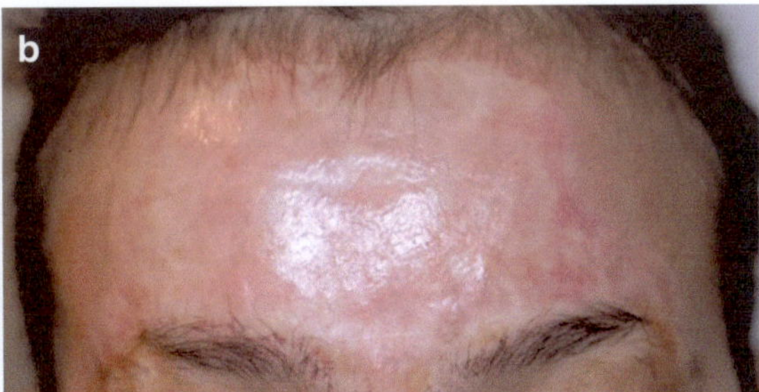

Fig. 45 (**a**) Burn sequellae of forehead before a classic resurfacing CO_2 laser. (**b**) Burn sequellae of forehead after classic resurfacing CO_2 laser. Courtesy of Thierry Fusade

Case 38 Scar Tissue After Skin Grafting
See Fig. 46a, b.

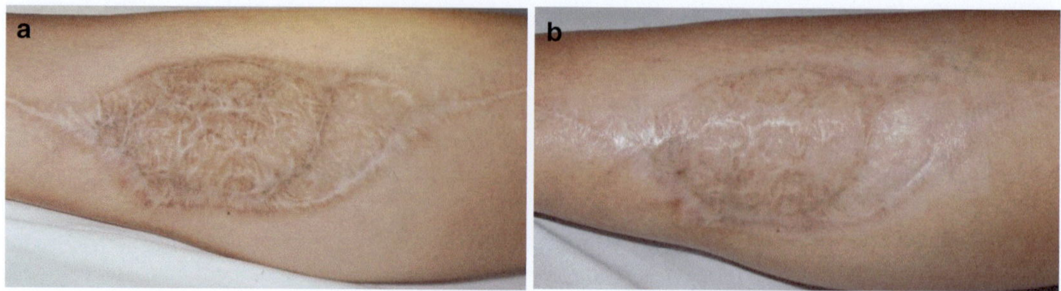

Fig. 46 (**a**) Combination of mixed AFL and AFL on skin grafting. (**b**) Result after 4 sessions and 1 year apart. Courtesy of Thierry Fusade

The combination of time, non-ablative laser, and pulsed dye laser allowed the opening of the mouth to be restored because the scar tissue became more pliable and flexible.

Treatment decision algorithm (Table 1)

Erythema stage: nothing, LEDs or corticoids tape/cream −/+ PDL 6 J/cm², 0.5–1.5 ms or 6 ms, 10 ms or KTP or IPL specific settings every 4–6 weeks.

Fresh surgery scar: 10 days to 3 weeks: PDL 6 J/cm² 3–6 ms or AFL5% or PDL + AFL 5% −/+ muscle injection of Botulinum Toxin.

Telangiectasia: any vascular laser.

Red Hypertrophic stage: corticoids tape/cream or LADD with fractional CO_2 density 5% every 6 weeks or PDL 6–10 J/cm², 1 ms, 5–3 or Nd: YAG or IPL or KTP +/− Botulinum Toxin in scars.

Keloids: complex situation PDL-LADD-AFL/corticoids-TAC +/− 5FU, cryosurgery-radiotherapy.

Mature hypertrophic stage: AFL +/− corticoids tape/LADD or MRF.

Atrophic stage: AFL CO_2/Er: YAG, density 10–15% or NAFL +/− Hyaluronic acid every 6–12 weeks or mechanical subcision/roller/MRF.

Texture/structure remodeling stage: with color PDL, IPL, KTP, Nd: YAG LP and if no red color AFL or pure ablative or NAFL, Pico-Nano Q-switched (pigmented or no) or MRF or micro-needling.

White scar: AFL/NAFL or cosmetic tattoo or melanocytes graft.

Post-inflammatory pigmentation: sunscreen and +/− corticoids +/− Depigmented cream +/− Laser if less and less red.

Mature pigmentated scar: depigmented cream-peels, NAFL or AFL/pure Ablative or Pico-Nano Q-switched.

Specific protocol for NAFL and AFL treatment of skin of color (III–VI Fitzpatrick scale)

Table 1 Decision algorithm according to the scar type

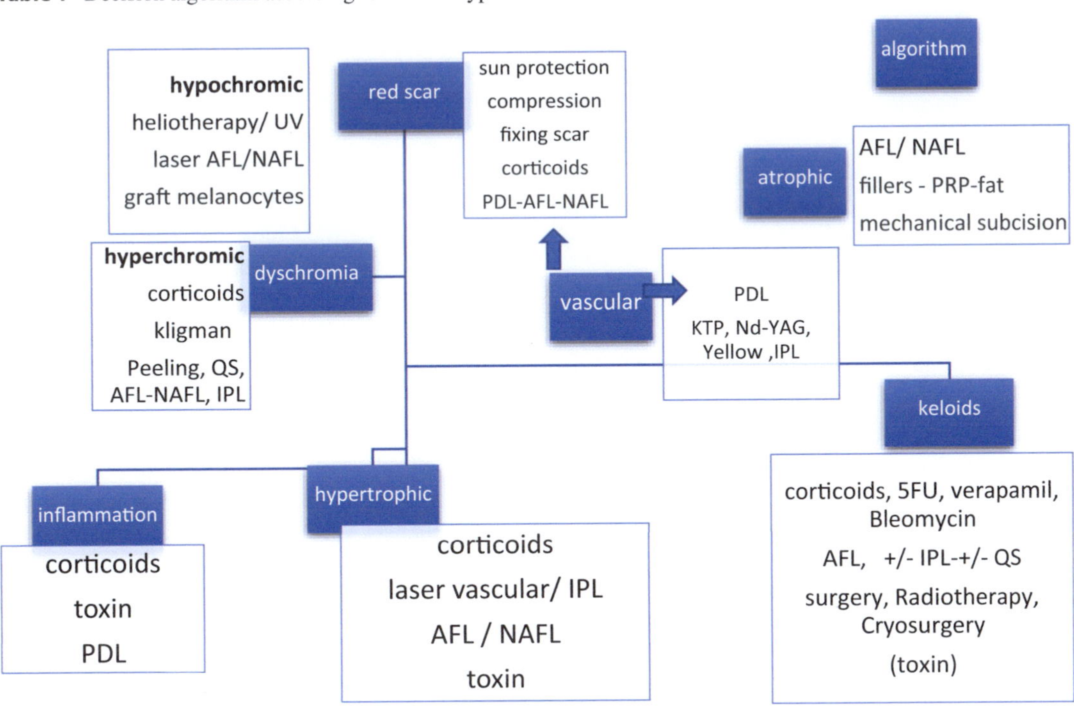

- Sun protection for at least 6 weeks before and after treatment.
- Pre-treatment regimens may include retinoic acid and/or hydroquinone for 2–6 weeks prior to treatment. It is also debated.
- Extend interval treatment from 6 weeks to 8/12 weeks.
- LADD with corticosteroids must be considered at the time of treatment and several days after the session.
- Post-treatment regimens include prophylactic or as needed topical azelaic acid 15–20%, hydroquinone 5% for 2–6 weeks after laser especially with AFL.
- If PIH, wait until it has resolved before the next treatment, at least 4 weeks or more.

Keep in mind the 2020 consensus recommendations [28]
- For smaller traumatic injuries, 90% of panelists would optimally begin laser treatment within 1 month, and over 70% within 1 week or less.
- For larger traumatic injuries such as burn, over 90% of panelists would optimally begin laser within 4 months or less and 76% within 2 months or less.

Current AFL devices have proven safe and effective, but the optimal settings are not yet known
- Tunable depth of penetration and density with the option to penetrate several mm.
- Narrow beam diameter (<300 μ).
- Appropriate surrounding coagulation (CO_2 more than Er: YAG).
- Short pulse duration to minimize thermal injury (1 ms).

Fractional lasers and MRF might apply to all skin types, though changes in medications regimen and procedure parameters may be considered for skin of color type (low density 1–5%, less 1 ms for a same energy as Caucasian type).

Laser and EBD treatment may be continued until the desired effect is obtained or improvement stabilizes. Complications rates associated with laser after scar treatment appear to be extremely low compared to scalpel surgery.

Conclusion

The management of scars really has no limit. The numerous types of scars are a source of debate. Lasers and other tools contribute to help the practitioner in his choices. Numerous publications and Consensus are regularly published and help in decision-making according to clinical practices [28–36].

Nevertheless, a personalization is necessary in agreement with the patient and often their entourage.

Helping the patient to learn to live with a scar, which we know will leave physical and psychological traces, is also a long learning process and a matter for the practitioner.

All laser physicians are asked to contribute this information
- Lasers and EBDs have become a real option for the treatment of scars, especially hypertrophic and keloid scars. It is never too late to initiate laser for scars particularly for traumatic scars.
- Most of them can be used early to treat any scars and complications, such as hypertrophic and keloid scars.
- Many devices work well alone or in combination such as AFL and PDL or with many topical products to increase efficacy.

References

1. Wenande E, Anderson RR, Haedersdal M. Fundamentals of fractional laser-assisted drug delivery: an in-depth guide to experimental methodology and data interpretation. Adv Drug Deliv Rev. 2020;153:169–84.

2. Laubach HJ, Tannous Z, Anderson RR, Manstein D. Skin responses to fractional photothermolysis. Lasers Surg Med. 2006;38(2):142–9. https://doi.org/10.1002/lsm.20254.

3. Gladsjo JA, Jiang SI. Treatment of surgical scars using a 595-nm pulsed dye laser using purpuric and non-purpuric parameters: a comparative study. Dermatol Surg. 2014;40(2):118–26.

4. Patel PM, Bakus AD, Garden BC, Lai O, Jones VA, Garden JM. Treatment of pain in keloids using only a long-pulsed 1064 nm Nd:YAG laser. Lasers Surg Med. 2021;53(1):66–9.

5. Koike S, Akaishi S, Nagashima Y, Dohi T, Hyakusoku H, Ogawa R. Nd:YAG laser treatment for keloids and hypertrophic scars: an analysis of 102 cases. Plast Reconstr Surg Glob Open. 2015;2(12):e272.

6. Cartier H. Use of intense pulsed light in the treatment of scars. J Cosmet Dermatol. 2005;4(1):34–40.

7. Park YJ, Kim SJ, Song HS, Kim SK, Lee J, Soh EY, Kim YC. Prevention of thyroidectomy scars in Asian adults with low-level light therapy. Dermatol Surg. 2016;42(4):526–34.

8. Alster TS, Li MKY. Micro-needling of scars: a large prospective study with long-term follow-up. Plast Reconstr Surg. 2020;145(2):358–64.

9. Zouboulis CC, Zouridaki E. Cryosurgery as a single agent and in combination with intralesional corticosteroids is effective on young, small keloids and induces characteristic histological and immunohistological changes: a prospective randomized trial. Dermatology. 2021;237(3):396–406.

10. Berman B, Nestor MS, Gold MH, Goldberg DJ, Weiss ET, Raymond I. A retrospective registry study evaluating the long-term efficacy and safety of superficial radiation therapy following excision of keloid scars. J Clin Aesthet Dermatol. 2020;13(10):12–6.

11. Kauvar ANB, Kubicki SL, Suggs AK, Friedman PM. Laser therapy of traumatic and surgical scars and an algorithm for their treatment. Lasers Surg Med. 2020;52(2):125–36.

12. Karmisholt KE, Wenande E, Thaysen-Petersen D, Philipsen PA, Paasch U, Haedersdal M. Early intervention with non-ablative fractional laser to improve cutaneous scarring—a randomized controlled trial on the impact of intervention time and fluence levels. Lasers Surg Med. 2018;50(1):28–36.

13. Friedman O, Gofstein D, Arad E, Gur E, Sprecher E, Artzi O. Laser pretreatment for the attenuation of planned surgical scars: a randomized self-controlled hemi-scar pilot study. J Plast Reconstr Aesthet Surg. 2020;73(5):893–8.

14. Casanova D, Alliez A, Baptista C, Gonelli D, Lemdjadi Z, Bohbot S. A 1-year follow-up of post-operative scars after the use of a 1210-nm laser-assisted skin healing (LASH) technology: a randomized controlled trial. Aesthet Plast Surg. 2017;41(4):938–48.

15. Alam M, Pon K, Laborde SV, Arndt KA, et al. Clinical effect of a single pulsed dye laser treatment of fresh surgical scars: randomized controlled trial. Dermatol Surg. 2006;32:21–5.

16. Yun JS, Choi YJ, Kim WS, Lee GY. Prevention of thyroidectomy scars in Asian adults using a 532-nm potassium titanyl phosphate laser. Dermatol Surg. 2011;37(12):1747–53.

17. Tierney E, Mahmoud BH, Srivastava D, Ozog D, Kouba DJ. Treatment of surgical scars with non-ablative fractional laser versus pulsed dye laser: a randomized controlled trial. Dermatol Surg. 2009;35(8):1172–80.

18. Choe JH, Park YL, Kim BJ, Kim MN, Rho NK, Park BS, Choi YJ, Kim KJ, Kim WS. Prevention of thyroidectomy scar using a new 1550-nm fractional erbium-glass laser. Dermatol Surg. 2009;35(8):1199–205.

19. Ibrahim SM, Saudi WM, Abozeid MF, Elsaie ML. Early fractional carbon dioxide laser intervention for postsurgical scars in skin of color. Clin Cosmet Investig Dermatol. 2019;12:29–34.

20. Shin JU, Gantsetseg D, Jung JY, Jung I, Shin S, Lee JH. Comparison of non-ablative and ablative fractional laser treatments in a postoperative scar study. Lasers Surg Med. 2014;46(10):741–9.

21. Kim DH, Ryu HJ, Choi JE, Ahn HH, Kye YC, Seo SH. A comparison of the scar prevention effect between carbon dioxide fractional laser and pulsed dye laser in surgical scars. Dermatol Surg. 2014;40(9):973–8.

22. Waibel JS, Wulkan AJ, Shumaker PR. Treatment of hypertrophic scars using laser and laser

assisted corticosteroid delivery. Lasers Surg Med. 2013;45(3):135–40.

23. Tapking C, Prasai A, Branski LK. Are hypertrophic scars and keloids the same? Br J Dermatol. 2020;182(4):832–3.

24. Ouyang HW, Li GF, Lei Y, Gold MH, Tan J. Comparison of the effectiveness of pulsed dye laser vs pulsed dye laser combined with ultrapulse fractional CO_2 laser in the treatment of immature red hypertrophic scars. J Cosmet Dermatol. 2018;17(1):54–60.

25. Vaccaro M, Borgia F, Guarneri B. Treatment of hypertrophic thyroidectomy scar using 532-nm potassium-titanyl-phosphate (KTP) laser. Int J Dermatol. 2009;48:1139–41.

26. Babu P, Meethale Thiruvoth F, Chittoria RK. Intense pulsed light vs silicone gel sheet in the management of hypertrophic scars: an interventional comparative trial in the Indian population. J Cosmet Laser Ther. 2019;21(4):234–7.

27. Manuskiatti W, Wanitphakdeedecha R, Fitzpatrick RE. Effect of pulse width of a 595-nm flashlamp-pumped pulsed dye laser on the treatment response of keloidal and hypertrophic sternotomy scars. Dermatol Surg. 2007;33(2):152–61.

28. Seago M, Shumaker PR, Spring LK, Alam M, Al-Niaimi F, Rox Anderson R, Artzi O, Bayat A, Cassuto D, Chan HH, Dierickx C, Donelan M, Gauglitz GG, Leo Goo B, Goodman GJ, Gurtner G, Haedersdal M, Krakowski AC, Manuskiatti W, Norbury WB, Ogawa R, Ozog DM, Paasch U, Victor Ross E, Tretti Clementoni M, Waibel J. Laser treatment of traumatic scars and contractures: 2020 international consensus recommendations. Lasers Surg Med. 2020;52(2):96–116.

29. Gao FL, Jin R, Zhang L, Zhang YG. The contribution of melanocytes to pathological scar formation during wound healing. Int J Clin Exp Med. 2013;6(7):609–13.

30. Park KY, Choi SY, Mun SK, Kim BJ, Kim MN. Combined treatment with 578-/511-nm copper bromide laser and light-emitting diodes for post-laser pigmentation: a report of two cases. Dermatol Ther. 2014;27(2):121–5.

31. Zaleski-Larsen LA, Fabi SG, McGraw T, Taylor M. Acne scar treatment: a multimodality approach tailored to scar type. Dermatol Surg. 2016;42(Suppl 2):S139–49.

32. Wiznia LE, Stevenson ML, Nagler AR. Laser treatments of active acne. Lasers Med Sci. 2017;32(7):1647–58. https://doi.org/10.1007/s10103-017-2294-7.

33. Artzi O, Koren A, Shehadeh W, Friedman O. Quasi long-pulsed 1064 nm Nd:YAG (micro pulsed) technology for the treatment of active acne: a case series. J Cosmet Dermatol. 2021;20(7):2102–7.

34. Sawcer D, Lee HR, Lowe NJ. Lasers and adjunctive treatments for facial scars: a review. J Cutan Laser Ther. 1999;1:77–85.

35. Cho SI, Kim YC. Treatment of atrophic facial scars with combined use of high-energy pulsed CO_2 laser and Er: YAG laser: a practical guide of the laser techniques for the Er: YAG laser. Dermatol Surg. 1999;25:959–64.

36. Anderson RR, Donelan MB, Hivnor C, Greeson E, Ross EV, Shumaker PR, Uebelhoer NS, Waibel JS. Laser treatment of traumatic scars with an emphasis on ablative fractional laser resurfacing: consensus report. JAMA Dermatol. 2014;150(2):187–93.

Surgical Scar Therapy

Eva Koellensperger and Guenter Germann

Core Messages
- Scar revision surgery often requires multiple sessions or one approach with a combination of different techniques.
- As scar revision surgery leads to new scarring it is only indicated if aesthetic or functional improvement can be achieved.
- Proper postoperative care is essential to achieve an optimal result after scar revision surgery.

Introduction

Scars are the final result of a dermal trauma. Irrespective of their cause, they cannot only disturb aesthetic harmony but also interfere with functional requirements. Examples for the latter include a loss in skin elasticity, mechanical stability, or disturbing adherence to underlying tissues. Both aesthetic and functional impairments might induce the need of surgical scar improvement.

Surgery offers different options for scar therapy, which, however, are not always suitable for the individual scar. Choosing an appropriate type of surgery in an individual situation not only requires extensive experience but also a broad knowledge of the different techniques and their effects, risks, and limitations.

> **Important to Know**
> Surgery always leads to new scarring, thus may be indicated for scar therapy only, if aesthetic and/or functional improvement can be achieved.

Prior to surgery, it is crucial to explore the characteristics of the scar and the local tissue environment. A thorough discussion of the different options with their respective requirements, risks, and limitations with special regard to the patients' needs and expectations is fundamental. The patient needs to understand that a complete removal of a scar is often not possible and camouflaging or reorientation techniques may be valid alternatives.

Relaxed skin tension lines (RSTLs) represent the direction with the lowest elasticity of the skin according to the orientation of the underlying collagen fibers in the dermal reticular layer. Respecting these RSTLs is important, especially when performing local flaps, to achieve cosmetically and functionally favorable results.

Surgical scar therapies can either focus on completely removing a scar or improving, camouflaging or modifying it for a better aesthetic or functional outcome. These are often staged, multi-step procedures.

E. Koellensperger (✉) · G. Germann
ETHIANUM Clinic for Plastic, Aesthetic and Reconstructive Surgery, Spine, Orthopedic and Hand Surgery, Preventive Medicine, Heidelberg, Germany
e-mail: eva.koellensperger@ethianum.de;
guenter.germann@ethianum.de

Performing surgery in active scar tissue might lead to a higher incidence of hypertrophic scarring and further postoperative complications. For this reason, it is often recommended to await scar maturation before beginning surgical therapy.

For optimal results, scar revision surgery should always be followed by proper postoperative care. This includes, but is not limited to, wearing compression garments, using adequate sun protection, and where appropriate adding additional nonsurgical applications, such as laser therapy or medical needling (see respective chapters).

Surgical Options for Scar Therapy

Deciding which surgical method promises the best results for a specific scar largely depends on the characteristics of the scar itself, the surrounding tissue, a potential lack of function induced by the scar, and the patient's expectations.

Hypo- or atrophic scars mandate different treatments compared to contracted, adherent, or hypertrophic scars.

Excision, Serial Excision

Excision

If a scar lies parallel to the RSTLs, is not contracted or otherwise functionally disturbing, and is surrounded by an adequate amount of unaffected healthy skin and soft tissue, a fusiform complete excision can be performed with primary closure (see Fig. 1). One needs to keep in mind that the ends of the fusiform excision should have an angle equal or smaller than 30° to prevent the formation of dog ears. Hypotrophic or dyspigmented scars can often be treated in this fashion. However, one has to keep in mind that the resulting scar is longer than the one before, and there always remains the risk of recurrence of the undesired characteristic.

Making sure that there is enough healthy adjacent soft tissue to close the wound without generating orthogonal tension is also important. Such tension might lead to excessive collagen production, which, in turn, can lead to hypertrophic scarring. If there is too much tension despite thorough undermining of the adjacent soft tissue and proper placing of an adequate number of subcutaneous sutures, performing serial excisions can help (see Serial Excision).

Serial Excision

Serial excision is the method of choice for scar correction or clearance if the scar is too large for a single-step procedure but the surrounding, unaffected skin allows for a multi-step approach (see Fig. 2). The adjacent healthy tissue has to have adequate elasticity. Depending on the individual laxity and elasticity of the surrounding skin, the amount of excised skin per serial step can vary.

Caution needs to be taken not to excise too much tissue in one step. Ignoring this, an excess of tension in wound closure may follow. This could promote broad and unaesthetic scarring or

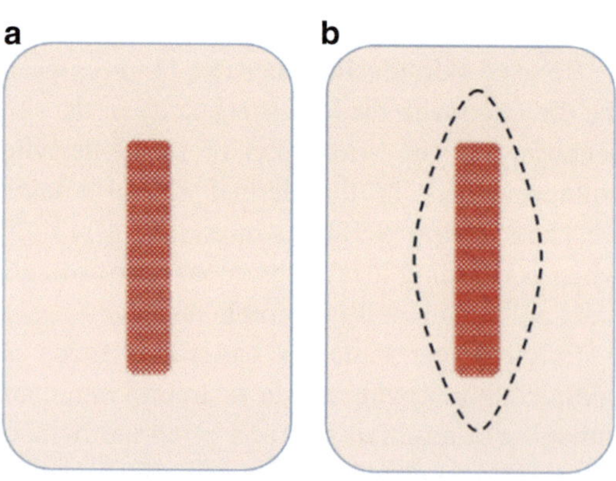
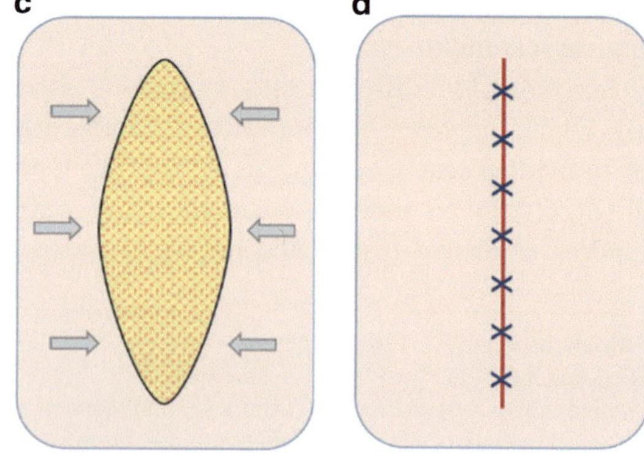

Fig. 1 Fusiform excision. If the scar lies parallel to the RSTLs, is not contracted or otherwise functionally disturbing, and is surrounded by an adequate amount of healthy skin and soft tissue, a fusiform complete excision can be performed with primary closure. The ends of the excision should have an angle equal or smaller than 30° to prevent the formation of dog ears

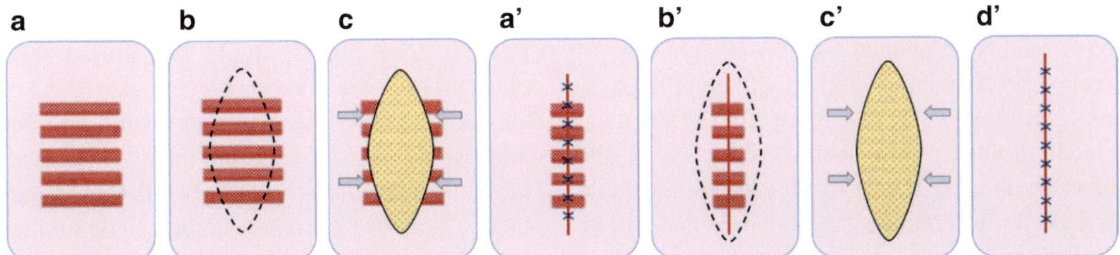

Fig. 2 Serial excision. If the scar is too large for a single-step procedure, serial fusiform excisions are performed with an angle of approximately 30° at the corners and the incision line being placed either within or parallel to a relaxed skin tension line. It is recommended to place the fusiform serial incisions in the central portion of the scar that has to be removed. (**a–c**) First step; (**a′–d′**): second step

even a lack of perfusion in underlying muscles leading to an iatrogenic compartment syndrome. Accordingly, it is recommended to evaluate and mark the amount of skin that can safely be excised before positioning the patient on the operating table and before applying local anesthesia.

> **Caution!**
> Do not excise too much tissue in one session. This can cause unwelcome scarring or low perfusion and subsequent loss of underlying or adjacent tissue, or possibly a dehiscent scar.

Mostly, serial excisions are performed by fusiform excision with an angle of approximately 30° at the corners and the incision line being placed either within or parallel to a relaxed skin tension line. It is recommended to place the fusiform serial incisions in the central portion of the scar that has to be removed (Fig. 2).

> **Clinical Tip**
> The multiple steps of serial excision should be performed approximately 6–9 months apart.

In our experience, the average latency between the multiple steps of serial excision is 6–9 months, depending on the elasticity of the skin and inter-individual differences.

Placing adequate multilevel sutures for closing is crucial for a favorable result. Subcutaneous or dermal sutures take most tissue tension while more superficial cutaneous sutures provide accurate alignment of wound borders supporting uncomplicated healing and preventing broad and unpleasant scarring.

Extensive scar tissue seen in, e.g., deep burn scars is generally not suited for serial excisions as wound healing issues related to reduced wound healing capacities and impaired microperfusion may arise.

Careful placement of larger excisions parallel to the axis of the extremity or the skin tension lines can help avoid subpar outcomes with respect to function and cosmetics.

> **Caution!**
> When placing wound margins and sutures in extensive scar tissue, impaired healing has to be expected due to reduced vascularization.

Use of Tissue Expanders

Inflatable or self-expanding tissue expanders can be used to activate a number of mechano-transduction pathways in the skin. Aims include cellular proliferation and development of excess new skin. The latter can be used to cover defects created when excising larger areas of adjacent skin tissue that could not be closed by primary suture [1].

Tissue expanders are inflatable silicon balloons mainly implanted subcutaneously next to tissue defects and then gradually filled with physiological saline. The subsequent mechanical stretch produces skin overgrowth to cover the adjacent defects. Tissue expanders are available in multiple different shapes and sizes that can be chosen according to the area in need of covering. In most instances, a rectangular tissue expander is a good choice [2]. Furthermore, osmotic, self-inflating expanders need to be distinguished from expanders that have to be filled manually through an external port or internal valve.

> **Important to Know**
> For the most part, the height of the chosen expander defines the possible gain in skin tissue.

The generated surplus skin matches the color, texture, and thickness of the surrounding skin very well and thus is a good replacement option for local defects after scar revision surgery.

The precise location of the incision for tissue expander placement has to be planned meticulously according to the prospective flap design. Generally, along this incision, the expander has to be removed, and it furthermore co-determines the axis of tissue transfer and possible relocation that can be performed. For rectangular expanders, an incision with half of the length of the base of the expander usually is sufficient for creating a suitable pocket [2]. The pocket is prepared slightly bigger than the full base size of the expander (0.5–1.0 cm), to enable a fully flat position after insertion [3].

The leak tightness and functionality of the tissue expander, its port, and the connecting tube should be tested by injection of a few milliliters of normal saline prior to the insertion into the prepared pocket.

Before insertion, the tissue expander is placed in a sterile solution with antibiotics. The port should be placed and fixed with subcutaneous non-resorbable sutures far enough away from the expander envelope. This helps to avoid accidental puncturing when injecting volume into the expander. The pouch should be sutured thoroughly in multiple layers with subcutaneous and skin sutures. Next, the expander should be filled with a small amount of saline (about 10% of its maximum capacity) to snuggly fill the created pouch. Negative-pressure drainage is applied routinely, and left until discharge is less than approximately 15 cc/24 h. A compressive bandage should be applied after the procedure. Antibiotics are recommended for 3–5 days postoperatively [3]. A case treated with tissue expander (among others) is depicted in Fig. 3.

After initial wound healing (3–4 weeks), the expander is inflated by injections of saline through the subcutaneous port in multiple small steps over several weeks leading to a slow stretching of the overlaying skin.

If the desired or maximum volume of inflation is reached, usually a phase of consolidation is needed. Then the expander is removed and the generated excess skin is ready for skin reconstruction in a second procedure.

The resulting capsule around the expander can either be removed or used to increase the stability and volume of the expanded tissue.

> **Important to Know**
> The expanded skin will retract to some degree as soon as the expander is removed. Thus, adequate overexpansion of the skin envelope is recommended as well as immediate reconstruction after removal of the tissue expander.

Major complications of tissue expander use can occur in 40% or more of cases. Problems include perforation of the skin, dehiscence of the wound or tissue pocket with exposure of the expander (2–25%), infection (6–13%), hematoma (13%), seroma (9%), perforation of the port or disconnection of the tubes (2%), and lack of adhesions of the expanded flap in the new wound bed (4%) [2–4]. Among independent risk factors for expander infection are the duration of the underlying disease for less than 1 year, expander

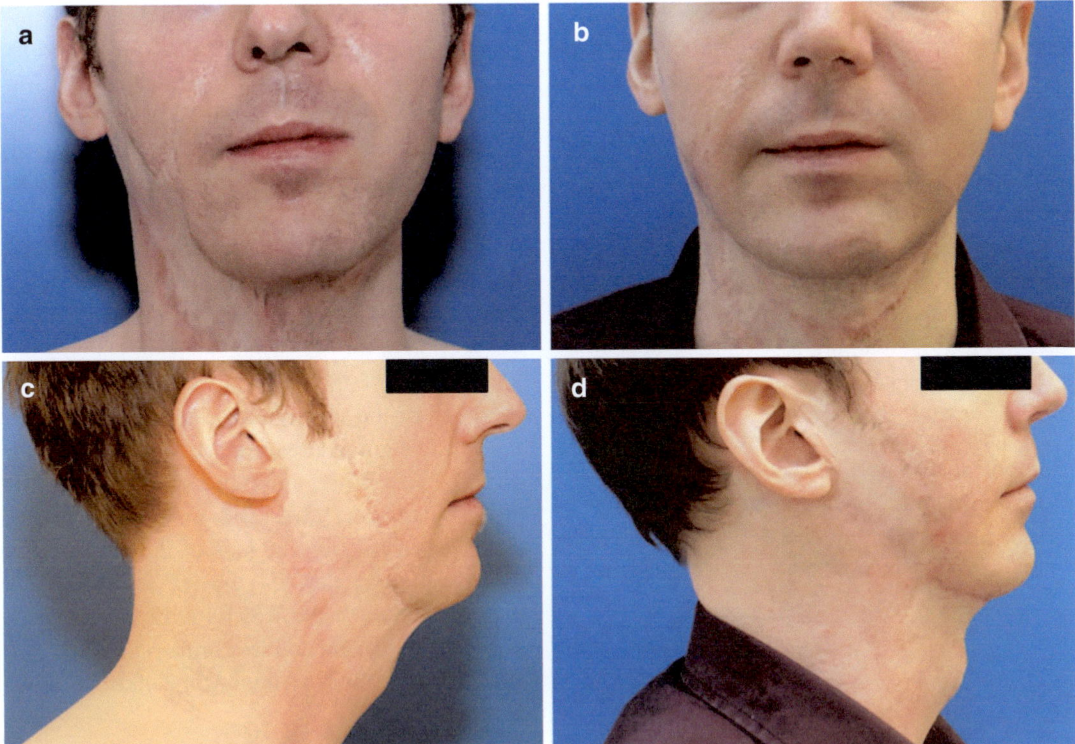

Fig. 3 Patient with mento-sternal contracture, destroyed jaw line, and a functionally and aesthetically disturbing areal scar in the neck, jowl, preauricular and paranasal area after third-degree burn injury during adolescence. (**a, c**) Preoperative frontal and lateral view. (**b, d**) Postoperative frontal and lateral view after tissue expansion in the right neck area with a 250 cc rectangular expander, Z-plasty on the frontal rim of the expanded tissue, full-thickness skin grafting to the mento-sternal area, split-thickness skin grafting to the right preauricular area, and lipofilling of the midface and jawline. The mento-sternal angle and the jaw line are reconstructed and facial symmetry is improved, especially in the frontal view

volume >200 mL, expander insertion at limb site, and prior necessity of hematoma evacuation from the wound bed [3]. In accordance with this, some authors recommend the use of smaller tissue expanders with subsequent, compensatory overexpansion by 30–50% [2]. Furthermore, meticulous hemostasis is essential as shown by these results. Some authors also found female gender and high blood pressure to be risk factors for expander complications [4].

Using tissue expanders can reduce the need of multiple procedures in serial scar excisions when removing larger scar areas. If a single-step procedure is preferred local vascularized pedicled flaps might be an alternative option. Tissue expansion is especially valuable in treating bald scars in hair-bearing areas of the scalp. The procedure can then serve as an alternative to hair transplantation, especially if the scar is not suitable for hair grafting because of low perfusion or low dermal and subcutaneous thickness [5].

> **Clinical Tip**
> Meticulous hemostasis should be performed to avoid formation of hematoma, which significantly increases the risk of postoperative complications and expander failure.

Flap Surgery

Local Flaps

The general principle of local flaps in scar revision surgery is to excise the disturbing scar and to reconstruct the resulting defect with local tissue rearrangement. In local flap surgery, one scar is traded for another. Thus, caution needs to be taken not to worsen the overall local aesthetic and functional situation.

Excisional and incisional techniques can be differentiated based on whether the scar tissue is removed or released in situ before neighboring tissue is rearranged in a variety of configurations [6]. In the following, a few flaps are presented due to their useful application in scar surgery. However, many more exist that might be suitable depending on the individual case.

> **Important to Know**
> It is important to handle soft tissue in an atraumatic fashion and being aware of relaxed skin tension lines to receive a pleasing and successful outcome.

> **Caution!**
> Be aware of reduced skin elasticity and vascularity in scarred areas.

Z-plasty

A Z-plasty is a local double transposition flap that is especially useful for lengthening and releasing restraining linear scar contractures. Examples may include areas over joints and the disruption and realignment of unfavorable running linear scars.

Z-plasties are used for the revision of scars that require alteration of their direction in relation to the RSTLs [6].

Z-plasties can also be used to reorient and disrupt impairing or contracted scar lines (see Fig. 4).

The axis of the original scar is used as the central portion of the "Z" while the parallel upper and lower limbs of the "Z" are placed obliquely on each end of the scar to rotate and reorient it (see Fig. 4). The procedure creates two triangular flaps of equal size in the adjacent skin undermined in the subcutaneous layer and transposed reciprocally. When rotating the axis of the original scar (central limb of the "Z") by 90° it can then be placed parallel to the RSTLs easily, making the scar less noticeable and less impairing. The linear scar is transformed to a nonlinear Z-like new structure [6] (Fig. 5).

> **Clinical Tip**
> Z-plasty makes scar lines less noticeable by reorientation and disruption. They are best used for contracted scars and those deviating more than 30° from the RSTLs.

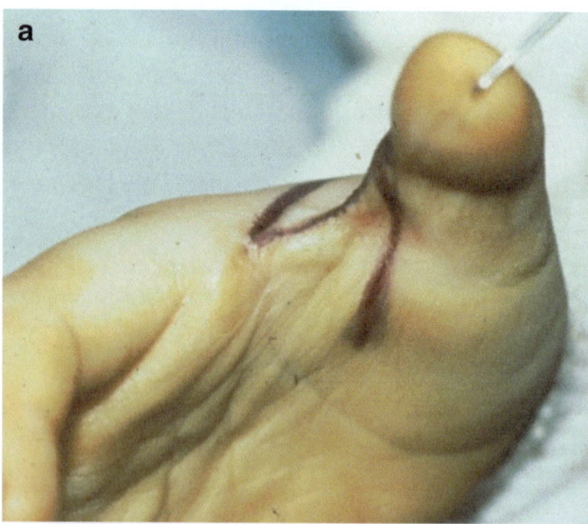
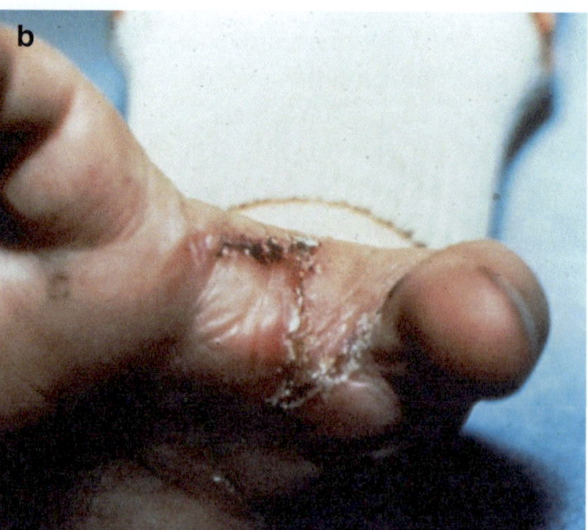

Fig. 4 Z-plasty to disrupt and realign a contracted and disturbing linear scar in the first web space of the right hand of a child. (**a**) Preoperative markings; the central portion of the Z is placed along the axis of the linear scar. (**b**) Result 2 weeks after the procedure with improved depth and motion range of the first web space

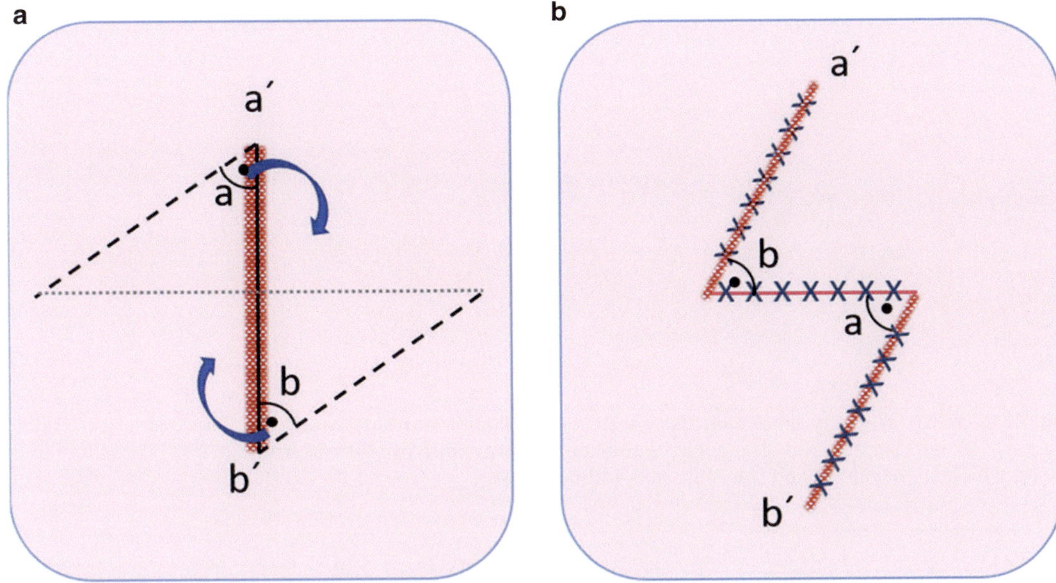

Fig. 5 Z-plasty. (**a**) The axis of the original scar is used as the central portion of the "Z" (**b**) while the parallel upper and lower limbs of the "Z" are placed obliquely on each end of the scar to rotate and reorient it

The angle between the central and the oblique portions of the "Z" determines how much the scar tissue is lengthened. Typically, angles of 60° between the central portion of the "Z" and its upper and lower oblique arms are used. The larger the angle, the greater the length gain. Theoretically, a 30° angle lengthens a scar by 25%, a 45° angle lengthens by 50%, a 60° angle lengthens by 75%, a 75° angle by 100%, and a 90° angle by 120–125% [7, 8]. However, scar lengthening might be impaired by reduced local scar skin elasticity. In contrast, when designing small angles, tip vascularity might be compromised. For this reason, an angle of 60° is most feasible in the majority of cases [8].

> **Clinical Tip**
> The larger the angles of the Z, the greater the length gain.

Instead of using a single large Z-plasty performing sequential smaller Z-plasties along an elongated scar can be favorable, making it less eye-catching with less lateral tension [8].

W-Plasty—Running W

A W-plasty breaks up the scar margins into small serial triangular components, which are advanced and interdigitated without rotation or transposition (see Fig. 6). This technique creates a new, more irregular scar that is less perceptible to the eye [6, 7].

An adequate amount of elastic and unaffected skin nearby is required to successfully perform a W-plasty. The reason for this is that not only the scar but also some adjacent skin has to be excised creating a defect that has to be covered by advancing surrounding tissue.

W-plasty design should be guided by the relaxed skin tension lines (RSTL) since the original, more perpendicular vector is changed into many small ones lying oblique or parallel to the RSTLs leading to less lateral tension force.

Bigger angles of the small "W"-triangles reduce the tension forces more effectively than a smaller ones would.

W-plasties can well be used on curved or concave surfaces [6, 8]. Goutos et al. recommend using isosceles triangles in areas with curved surfaces lacking clear RSTLs with one side of the triangles being placed parallel to the RSTLs. In

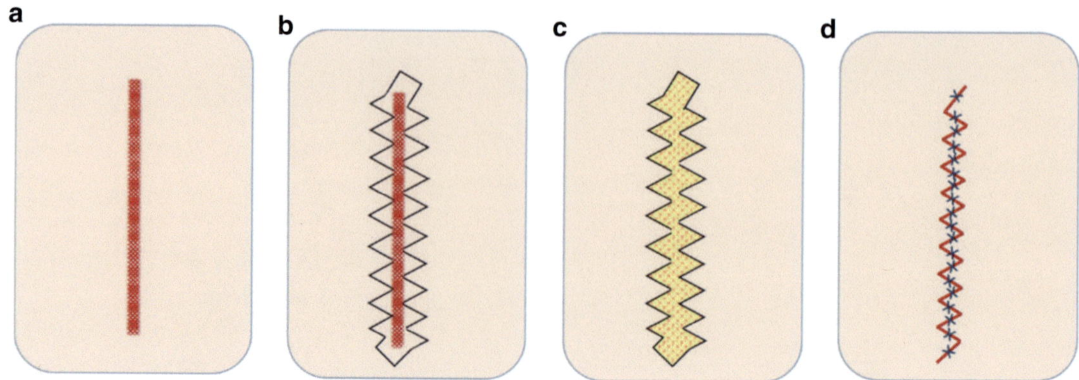

Fig. 6 W-plasty. W-plasty breaks up the linear scar margins (**a**) into small serial triangular components (**b, c**), which are advanced and interdigitated without rotation or transposition (**d**). This technique creates a new, more irregular scar that is less perceptible to the eye

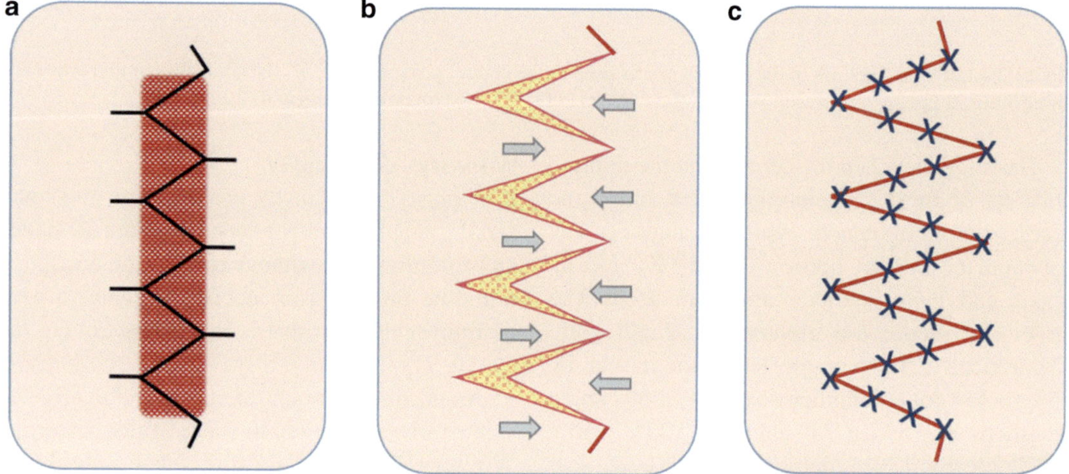

Fig. 7 (**a**) Multiple Y-V plasties. (**b**) Multiple consecutive Y-V-plasties can be used to release skin tension and to gain adjacent soft tissue. (**c**) The longer the straight limb of the "Y" is designed, the more advancement can be achieved

areas with well-defined RSTLs scalene triangles can be used with the smaller side of the triangle being placed along the wrinkle lines [6].

Multiple Y-V-Plasties

Multiple consecutive Y-V-plasties can be used to release skin tension and to gain adjacent soft tissue [9]. The longer the straight limb of the "Y" is designed, the more advancement can be achieved (see Fig. 7).

Vascularized Pedicled Regional Flaps

If no or not enough healthy and mobile adjacent tissue is available for coverage of defects after scar excision a local vascularized pedicled flap might be an option.

Vascularized pedicled flaps can also be a single-step alternative to multi-step procedures like tissue expanders or serial excisions.

However, the length and versatility of the vascular pedicle limit the possible distance between flap origin and the scar that needs to be reconstructed. Furthermore, it is crucial to think about the necessary incision lines and resulting scars of a potential flap in detail ahead of the procedure. This helps to avoid the generation of new unfavorable or debilitating scars in an area that is already limited in function and aesthetics.

For instance, while a pedicled latissimus dorsi flap (LDF) might cover defects from scars on the lateral or frontal chest a pedicled radial forearm flap could help reconstruct a defect on the dorsum of the hand. Both flaps can also be used as microvascular free flaps. For more detailed information check the recommendations in the "suggested reading" section at the end of this chapter.

Free Flaps

Local flaps are dependent on the availability of healthy and mobile adjacent skin, which is often rare for large areal scars. In such cases, microvascular free flaps might pose a valuable option for reconstruction.

A free flap is considered a free microvascular autologous tissue transfer with inherent vascular structures that has to be reconnected to blood supply by anastomosis to blood vessels in the recipient region.

Free flaps might be considered for covering defects after excision of large-scale scars, or for scars with no or not enough healthy adjacent tissue (see Fig. 8). Furthermore, if a complex reconstruction is needed, including more than skin and subcutaneous tissue, free flaps might also be the right choice.

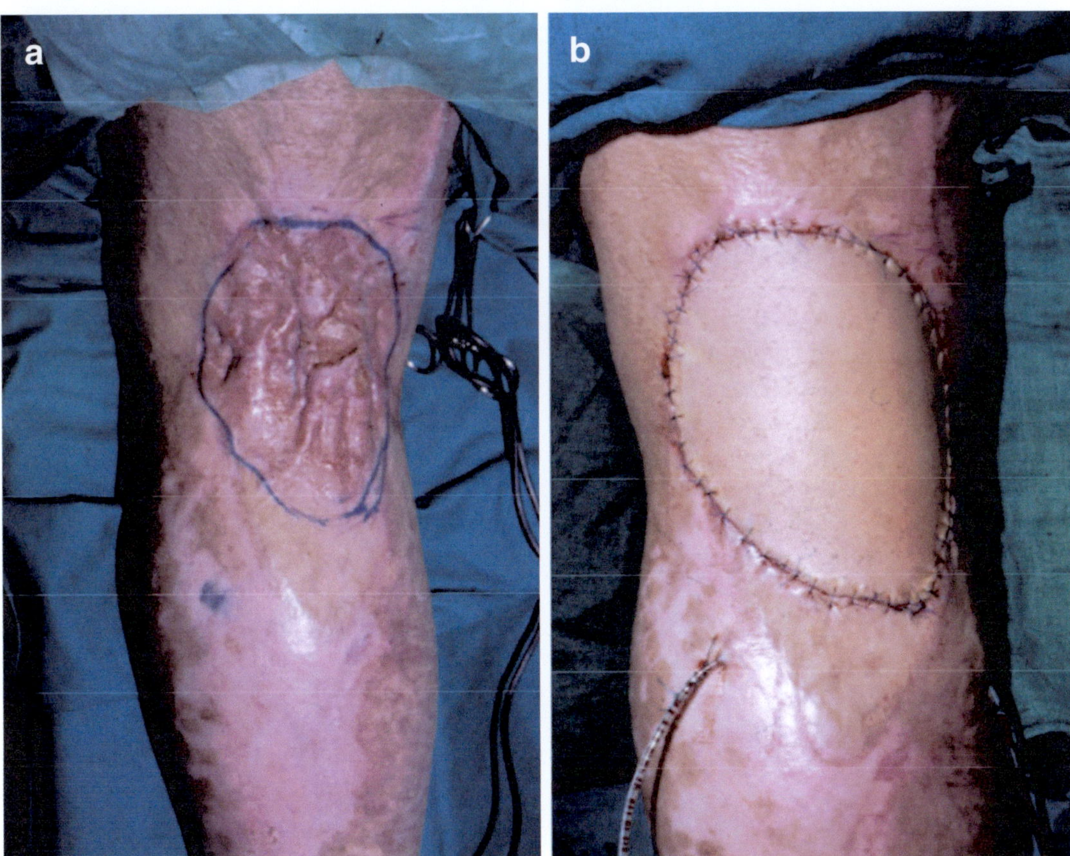

Fig. 8 Free microvascular scapula flap for reconstruction of a chronic wound in a contracted scar area in the Fossa poplitea. (**a**) Preoperative view. (**b**) Immediate postoperative view

There are multiple different options in choosing the perfect tissue match and flap size for the reconstruction of each individual scar situation. For instance, in situations with large scar areas, the anterior lateral thigh perforator flap (ALT) or the latissimus dorsi musculocutaneous free flap can prove a good choice due to the broad amount of available tissue.

The two main disadvantages of free flaps are their dependence on the patency of the underlying microvascular anastomosis and the general necessity of microvascular technique. The latter is not always available and requires extensive training. Furthermore, free flap surgery is often time-consuming and creates a second wound site in a new area with its potential complications. However, if a microvascular flap promises the best aesthetic and functional result, one should not hesitate to select this option.

For more detailed information check the recommendations in the "suggested reading" section at the end of this chapter.

Dermabrasion

Dermabrasion is a mechanically ablative surgical therapy in which the upper skin layers and the surrounding tissue of a scar are removed. This is achieved by a high-frequency rotating device, typically diamond drills. Dermabrasion can also be applied to blend scar lines with the surrounding tissue by smoothing sharp scar lines. The depth of ablation is an important parameter as it affects (1) the degree of new and/or hypertrophic scarring, (2) the likelihood of a fast and uncomplicated healing, and (3) the degree of aesthetic improvement of the scar.

Important to Know
New and stronger scarring and the camouflaging effect increase with the depth of the dermabrasion.

Often, multiple dermabrasion steps need to be performed to accomplish a satisfying result. In our experience, one should wait on average 6–12 months between each step. The waiting interval is determined by the depth of the treatment and interindividual differences.

Especially for deeper dermabrasions, it is recommended to wear compression garments and silicone scar pads for best results after the initial postoperative period.

Dermabrasion can be combined with different types of skin grafting, e.g., split thickness, suction blisters, or fluid spray-on cellular skin grafts [10].

Lipofilling—Fat Grafting

Fat grafts have been shown to improve a variety of symptoms related to scar tissue such as scar appearance, skin characteristics, and pain [11].

Adipose tissue offers multiple favorable properties and functions in scar revision surgery. First, it provides volume, which is essential to fill retracted, adherent, or hypovolemic scars and to restore contour (see Fig. 3). Second, it not only consists of volume-bearing adipocytes but also a multitude of stromal cells, the so-called stromal vascular fraction, which includes mesenchymal stem cells (MSCs). MSCs are known to have a number of modulating and positive effects on the skin. These include the stimulation of collagen synthesis and increase in dermal thickness, the support of neovascularization, the reduction of UVB-induced skin cell apoptosis and UVB-induced wrinkles, the protection of dermal fibroblasts from oxidative stress, and the inhibition of melanin synthesis and tyrosine kinase activity in melanocytes causing a "whitening" effect. Furthermore, fat grafting is thought to remodel the scar tissue from inside [12–16].

Fat grafting is often used to "reconstruct" a lost subcutaneous tissue layer below adherent scar tissue. Jasper et al. could show that a single-step procedure of autologous fat grafting leads to a significant improvement of skin elasticity and maximal extension. They could also show a significant reduction of pain after 3 months in patients treated for adherent scars after severe burn trauma, degloving injuries, or necrotizing fasciitis [17].

Subcutaneous liposuction is most commonly used for adipose tissue harvest with the abdomen and the trochanteric region being the most common sites. This can either be performed with power assistance or manually. For manual liposuction, Coleman harvesting cannula and Luer Lock syringes are used with a gradual negative suction being applied. After fat harvest, different methods can be employed to prepare the adipose tissue for transplantation into the recipient area. These include decantation, centrifugation, emulgation, use of strainers, and adding platelet-rich plasma (PRP). PRP is thought to influence adipose tissue performance at recipient sites and overall outcome [17, 18].

Proceeded adipose tissue is most commonly reinjected at the recipient site manually with blunt cannula during withdrawal in a fan-like manner. This method can also be used for adhesiolysis of adherent scar tissue. Since adipocytes are sensitive to mechanical stress and pressure it is recommended to thoroughly undermine retraced scars and release possible adhesions. Prior to applying, the fat transplant performing a subcision can help achieve this and prevent common problems such as low graft take and the development of oil cysts.

Multiple sessions are recommended to fill deeper defects instead of using a larger amount of adipose tissue in one session.

Volume retention and take rate of fat grafts vary from 30 to 90% and seem to depend largely on the application technique as well as on the use of additional supplements. These include the stromal vascular fraction, platelet-rich plasma, or insulin [11]. A 3D-multi-depot approach with application of many small doses of adipose tissue in different layers is favorable compared to the application of a large single depot at one site. Slow injection and the use of blunt cannulas are recommended [18]. To date, no single technique can be recommended unequivocally.

Among others, possible complications of fat grafting are swelling, bruising, infections at donor and recipient site, low graft take/fat necrosis, contour irregularities, formation of oil cysts or calcifications, and fat thrombosis or embolism [18].

Skin Grafting

Skin grafting might be useful in scar reconstruction to enable skin coverage after scar release, to deal with hypopigmentation, or to improve overall skin appearance. Among others, skin grafting includes split-thickness skin grafts, full-thickness skin grafts, transplantation of epidermal microdomes, and liquid skin grafts.

Autologous skin grafts are in general classified according to the depth of the skin harvest and the thickness of the explant. Split-thickness skin grafts include the epidermis and a small portion of the dermis leaving the deeper, reticular dermis intact. Depending on the amount of dermis included they can be further subclassified as thin (0.13–0.32 mm), intermediate (0.33–0.45 mm), and thick (0.46–0.76 mm). Full-thickness skin grafts consist of the epidermis and the entire thickness of the dermis, and are usually thicker than 0.6 mm [19, 20].

Split-thickness skin grafts are usually harvested using a dermatome in which the thickness of the harvested skin can be adjusted.

Full-thickness grafts are usually harvested by surgical excision in areas with sufficient skin laxity to enable primary closure of the created defect.

Split-thickness skin grafts are more often and intensely subject to graft contraction during healing compared to full-thickness skin grafts. The latter show less contraction and more elasticity since contraction is related to the amount of dermis. Split-thickness skin grafts are therefore often less cosmetically appealing and also less durable [20]. However, graft take is often easier and more reliable in split-thickness skin grafts. This is especially true when the vascular supply of the recipient site is limited. Split-thickness skin grafts are also more suitable for larger areas in need of covering compared to a full-thickness skin graft, due to the higher availability of donor sites. Another advantage of full-thickness skin grafts on the other hand is that they show only minimal wound contraction and supply further dermal adnexal structures. However, these grafts require a rich vascular supply for successful graft take. Often best results are achieved by choosing a donor site in the same region as the recipient site with a good color and texture match. To accommodate for graft shrinkage, full-thickness skin grafts should be about 3–5% larger than the defect to be covered [20].

> **Important to Know**
> Split-thickness skin grafts tend to contract more than full-thickness skin grafts but they also show easier and more reliable graft take especially in recipient sites with impaired vascular supply.

Since skin grafts lack an autonomous blood supply at the time of transplantation into the recipient site, close contact with the underlying, well-vascularized wound bed is crucial for revascularization and reliable take of the graft. Therefore, hematoma or other fluid collections in the wound bed hinder graft take and need to be avoided. In split-thickness skin graft sheets, drainage of wound fluid is facilitated by adding multiple small slits or holes in the graft before applying it to the recipient site.

Meshing a graft allows the graft to stretch, which might be useful to cover larger areas but also impairs aesthetic outcomes.

Additionally, immobilization of the affected area, as well as fixating compression of the graft into the wound bed, is recommended to minimize shearing forces and the risk of fluid collection beneath the graft and recipient site. Vascular proliferation into the graft mostly occurs 3–7 days after the procedure [19, 20].

> **Clinical Tip**
> Close contact between skin graft and recipient site is crucial for graft take. Avoid hematoma or fluid collection underneath the skin graft by meticulous hemostasis and by installing a compressive garment on the skin graft.

For scar reconstruction and especially treatment of hypopigmentation, split-thickness skin grafts should be preferentially placed as full sheet and not as meshed graft. This is because a full-sheet skin graft offers a more aesthetical outcome than a meshed or otherwise structured skin graft, since in meshed skin grafts, the wound healing in between the mesh occurs as secondary healing.

If only hypopigmentation needs to be addressed split-thickness skin-graft sheets or epidermal micrografts harvested via suction of blister microdomes can be considered. Epidermal micrografts offer the advantages of a harvest procedure without general need for anesthesia and donor site healing without visible scarring in most cases [21, 22].

Dermal substitutes for reconstruction can complement split-thickness skin grafts with positive effects, e.g., on the pliability of the grafts after the excision of full-thickness scars or for the treatment of postburn scar contractures and hypopigmentation [23–25].

Hair Transplantation

The restoration of hair-bearing skin areas in scalp or facial scars can improve aesthetic outcome and individual self-esteem tremendously. Typical situations include scars from burn, trauma, or surgical procedures such as cleft lip repair, brow, forehead, or scalp surgeries [26, 27].

Hair restoration can either be performed with autologous hair transplantation or by excision, use of tissue expanders, or local flaps originating in adjacent healthy tissue with high hair density [5, 28].

There are two main different methods to gain hair follicles for transplantation, follicular unit extraction (FUE), and follicular unit transplantation (FUT). FUT is also known as "strip method" and relies on the subcutaneous excision of a fusiform, horizontal strip from the occipital hair-bearing scalp. This strip is then further dissected into multiple follicular units. These are naturally occurring groups of one to four hair roots with surrounding sebaceous glands, nerves, erector pili muscle, and supporting fat and stroma. The follicular units can later be retransferred into the recipient area. The donor site is closed by primary suture [29].

To avoid the linear scar after excision of the fusiform FUT strip, FUE was developed. FUE uses small circular punches with outer diameter sizes mostly from 0.8 to 1.05 mm to remove individual follicular units from the donor area without creating a visible linear scar (see Fig. 9). The extraction sites heal with small, diffusely scattered circular scars that are often easier to camouflage. This is especially important for patients who prefer short haircuts. Furthermore, postoperative pain is reduced compared to FUT [29].

Benefits of autologous hair transplantation include the lack of additional tissue excision, no creation of major visible scars and incision lines (when performing FUE), and the possibility of placing the grafts in the natural hair growth direction. However, FUE is a delicate procedure that requires prior thorough technical training.

> **Clinical Tip**
> Follicular unit extraction (FUE) can improve aesthetic outcome in facial or scalp scar without creation of major visible scars and incision lines.

Lipofilling to restore the subcutaneous fat layer prior to hair transplantation in deeply scarred tissue is often needed at the recipient site for the hair grafts. This might also be a useful combination to cover up philtral scars and alopecia after cleft lip repair [30]. Furthermore, it might be necessary to perform a second session of hair transplantation 1 year after the first procedure to obtain the desired hair density [26].

Due to a lack of subcutaneous tissue, vascularization and regular skin structure, the regrowth of the transplanted hair and the take of the follicular grafts might be considerably reduced compared to regular unscarred skin.

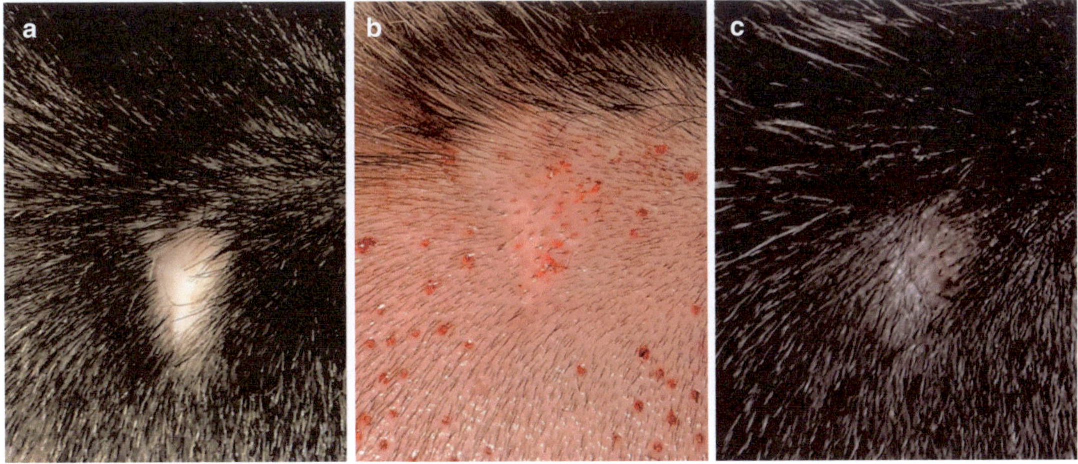

Fig. 9 FUE hair transplantation to a scar in the hair-bearing scalp. (**a**) Burn scar from early childhood with disturbing alopecia. (**b**) Situs immediately after transplantation of autologous FUE grafts with an extraction punch size of 0.8 mm. The small extraction wholes (**b**) will heal without major scarring. (**c**) 2 weeks after the procedure

> **Important to Know**
> Graft take and hair regrowth might be impaired in scarred areas.

Postoperative Care

Achieving the optimal result after scar revision surgery always includes proper postoperative care such as wearing compression garments with or without additional silicone scar pads, using UV/sun protection, and adding additional non-surgical applications (e.g., lasers when appropriate; see respective chapters).

Conclusion

Surgical scar therapy includes a multitude of different techniques from microsurgical to local flaps, from dermabrasion to serial excisions, from lipofilling or skin grafts to hair transplantation. Not all techniques are suitable for every type of scar. Minimal new scarring and preventing problematic scars from the start should be standard in every surgical procedure. Before any intervention, however, thorough consultation of the patients' wishes is required to align expectations with possibilities.

References

1. De Filippo RE, Atala A. Stretch and growth: the molecular and physiologic influences of tissue expansion. Plast Reconstr Surg. 2002;109(7):2450–62.
2. Karimi H, Latifi NA, Momeni M, Sedigh-Maroufi S, Karimi AM, Akhoondinasab MR. Tissue expanders; review of indications, results and outcome during 15 years' experience. Burns. 2019;45(4):990–1004.
3. Dong C, Zhu M, Huang L, Liu W, Liu H, Jiang K, et al. Risk factors for tissue expander infection in scar reconstruction: a retrospective cohort study of 2374 consecutive cases. Burns Trauma. 2020;8:tkaa037.
4. Smolle C, Tuca A, Wurzer P, Spendel SM, Forbes AA, Spendel S, et al. Complications in tissue expansion: a logistic regression analysis for risk factors. Burns. 2017;43(6):1195–202.
5. Shin H, Shin J, Lee JY. Scarred scalp reconstruction with a rectangular expander. Arch Craniofac Surg. 2020;21(3):184–7.
6. Goutos I, Yousif AH, Ogawa R. W-plasty in scar revision: geometrical considerations and suggestions for site-specific design modifications. Plast Reconstr Surg Glob Open. 2019;7(4):e2179.
7. Kadakia S, Ducic Y, Jategaonkar A, Chan D. Scar revision: surgical and nonsurgical options. Facial Plast Surg. 2017;33(6):621–6.
8. Sharma M, Wakure A. Scar revision. Indian J Plast Surg. 2013;46(2):408–18.
9. Shaw DT, Li CS. Multiple Y-V plasty. Ann Plast Surg. 1979;2(5):436–40.
10. Driscoll DN, Levy AN, Gama AR. Dermabrasion and thin epidermal grafting for treatment of large and small areas of postburn leukoderma: a case series and review of the literature. J Burn Care Res. 2016;37(4):e387–93.
11. Negenborn VL, Groen JW, Smit JM, Niessen FB, Mullender MG. The use of autologous fat grafting for treatment of scar tissue and scar-related conditions: a systematic review. Plast Surg Nurs. 2016;36(3):131–43.
12. Gargano F, Schmidt S, Evangelista P, Robinson-Bostom L, Harrington DT, Rossi K, et al. Burn scar regeneration with the "SUFA" (subcision and fat grafting) technique. A prospective clinical study. JPRAS Open. 2018;17:5–8.
13. Kim WS, Park BS, Sung JH. The wound-healing and antioxidant effects of adipose-derived stem cells. Expert Opin Biol Ther. 2009;9(7):879–87.
14. Forcheron F, Agay D, Scherthan H, Riccobono D, Herodin F, Meineke V, et al. Autologous adipocyte derived stem cells favour healing in a minipig model of cutaneous radiation syndrome. PLoS One. 2012;7(2):e31694.
15. Kim WS, Park BS, Park SH, Kim HK, Sung JH. Antiwrinkle effect of adipose-derived stem cell: activation of dermal fibroblast by secretory factors. J Dermatol Sci. 2009;53(2):96–102.
16. Si Z, Wang X, Sun C, Kang Y, Xu J, Wang X, et al. Adipose-derived stem cells: sources, potency, and implications for regenerative therapies. Biomed Pharmacother. 2019;114:108765.
17. Jaspers MEH, Brouwer KM, van Trier AJM, Middelkoop E, van Zuijlen PPM. Sustainable effectiveness of single-treatment autologous fat grafting in adherent scars. Wound Repair Regen. 2017;25(2):316–9.
18. Simonacci F, Bertozzi N, Grieco MP, Grignaffini E, Raposio E. Procedure, applications, and outcomes of autologous fat grafting. Ann Med Surg (Lond). 2017;20:49–60.
19. Andreassi A, Bilenchi R, Biagioli M, D'Aniello C. Classification and pathophysiology of skin grafts. Clin Dermatol. 2005;23(4):332–7.
20. Wanner A, Adams C, Ratner D. Skin grafts. In: Rohrer TE, Cook JL, Migden MR, editors. Flaps and grafts in dermatologic surgery. Amsterdam: Elsevier; 2008. p. 107–16.
21. Herskovitz I, Hughes OB, Macquhae F, Rakosi A, Kirsner R. Epidermal skin grafting. Int Wound J. 2016;13(Suppl 3):52–6.

22. Maderal AD, Kirsner RS. Clinical and economic benefits of autologous epidermal grafting. Cureus. 2016;8(11):e875.
23. Lebo PB, Grohmann M, Kamolz L. Delayed post-burn scar reconstruction of the dorsum of the hand with a collagen-elastin-based dermal substitute and split-skin graft. Handchir Mikrochir Plast Chir. 2017;49(2):127–31.
24. Oh SJ, Kim Y. Combined AlloDerm(R) and thin skin grafting for the treatment of postburn dyspigmented scar contracture of the upper extremity. J Plast Reconstr Aesthet Surg. 2011;64(2):229–33.
25. Yi JW, Kim JK. Prospective randomized comparison of scar appearances between cograft of acellular dermal matrix with autologous split-thickness skin and autologous split-thickness skin graft alone for full-thickness skin defects of the extremities. Plast Reconstr Surg. 2015;135(3):609e–16e.
26. Jung S, Oh SJ, Hoon KS. Hair follicle transplantation on scar tissue. J Craniofac Surg. 2013;24(4):1239–41.
27. Kilic A, Kilic A, Emsen IM, Ozdengil E. Lip scars camouflaged using microhair transplantation on male patients. Plast Reconstr Surg. 2000;106(6):1340–1.
28. Yoo H, Moh J, Park JU. Treatment of postsurgical scalp scar deformity using follicular unit hair transplantation. Biomed Res Int. 2019;2019:3423657.
29. Lee LN. Hair transplant surgery and platelet rich plasma. 1st ed. Cham: Springer International; 2020.
30. Akdag O, Evin N, Karamese M, Tosun Z. Camouflaging cleft lip scar using follicular unit extraction hair transplantation combined with autologous fat grafting. Plast Reconstr Surg. 2018;141(1):148–51.

Further Reading

Hierner R, Putz R, Bishop AT, Shen Z, Wilhelm K. Flaps in hand and upper limb reconstruction: surgical anatomy, operative techniques and differential therapy. Amsterdam: Elsevier; 2016.
Strauch B, Yu H. Atlas of microvascular surgery: anatomy and operative techniques. Stuttgart: Thieme; 2006.
Wanner A, Adams C, Ratner D. Chapter 9: Skin grafts. In: Flaps and grafts in dermatologic surgery. Amsterdam: Elsevier; 2008. p. 107–16.
Zenn MR, Jones G. Reconstructive surgery: anatomy, technique, and clinical application. Stuttgart: Thieme; 2012.

Oral Medication

Prevention and Therapy—Neurobiological Management of Scars

Varitsara Mangkorntongsakul, Alan J. Cooper, and Saxon D. Smith

Core Messages
- Neuropathic pain and itch arise as a consequence of pathological processes within the central nervous system (CNS) or through sensitisation of both CNS and the peripheral nervous system (PNS), resulting in chronic and persistent symptoms.
- Tricyclic antidepressants (TCAs), duloxetine and gabapentinoids are recommended as the first-line treatment for neuropathic pain based on Grading of Recommendations Assessment, Development, and Evaluation (GRADE) recommendation.
- Antihistamines, including cetirizine, cimetidine and loratadine, are recommended as the first-line oral agents for both adult and paediatric patients based on GRADE classification.
- Ondansetron is recommended as a second-line medication for the treatment of pruritus in both adult and paediatric patients based on GRADE classification.

Introduction

Pathological wound healing and scar formation are major medical challenges causing significant psychological and physical distress. Not only do they give rise to functional and aesthetic disadvantages, but scars can also result in various degrees of sensation disturbances. The sensation of itch and pain is closely related but also clearly distinct. Dysfunction of the nervous system and immune response will consequently lead to the development of chronic symptoms of itchy and painful scars, which have the capacity to become increasingly complex and potentially more difficult to treat over time. Recent advances in pharmaceutical drug design and medical treatment reveal numerous preventative and therapeutic modalities to manage these chronic and disabling symptoms. In this chapter, the authors reviewed the current literature on oral pharmacological approaches to symptoms of scar neuropathy, mainly related to burn hypertrophic and keloid scars, and prevention of acne scarring.

V. Mangkorntongsakul (✉)
Northern Clinical School, Sydney Medical School, University of Sydney, Sydney, NSW, Australia

Gosford Hospital, Central Coast Local Health District, Gosford, NSW, Australia

A. J. Cooper
Northern Clinical School, Sydney Medical School, University of Sydney, Sydney, NSW, Australia

Department of Dermatology, Royal North Shore Hospital, St Leonards, NSW, Australia

S. D. Smith
Northern Clinical School, Sydney Medical School, University of Sydney, Sydney, NSW, Australia

Sydney Adventist Hospital Clinic School, ANU Medical School, ANU College of Health and Medicine, The Australian National University, Canberra, ACT, Australia

The Dermatology and Skin Cancer Centre, St Leonards, Sydney, NSW, Australia

S. P. Nischwitz et al. (eds.), *Scars*, https://doi.org/10.1007/978-3-031-24137-6_13

Pathophysiology of Pain and Itch in Dermal Scar Tissues

Pain is defined as a distressing sensory and emotional experience associated with potential or actual tissue damage [1]. Physiologically, this is described as the activation of specialised primary afferent neurons originating as free nerve endings in the cutaneous tissues, namely myelinated A-delta fibres and subtypes of unmyelinated C fibre by a broad spectrum of painful neuromodulators. These include but are not limited to acetylcholine, bradykinin, adenosine triphosphate and prostaglandin [2].

Following the depolarisation and activation of action potentials, A-delta fibres and C-fibres release the neurotransmitters (L-glutamate) and neuropeptides (glutamate, substance P and calcitonin gene-related peptide [CGRP]), respectively. The impulse is then carried to the dorsal column through the ascending pathway and forms a synapse with second-order neurons, which subsequently cross over to the contralateral side of the ascending spinothalamic tract to reach the thalamus and pons and onto different parts of the brain, evoking a withdrawal reflex. Although they play no role in acute pain activation, A-beta fibres are involved in the basis of chronic neuropathic pain by modulating peripheral nociceptors under the gate control theory of pain [3].

Pain can be categorised as acute or chronic as determined by the duration of the symptoms or nociceptive or non-nociceptive pain (neuropathic or psychogenic) as determined by the underlying pathophysiology [3].

Acute pain serves a protective purpose to prevent individuals from potentially hazardous situations. Chronic pain, however, has little protective significance and can cause distress if the pain persists for three or more months despite normalisation after injury [4].

Nociceptive pain is a natural physiological response towards a noxious stimulus through activation or sensitisation of peripheral nociceptors. Once the stimuli are removed, the symptom then subsides. Neuropathic pain, on the other hand, arises as a consequence of pathological processes within the central nervous system (CNS) or through sensitisation of the peripheral nervous system (PNS), resulting in chronic and persistent pain—a frequently observed symptom of scar tissues [2].

Itch (pruritus) is defined as an unpleasant cutaneous sensation that provokes the desire to scratch [5]. Itch can be a symptom of distinct skin conditions or of occult underlying systemic diseases [6]. Itch can be classified into acute and chronic with acute itch lasting less than 6 weeks and chronic itch lasting longer than 6 weeks. However, in burn survivors, acute itch was proposed to last less than 3–6 months and chronic itch can last up to 6 months postburn injury [2, 7]. Itch can be further categorised into four subtypes according to their underlying pathophysiology: pruritoceptive, neuropathic, neurogenic and psychogenic [2, 6, 7].

Similar to pain, the mechanisms of itch can originate from the CNS or peripheral nervous system (PNS) [6]. The precise mechanism of pruritic scars is not well understood, but it has been suggested to display a mixture of pruritogenic and neuropathic features such as ongoing paresthesia [8]. Postburn pruritus has been shown to be intractable to traditional treatment of antihistamine but is instead noted to be responsive to neuroleptic agents [9].

Following an injury, pruritoceptive itch arises from pruritogenic neuromediators released from cutaneous inflammation and C-fibres which are mediated by various endogenous pruritogens. These neuromediators work by directly stimulating nerve endings, activating the release of cytokines responsible for pruritic sensation or sensitising the specialised C-fibres [2, 6]. These unmyelinated C-fibres are anatomically identical to those associated with the mediation of pain but are functionally distinct [6].

C-fibres are broadly categorised into two groups based on mechanosensitivity: mechanically sensitive polymodal nociceptors (C mechano-heat (CMH) nociceptor) and mechanically insensitive C-fibres (C-MIAs) [10]. The CMH nociceptor is the most common type of C-fibre which is associated with non-histaminergic mechanisms as this fibre is either insensitive to histamine or comparatively weak in response to it. The fibre also plays a role in a mechanism of poor localisation and dull pain sensation [6, 11]. C-MIAs, consisting of 5% of all afferent C-fibres, are thought to mediate histamine-induced itch pathway. This is because they vigorously respond to histamine and other pruritogenic neuromediators but are unresponsive to mechanical stimuli [11]. They convey pruritic impulses to the dorsal horn of the spinal cord and form a synapse with secondary neurons that cross to the contralateral spinothalamic tract. C-MIAs then ascend to the ventromedial and dorsomedial nuclei, and on to the somatosensory cortex, producing the desire to scratch [6, 9, 11].

After an acute phase of wound healing, histamine is known to be less important to the pruritic mechanism. At the chronic stage, neuropathic itch is proposed to be the main underlying pathophysiology which is characterised by antihistamine-resistant wound with neural sensitisation [9].

While the differences in pain and itch are apparent in acute settings, they share many similar mechanisms in chronic wounds involving peripheral sensitisation as well as central sensitisation [13]. There are two mechanisms that have been postulated to cause peripheral sensitisation in chronic sensory phenomena in burn survivors: the injured afferent hypothesis and the intact nociceptor hypothesis.

The concept of **injured afferent hypothesis** posits that neuropathic pain and itch may arise from a neuroma, which is an injured primary peripheral afferent nerve fibre, resulting in disorganised growth of unmyelinated C fibres from injured axons. This leads to spontaneous excitability secondary to enhanced sensitivity to mechanical, thermal and chemical stimuli [9, 14]. In the **intact nociceptor hypothesis**, it has been suggested that uninjured nociceptors that innervate the area affected by the transacted nerve fibres become sensitised and develop spontaneous activity [2, 14].

In established central sensitisation, there is a persistent autonomous activity in the CNS related to aberrant somatosensory processing which shifts maintenance into a chronic phase. Several mechanisms have been hypothesised as the basis of central sensitisation in neuropathic phenomena, namely increased activity of dorsal horn projection neurons, deafferentation theory, loss of CNS inhibitory neurons, loss of descending inhibition and synaptic reorganisation (Fig. 1) [9].

The repetitive stimulation of the peripheral nociceptor amplifies nociceptive information, which then causes an **increase in activity of dorsal horn projection neurons** of the spinal cord. The afferent terminal then releases excitatory neurotransmitter glutamate and substance P [1, 9]. A-beta fibres are responsible for modulation of nociceptor impulses and indirect interruption of sensory transmission by inhibiting the effect of nociceptive afferents. Following tissue injury, **loss of myelinated A-beta fibres (deafferentation theory)** input allows excess disinhibited noxious stimuli to reach the CNS. Inhibitory effects in the CNS are modulated by γ-aminobutyric acid (GABA) interneurons in the dorsal horn and descending pathway, which when stimulated lead to inhibitory effects of nociceptors in laminae of the spinal cord [2, 9]. Thus, **loss of CNS inhibitory neurons and descending inhibition** are linked to chronic sensory disturbances through decreasing inhibition of nociceptive pathway and increasing excitability and sensitivity of the CNS. Furthermore, an injury to the skin can lead to **synaptic reorganisation** where neuronal loss or loss of synaptic connection as deafferentation causes alterations to the functional topography in the primary somatosensory cortex. Thus, injured afferent neurons mediate reorganisation that creates a distorted mapping of the skin [9, 15].

In neuropathic pain, prolonged repetitive activation of nociceptors not only leads to pain at the site of the wound but also sensitises second-order neurons in the dorsal horn. This combination enhances the perception of cutaneous somatosensation due to a decrease in the threshold of pain-evoking stimuli. This is a natural phenomenon known as primary hyperalgesia, which is largely

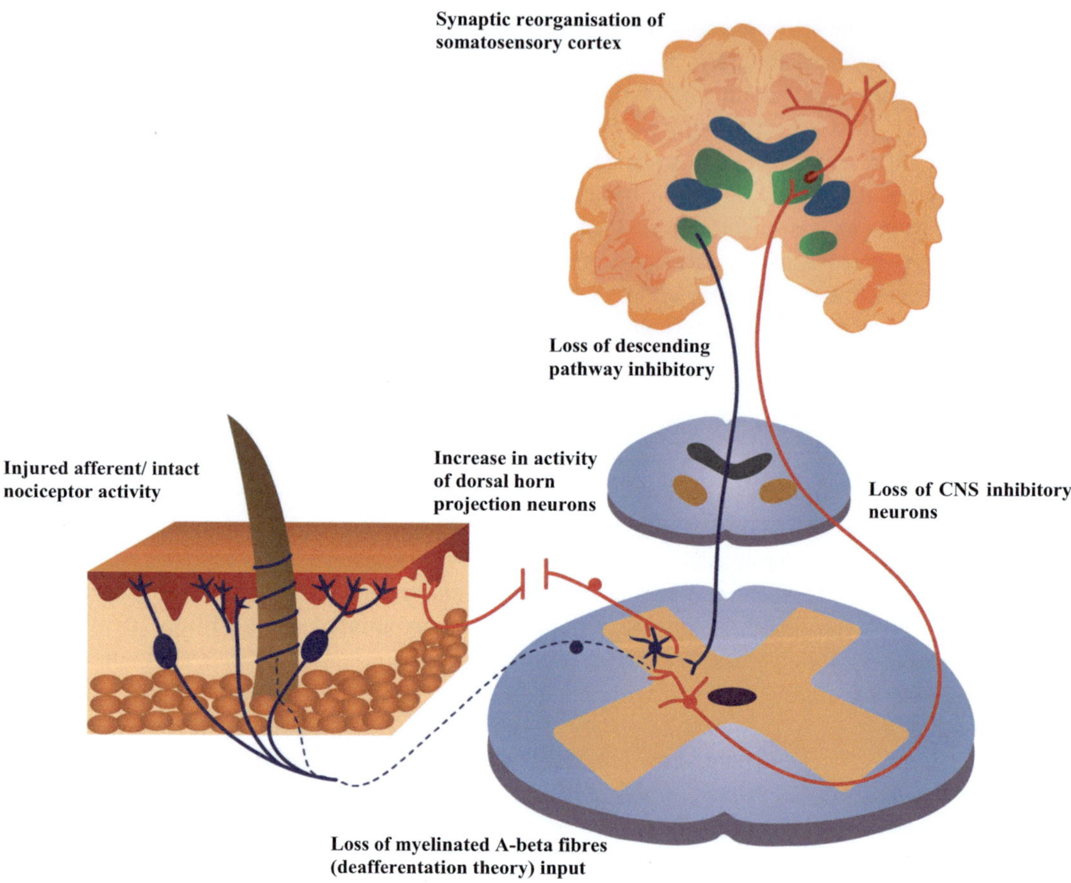

Fig. 1 Schematic diagram of mechanisms underlying peripheral and central nervous system neuropathies. Adapted from [2, 12]

related to the peripheral component of the nervous system.

Secondary hyperalgesia or allodynia, on the other hand, is due to central sensitisation. The sensation is characterised by touch or brush-evoked pain induced by typically innocuous mechanical stimuli in the uninjured regions of an injury. This occurs as a result of anatomical reorganisation in which the primary afferent A-fibres that normally carry non-noxious stimuli gain access to activate the pain pathway in dorsal horn neurons [1, 11]. These pain sensitisation phenomena are analogous to the itch dysesthesias, such as allokenesis and hyperkinesis, where itch is evoked by non-pruritic stimuli and itch perception is intensified in response to itch-induced stimuli, respectively [11, 16].

Pharmacological Therapy for Scar Tissue Pain

Neuropathic pain arises from scar tissues and is caused by injury to the afferent nerve resulting in dysfunction of the somatosensory system [17]. To provide optimal therapeutic approach to painful scars, the management often involved a combination modality including both pharmacological and non-pharmacological therapies. The current evidence for oral pharmacotherapy of neuropathic painful scars, which is mainly related to burn hypertrophic and keloid scars, supports the use of tricyclic antidepressants (TCAs), serotonin-norepinephrine reuptake inhibitors (SNRIs), gabapentin and pregabalin. There is no consensus on the best therapeutic approach to neuropathic pain due to scar tissues; thus there is a need for a more comprehensive study, specifically regarding neuropathic pain in scar tissues.

Antidepressants

Antidepressants are commonly prescribed for the management of chronic neuropathic pain. However, there have been limited studies investigating the efficacy of antidepressants in the management of scar pain. Chronic scar pain has a component of neuropathic pain; thus, it can be hypothesised that effective agents for neuropathic pain may provide analgesic properties to attenuate pain in scar tissues. The coexistence of pain and depression may be due to altered neuroplasticity and neurobiological mechanisms in the CNS regions, which may be responsible for both mood and peripheral pain [18]. Therefore, antidepressants can be a useful option in the treatment of neuropathic pain in individuals with coexisting mood disorders.

Although the underlying mechanisms of antidepressant properties in neuropathic pain have not been clearly delineated, the dosage of these drugs for analgesia is lower than that for treating depression, suggesting plausible different mechanisms of action. Increasing evidence has shown that noradrenaline plays a vital role in the reduction of neuropathic pain. Inhibition of noradrenaline reuptake in the spinal cord has been shown to have a direct analgesic effect on neuropathic pain through α2-adrenergic receptors. It has been observed that increasing the level of noradrenaline around the locus coeruleus improves the impaired activity of the descending noradrenergic inhibitory system. Moreover, studies have found that serotonin and dopamine may facilitate the anti-neuropathic effects of noradrenaline [19].

Tricyclic antidepressants (TCAs) and serotonin-norepinephrine reuptake inhibitor (SNRIs), such as duloxetine, were recommended as the first-line treatment for neuropathic pain based on strong Grading of Recommendations Assessment, Development, and Evaluation (GRADE) recommendations for use [20].

Tricyclic Antidepressants

Due to their lack of selectivity, TCAs have shown to have superior therapeutic effects in the treatment of neuropathic pain compared to that of SNRIs. However, the clinical use of TCAs is limited, in particular in elderly subjects, due to significant side effects including potent anticholinergic effects, sedation, postural hypotension and heart block as well as fatal cardiac arrhythmia [21, 22].

Amitriptyline is believed to provide analgesic control through inhibition of voltage-gated sodium channels and serotonin-norepinephrine reuptake. It may also have a direct effect on central sensitisation by blocking NMDA receptors in the spinal cord which induces hyperalgesia [22, 23].

In 2017, an animal study conducted by Hiroki et al. demonstrated that despite the suppression of inhibitory descending noradrenergic system, amitriptyline still provides significant anti-hyperalgesic properties through mediating neurons in locus coeruleus and enhances noradrenergic fibre density. These findings suggest that amitriptyline may enhance the analgesic effect of other neuropathic medications which requires an intact descending noradrenergic inhibition pathway. Thus, this property makes amitriptyline a potential effective analgesic option for combination therapy with SNRI and gabapentinoids [24].

These findings may explain Gilron et al. (2009)'s observation in their double-blind, randomised controlled, crossover trial with 56 subjects comparing the efficacy of nortriptyline and gabapentin as monotherapy versus combination therapy for neuropathic pain. A combination therapy was found to be more efficacious than either drug as monotherapy [25].

Nortriptyline, a secondary amine TCAs, has shown equivalent benefits to amitriptyline but was found to be better tolerated with fewer toxicity profiles [26, 27]. However, the available evidence to support the claim that nortriptyline has less associated adverse effects remains inconsistent [27].

Serotonin-Norepinephrine Reuptake Inhibitor

Duloxetine, a serotonin-norepinephrine reuptake inhibitor (SNRI), also has been recommended as a first-line treatment based on GRADE recommendations due to consistent reports of its effective use in several neuropathic conditions namely diabetic neuropathy, chronic lower back pain and chemotherapy-induced peripheral neuropathy [20, 28].

Minami et al. (2017) observed that duloxetine may elicit analgesic effects mainly through the activity in the monoamine system in the spinal cord [29]. In their animal study, Ito et al. (2018) also noted that duloxetine provided analgesic effects against neuropathic pain by inhibiting the accumulating effect of noradrenaline in the spinal cord [30].

In 2019, Najafi et al. conducted an open-label randomised controlled trial that investigated the analgesic effects of duloxetine dosed at 60 mg/day as a combination therapy to usual analgesic regimens of morphine ± acetaminophen ± gabapentin in 46 burn survivors. Duloxetine was found to enhance analgesic effects of other analgesic medications [21].

Selective Serotonin Reuptake Inhibitors

The GRADE recommendations for SSRIs as the treatment of neuropathic pain are inconclusive due to contradictory findings [20]. Lacking norepinephrine activity, SSRIs exert low analgesic property in the inhibition of neuropathic pain. However, there have been suggestions that SSRIs may have auxiliary actions when given with nor-adrenaline reuptake inhibitors [31]. Due to their receptor selectivity, SSRIs elicit less side effects compared to other antidepressants. It can still be a drug of choice for neuropathic pain patients with mood disorder due to their better tolerability and favourable side effect profile [32].

Neuroleptics

Pregabalin and gabapentin are classified as gabapentinoids due to their structural resemblance to the inhibitory neurotransmitter gamma-aminobutyric acid (GABA); however, neither agent has activity in GABAergic neuronal systems [33, 34]. Gabapentinoids are calcium channel antagonists that are characterised by high-affinity binding, selectively to alpha-2delta subunit voltage-gated calcium channels. Through suppressing excitatory neurotransmitters, pregabalin and gabapentin produce antiepileptic, analgesic and anxiolytic properties [34–36]. They have been recommended as a first-line treatment for various neuropathic pain syndrome such as diabetic neuropathy, post-herpetic neuralgia and burn injury [33, 37, 38].

Gabapentin

Gabapentin specifically affects the nociceptive process involving in central sensitisation by suppressing glutamate and substance P transmission as well as modulating GABA receptors [39]. The evidence of the efficacy of gabapentin in the management of acute burn pain and opioid consumption remains conflicting. Several studies reported the potential benefit of gabapentin as an adjunct to opioid analgesic therapy in the treatment of acute burn pain.

A double-blind randomised controlled trial performed by Rimaz et al. (2012), assessing 50 burn patients with a single oral dose of gabapentin (1200 mg) or placebo 2 h prior to surgery, demonstrated a statistically significant overall reduction in morphine requirement (52.45 ± 10.4 mg in the placebo group to 33.8 ± 18 mg in the gabapentin group [p <0.05]) and pain scores (p <0.05) in gabapentin group after surgical debridement in burn survivors [40].

The report was further supported by a retrospective observational study performed in Belgium that investigated the opioid-sparing and analgesic effects of gabapentin (2400 mg in three divided doses) in 10 severely burned patients (mean total body surface area [TBSA] 25%) from days 3 to 24. The study found an improvement in mean daily pain scores and a reduction in opioid requirements in patients receiving gabapentin both during treatment (21 days) and 21 days post-treatment [39].

Notably, the analgesic effect of gabapentin was exceeding the pharmacologic duration, which was likely due to its ability to prevent central hyperalgesia [39, 41]. Consistent observation of an improvement of acute burn pain in patients receiving gabapentin was also made by another case series study [42].

However, Gustorff et al. (2004) conducted a double-blinded placebo-controlled, crossover study in 16 participants, evaluating the effects of remifentanil and gabapentin on hyperalgesia in an experimental superficial burn model and observed neither anti-hyperalgesic nor opioid-enhancing properties in gabapentin [43].

In 2014, a more recent randomised controlled study assessed the efficacy of gabapentin in 50 burn survivors with TBSA of 5% and found that gabapentin was ineffective as an analgesic adjunct as its use did not reduce pain scores (rest and procedural) or lessen opioid consumptions in the acute burn period [44].

Pregabalin

Pregabalin is a newer analogue of gabapentin with comparatively better pharmacokinetic profiles including linear and dose-independent absorption and a narrow therapeutic dosing range [34, 45].

In 2010, Wong et al. conducted a retrospective study of 13 outpatients with TBSA of 5% or more receiving pregabalin in variable doses (maximum 600 mg). In this series, a reduction of pain scores up to 69% was noted in their treated participants [46].

An Australian double-blind, randomised placebo-controlled trial evaluated the efficacy and tolerability of pregabalin in 90 inpatients with moderate to severe burn injury and found positive outcomes of pregabalin in the treatment of postburn pain. Pregabalin was observed to be well tolerated and effective with the starting dose at 75 mg twice daily and progressively increased to 300 mg twice per day in severe burn individuals who have features of acute neuropathic pain. Interestingly, it was noted that an overall improvement of procedural pain was increased. The effect was shown to be greatest during 3 weeks of treatment with a reduction in pain score up to 40% in the pooled data [47].

A retrospective review of pharmacy records and charts noted pregabalin and gabapentin being dispensed in variable doses starting at 50 mg thrice daily for the management of neuropathic pain and itch. The study included a total of 136 burn patients aged 10 months to 20 years old. Of these 136 patients, 112 received only gabapentin, none received only pregabalin while 24 received both agents. Of the patients who only received gabapentin, adequate response reported for pruritus and pain was 91.4% and 100%, respectively while only 43.3% was reported for both symptoms. Of patients who received both gabapentin and pregabalin, 88.2% noted adequate relief for both symptoms [48].

In 2019, Jones et al. performed a prospective, randomised, double-blinded, placebo-controlled trail with 51 participants, comparing the efficacy of 300 mg pregabalin versus 600 mg pregabalin versus a placebo on acute postburn pain. In both noncritical partial and full-thickness burn injuries, pregabalin was observed to be well tolerated and dosing 600 mg of pregabalin per day provided superior pain control compared to 300 mg pregabalin per day ($p < 0.260$). An overall opioid consumption and pain values were lessened across time, suggesting dosage amount of pregabalin may play a role in adequate pain management in burn care [47].

Clinical Tip

- Psychiatric patients who experience neuropathic pain may benefit from antidepressants.
- Combination therapy of TCA and pregabalin/gabapentin can be used in patients who are unresponsive to monotherapy or have intolerance to higher doses of either drug.
- Combination of SNRIs and pregabalin/gabapentin/morphine has been shown to reduce intensity of neuropathic pain and fewer side effects compared to monotherapy [49].
- Apart from combination therapy with antidepressants, pregabalin/gabapentin coupled with opioid has also shown to be more effective in neuropathic pain.

> **Caution!**
> - Tricyclic antidepressants (TCAs) such as amitriptyline and nortriptyline should be used cautiously in elderly and cardiac patients due to associated side effects.
> - Treatment of gabapentinoids should be taken with caution in particular in elderly patients given its adverse effects of dizziness and somnolence [45].
> - TCAs have superior analgesic property but carry more side effects compared to those of SNRIs.
> - Following the commencement of antidepressant, patients should be monitored for emergence of suicidal ideation.

Pharmacological Therapy for Scar Tissue Itch

Goutos et al. (2010) demonstrated that early treatment with combination therapy consisting of peripherally and centrally acting agents is often required to achieve satisfactory relief in most pruritic scar symptoms [50]. Oral therapy which has been shown to improve the symptoms of pruritic scars to date includes antihistamine, naltrexone, antidepressants, neuroleptic agents and ondansetron.

Antihistamine

Antihistamines are recommended as first-line pharmacological management of scar pruritus [51]. H1-antihistamines are inverse agonists of histamine H1-receptors, leading to the inactive state of the H1-receptor. Antihistamines demonstrate anti-inflammatory and anti-fibrotic properties on scars, reducing scar formation and improving symptoms of pruritus [51].

Adverse drug reactions, commonly CNS related, are mostly associated with first-generation H1-antihistamines due to their ability to readily cross blood-brain barriers and interfere with histaminergic transmission. Hence, this restricts daytime use of sedating antihistamines, but they may have a role in nocturnal pruritus. Second-generation H1-antihistamines have become a preferable option given they are highly selective for the H1-receptor with no anticholinergic effects. Thus, they are more efficacious with a longer duration of action and favourable safety profiles [52, 53].

In adult postburn pruritus, the response rate of antihistamines was varied, which could be attributable to the complexity of itch and multifactorial pathophysiology that contribute to it in burn individuals. In participants who were treated with antihistamines, 20% had their symptoms completely relieved, while 60% had partial relief and 20% had no relief of symptoms [15, 54]. A tolerance may develop in prolonged use of antihistamine therapy, although an increased dose and temporary discontinuation of drug have shown to effectively restore a response [8, 54].

Opioid Receptor Agonists or Antagonists

Naltrexone, a μ-opioid antagonist, has been used in the treatment of pruritus associated with different conditions including cholestasis, end-stage renal disease and atopic dermatitis [55]. However, the evidence regarding antipruritic effects on postburn scars is yet to be established.

LaSalle et al. (2007) and Jung et at. (2009) found a positive outcome of naltrexone in the management of refractory pruritus with a high percentage of patient satisfaction and associated improvement in their quality of life [56, 57]. The mechanism of action of naltrexone is unclear. It was observed that μ-opioid receptor agonists induced the symptoms of pruritus which can be revered by μ-opioid receptor antagonists, suggesting an imbalance of endogenous opioidergic system, in particular central origin, may link to the underlying pathophysiology of pruritus [56].

A randomised crossover trial by Peer et al. (1996) demonstrated a significant reduction of plasma histamine in uremic patients who were treated with naltrexone. In their experiment, naltrexone was observed to inhibit histamine release from basophils. Thus, this may explain the mechanism of naltrexone's antipruritic action which was most likely through the modulation of histamine release rather than by the influence of opioid antagonist effect [58].

Pruritus is a well-documented side effect of opiates analgesia, for instance, morphine, which is commonly used in burn pain management [59]. Opioid antagonists have been recommended in the case of pruritus related to opiate administration; however, the use has not been investigated in burn survivors [56].

Low-dose naltrexone elicits anti-inflammatory properties and is a promising therapeutic option for chronic pain conditions in particular neuroinflammatory diseases, namely fibromyalgia, inflammatory bowel diseases, complex regional pain syndrome and multiple sclerosis. At low dosage, naltrexone was observed to modulate neuroinflammatory process, including glial cells and the release of CNS inflammatory substances [60, 61].

Antidepressants

Antidepressants have been prescribed in patients with psychogenic pruritus and paraneoplastic pruritus that are intractable to conventional therapy [55]. Kouwenhoven et al. (2017) conducted a systematic review on the use of oral antidepressants in patients with chronic pruritus particularly in patients with uremic pruritus, cholestatic pruritus and paraneoplastic pruritus and found a significant improvement of symptoms of itch in their participants during antidepressant therapy [62]; however, data regarding the effectiveness of antidepressants in pruritic scars remains lacking.

Selective Norepinephrine Re-uptake Inhibitor

Mirtazapine, a selective norepinephrine re-uptake inhibitor (SNRI) with both noradrenergic and serotonergic activity, has been observed to alleviate itch in patients with atopic dermatitis and malignancy. As a unique antagonist, mirtazapine selectively inhibits noradrenergic α_2-receptors, serotonin 5-HT_2 and 5-HT_3 receptors and indirectly enhances central noradrenergic and 5-HT_1 serotonergic neurotransmission. Subsequently, it prevents unwanted side effects associated with non-selective 5-HT receptors activation. Through its sedative effect of H_1-antihistamine properties, mirtazapine may offer a promising treatment agent for nocturnal pruritus when accompanied with anxiety and depression [63, 64].

Selective Serotonin Re-uptake Inhibitors

Selective serotonin re-uptake inhibitors (SSRIs) have shown to provide antipruritic effects in chronic itch of different aetiology which are refractory to traditional therapy. Paroxetine and fluvoxamine were administered in a total of 72 patients with pruritus in an open-label study by Stander et al. (2009). They observed an overall response rate to the intervention of up to 68%, with the most favourable outcomes being observed in pruritus due to atopic dermatitis, systemic lymphoma and solid carcinoma [65]. Several studies have reported a significant reduction or complete resolution of chronic pruritus in liver disease and chronic kidney failure patients when treated with sertraline [62].

Tricyclic Antidepressants

Doxepin and amitriptyline, tricyclic antidepressants (TCAs), act as an antagonist to histaminergic and cholinergic receptors and have been reported to provide relief from itch in chronic pruritus. Due to associated adverse effects, treatment with TCA, however, should be used with caution especially in the elderly patients [9].

Neuroleptics

Partial responses to antihistamines that are associated with neuropathic-type symptoms including pins and needles, burning sensation, numbness and stinging were noted in subgroups of burn survivors, suggesting that burn-related itch may be linked to neuropathy. Widely used for neuropathic pain, gabapentin and pregabalin also demonstrated an antipruritic property [66–70]. They have been prescribed in intractable pruritic scars and have shown to lead to marked reduction of itch in burned individuals [9, 71].

Gabapentin and pregabalin work by modulating the release of sensory neuropeptides, including reduction of calcitonin gene-related peptide (CGRP) and substance P (SP) release from primary afferent neurons. Increasing evidence shows that SP and CGRP play vital roles in the mediation of itch [72–75]. SP mediates inflammatory and pruritic pathways through activation of Mas-related G protein-coupled receptors expressed on human mast cells as well as sensory neurons [73].

It was proposed in an animal study that CGRP is central for the activation of itch regulated by VGLUT2-mediated transmission from Trpv1–Cre neurons [72]. By suppressing the release of these neurotransmitters, these neuroleptic agents may resolve the stimulated state in these patients, resulting in the attenuation of itch.

Neuropathic itch was found to be intractable to conventional treatment such as cetirizine and pheniramine maleate but rather responds to pregabalin [75–77]. A reduction of itch in mild or moderate pruritus with pregabalin or by a combination of pregabalin and antihistamine was observed in a double-blind, randomised and placebo-controlled study [77]. In patients with refractory to single neuroleptic medication, the combination of gabapentin and pregabalin was shown to provide better relief than monotherapy [76].

Serotonin Antagonist

Although relatively weak pruritogen, serotonin was shown to mediate the sensation of itch by stimulating action potential in cutaneous C-fibres [78]. It was postulated that serotonin may cause pruritus through indirect peripheral mechanisms involving the release of histamine from mast cells in the skin as well as through central mechanisms involving the opioid neurotransmitter system [6].

Ondansetron, a centrally acting serotonin antagonist, has been shown to improve symptoms of opioid-induced pruritus but is observed to have negligible effects on uremic pruritus [79, 80]. In a double-blinded, randomised, crossover trial comparing diphenhydramine to ondansetron in postburn patients, ondansetron was observed to have a greater antipruritic effect compared to antihistamine [79].

Clinical Tip
- Sedating antihistamines (first-generation) may be helpful when pruritus is exacerbated at night.
- Mirtazapine can be a drug of choice for nocturnal pruritus due to its sedative effect.
- Ondansetron can be used as prophylaxis and treatment of morphine-induced pruritus [81].
- Similar to pain, antidepressant is noted to be helpful in patients who have coexisting symptoms of pruritus.
- In intractable itch, combination therapy of low-dose mirtazapine and gabapentinoids can be the drug of choice.

Caution!
- First-generation antihistamines should be avoided for daytime use especially in elderly patients due to their soporific effects.
- Ondansetron can cause significant side effects with long-term use.

Acne Scar Prevention

Acne scarring is a common complication of acne vulgaris but remains a major therapeutic challenge for dermatologists. Acne scarring can be classified into three different categories: atrophic, hypertrophic and keloidal [82]. The majority of post-acne scarring is atrophic, which is likely associated with inflammatory mediators and enzyme-induced collagen fibre and subcutaneous fat degradation [83]. Current treatment modalities of atrophic acne largely involve non-pharmacological approaches, in which certain interventions and procedures can be invasive. To tackle acne scarring sequelae, early treatment of active acne is the most effective strategy.

Oral Isotretinoin

Isotretinoin, a synthetic vitamin A derivative (13-*cis*-retinoic acid), has remarkable clinical effectiveness, which targets simultaneously all the major aetiological factors that contribute to acne. The clinical course of isotretinoin showed a significant reduction of sebum production and comedogenesis in acne patients. Isotretinoin also exhibits potent anti-inflammatory and immune-modulating properties through inhibition of monocyte and neutrophil chemotaxis and enhances host immune response. Although systemic isotretinoin does not have direct antimicrobial properties, it has been shown to effectively reduce and eradicate Propionibacterium acnes by altering the microenvironment within the pilosebaceous duct, which is a less favourable environment for colonisation [84].

Early implementation of isotretinoin therapy in acne management is shown to reduce the likelihood of acne scar formation [85]. While originally only recommended for severe cystic acne, the indications for isotretinoin have now broadened, which includes less severe forms of acne to prevent complications of physical and psychological scarring [86].

Layton et al. (1997) reported their positive experience in early administering isotretinoin to 107 patients with facial acne. Patients who received early therapy of isotretinoin were noted to have significantly lesser degree of acne scarring compared to patients who received therapy later in their course of acne [85].

Isotretinoin has several side effects and acute flares of acne are commonly reported during the initial phase of treatment. To avoid undesirable therapeutic effects, the treatment of isotretinoin should be carried out with appropriate patient selection, careful dose modification, routine monitoring for plausible toxicity and, in severe cases, discontinuation of the drug [87]. Majority of common side effects are dose dependent and can be rendered tolerable by adjustment of the dosage. Lower starting dose or concurrent use of prednisolone has been recommended to reduce the risk of acute flares [84].

Mandekou-Lefaki et al. (2003) performed a study comparing high- and low-dose regimens of isotretinoin to evaluate the therapeutic efficacy and dose-related side effects of isotretinoin for the treatment of acne vulgaris. Lower dose of isotretinoin was found to be more tolerable and effective in preventing acne relapse and scarring [88].

It is important to know that isotretinoin is recommended only to be used for severe acne cases that are unresponsive to appropriate antibiotics and topical therapies [89]. Acute flare following isotretinoin therapy is common which can be severe and may last for several months.

Clinical Tip
- Start at a low dose of 0.5 mg/kg/day and titrate the dose according to clinical response and tolerance.
- Dose and duration of the treatment have been shown to affect the remission and cure rates. Relapse rate post-therapy can be minimised by a course of treatment with a total amount of at least 120 mg/kg. No benefit was found when a dose of 150 mg/kg is exceeded.
- Acute flare can be managed by dose adjustment. In severe cases, concurrent use of prednisolone at a dose of 0.5–1 mg/kg/day for 2–3 weeks, with a weaning dose over the next 6 weeks, has been recommended.

Caution!
- Pregnancy and breastfeeding are absolute contraindications. Patients should be made fully aware of the high risk of teratogenicity.

Conclusion

Pain and pruritus are common and serious complications of scars that can have a significant impact on patients' quality of life. The management of scars' symptoms can be extremely challenging which often requires multimodal approaches to target different origins of the neuropathy. The therapy should be tailored to the need of an individual patient as an essential part of holistic multidisciplinary approach. While there remains a need for comprehensive research into the precise mechanisms of itch and pain in dermal scar tissues to identify novel targeted therapies, a deeper understanding of currently available drugs is necessary to provide a guideline for effective clinical approaches. The development of standardised classification systems is important to assist appropriate management of refractory scar symptoms in clinical settings.

Early implementation of isotretinoin therapy in acne management has been shown to prevent the development of acne scarring. However, due to several associated undesirable therapeutic effects of isotretinoin, the treatment should be carried out with appropriate patient selection, careful dose modification and routine monitoring to reduce the likelihood of potential toxicity.

Funding None.

Conflicts of Interest The authors have no conflicts of interest to disclose.

Disclosures The authors have no disclosures.

References

1. Yam MF, Loh YC, Tan CS, Khadijah Adam S, Abdul Manan N, Basir R. General pathways of pain sensation and the major neurotransmitters involved in pain regulation. Int J Mol Sci. 2018;19(8):2164.
2. Farrukh O, Goutos I. Scar symptoms: pruritus and pain. In: Téot L, Mustoe TA, Middelkoop E, Gauglitz GG, editors. Textbook on scar management. Cham: Springer; 2020. p. 87–101.
3. Bechert K, Abraham SE. Pain management and wound care. J Am Col Certif Wound Spec. 2009;1(2):65–71.
4. Cole BE. Pain management: classifying, understanding, and treating pain. Hosp Physician. 2002;23:1–8.
5. Rothman S. Physiology of itching. Physiol Rev. 1941;21(2):357–81.
6. Twycross R, Greaves M, Handwerker H, Jones E, Libretto S, Szepietowski J, et al. Itch: scratching more than the surface. QJM. 2003;96(1):7–26.
7. Parnell LK. Itching for Knowledge About Wound and Scar Pruritus. Wounds. 2018;30(1):17–36.
8. Dannenberg TB, Feinberg SM. The development of tolerance to antihistamines: a study of the quantitative inhibiting capacity of antihistamines on the skin and mucous membrane reaction to histamine and antigens. J Allergy Ther. 1951;22(4):330–9.
9. Zachariah JR, Rao AL, Prabha R, Gupta AK, Paul MK, Lamba S. Post burn pruritus—a review of current treatment options. Burns. 2012;38(5):621–9.
10. Wooten M, Weng H-J, Hartke TV, Borzan J, Klein AH, Turnquist B, et al. Three functionally distinct classes of C-fibre nociceptors in primates. Nat Commun. 2014;5(1):1–12.
11. Binder A, Koroschetz J, Baron R. Disease mechanisms in neuropathic itch. Nat Clin Pract Neurol. 2008;4(6):329–37.
12. Chung BY, Kim HB, Jung MJ, Kang SY, Kwak I-S, Park CW, et al. Post-Burn Pruritus. Int J Mol Sci. 2020;21(11):3880.
13. Liu T, Ji R-R. New insights into the mechanisms of itch: are pain and itch controlled by distinct mechanisms? Pflugers Arch. 2013;465(12):1671–85.
14. Campbell JN, Meyer RA. Mechanisms of neuropathic pain. Neuron. 2006;52(1):77–92.
15. Nedelec B, LaSalle L. Postburn Itch: a review of the literature. Wounds. 2018;30(1):E118–E24.
16. Andersen HH, Akiyama T, Nattkemper LA, Van Laarhoven A, Elberling J, Yosipovitch G, et al. Alloknesis and hyperknesis—mechanisms, assessment methodology, and clinical implications of itch sensitization. Pain. 2018;159(7):1185–97.
17. Huang S-H, Wu S-H, Chang K-P, Lin C-H, Chang C-H, Wu Y-C, et al. Alleviation of neuropathic scar pain using autologous fat grafting. Ann Plast Surg. 2015;74:S99–S104.
18. Sheng J, Liu S, Wang Y, Cui R, Zhang X. The link between depression and chronic pain: neural mechanisms in the brain. Neural Plast. 2017;2017:1.
19. Obata H. Analgesic mechanisms of antidepressants for neuropathic pain. Int J Mol Sci. 2017;18(11):2483.
20. Finnerup NB, Attal N, Haroutounian S, McNicol E, Baron R, Dworkin RH, et al. Pharmacotherapy for neuropathic pain in adults: a systematic review and meta-analysis. Lancet Neurol. 2015;14(2):162–73.
21. Najafi A, Nejad HZ, Nikvarz N. Evaluation of the analgesic effects of duloxetine in burn patients: an open-label randomized controlled trial. Burns. 2019;45(3):598–609.
22. Fornasari D. Pharmacotherapy for neuropathic pain: a review. Pain Ther. 2017;6(1):25–33.

23. Moulin D, Clark A, Gilron I, Ware M, Watson C, Sessle B, et al. Pharmacological management of chronic neuropathic pain–consensus statement and guidelines from the Canadian Pain Society. Pain Res Manag. 2007;12(1):13–21.

24. Hiroki T, Suto T, Saito S, Obata H. Repeated administration of amitriptyline in neuropathic pain: modulation of the noradrenergic descending inhibitory system. Anesth Analg. 2017;125(4):1281–8.

25. Gilron I, Bailey JM, Tu D, Holden RR, Jackson AC, Houlden RL. Nortriptyline and gabapentin, alone and in combination for neuropathic pain: a double-blind, randomised controlled crossover trial. Lancet. 2009;374(9697):1252–61.

26. Mu A, Weinberg E, Moulin DE, Clarke H. Pharmacologic management of chronic neuropathic pain: review of the Canadian Pain Society consensus statement. Can Fam Physician. 2017;63(11):844–52.

27. Derry S, Wiffen PJ, Aldington D, Moore RA. Nortriptyline for neuropathic pain in adults. Cochrane Database Syst Rev. 2015;1:CD011209.

28. Urits I, Li N, Berardino K, Artounian KA, Bandi P, Jung JW, et al. The use of antineuropathic medications for the treatment of chronic pain. Best Pract Res Clin Anaesthesiol. 2020;34:493.

29. Minami K, Tamano R, Kasai E, Oyama H, Hasegawa M, Shinohara S, et al. Effects of duloxetine on pain and walking distance in neuropathic pain models via modulation of the spinal monoamine system. Eur J Pain. 2018;22(2):355–69.

30. Ito S, Suto T, Saito S, Obata H. Repeated administration of duloxetine suppresses neuropathic pain by accumulating effects of noradrenaline in the spinal cord. Anesth Analg. 2018;126(1):298–307.

31. Leventhal L, Smith V, Hornby G, Andree TH, Brandt MR, Rogers KE. Differential and synergistic effects of selective norepinephrine and serotonin reuptake inhibitors in rodent models of pain. J Pharmacol Exp Ther. 2007;320(3):1178–85.

32. Hoffelt C, Zwack A. Assessment and management of chronic pain in patients with depression and anxiety. Ment Health Clin. 2014;4(3):146–52.

33. Mathieson S, Lin C-WC, Underwood M, Eldabe S. Pregabalin and gabapentin for pain. BMJ. 2020;369:m1315.

34. Bockbrader HN, Wesche D, Miller R, Chapel S, Janiczek N, Burger P. A comparison of the pharmacokinetics and pharmacodynamics of pregabalin and gabapentin. Clin Pharmacokinet. 2010;49(10):661–9.

35. Verma V, Singh N, Singh JA. Pregabalin in neuropathic pain: evidences and possible mechanisms. Curr Neuropharmacol. 2014;12(1):44–56.

36. Yu J, Wang D-S, Bonin RP, Penna A, Alavian-Ghavanini A, Zurek AA, et al. Gabapentin increases expression of δ subunit-containing GABAA receptors. EBioMedicine. 2019;42:203–13.

37. Kukkar A, Bali A, Singh N, Jaggi AS. Implications and mechanism of action of gabapentin in neuropathic pain. Arch Pharm Res. 2013;36(3):237–51.

38. Wang Y, Beekman J, Hew J, Jackson S, Issler-Fisher AC, Parungao R, et al. Burn injury: challenges and advances in burn wound healing, infection, pain and scarring. Adv Drug Deliv Rev. 2018;123:3–17.

39. Cuignet O, Pirson J, Soudon O, Zizi M. Effects of gabapentin on morphine consumption and pain in severely burned patients. Burns. 2007;33(1):81–6.

40. Rimaz S, Alavi CE, Sedighinejad A, Tolouie M, Kavoosi S, Koochakinejad L. Effect of gabapentin on morphine consumption and pain after surgical debridement of burn wounds: a double-blind randomized clinical trial study. Arch Trauma Res. 2012;1(1):38.

41. Werner MU, Perkins FM, Holte K, Pedersen JL, Kehlet H. Effects of gabapentin in acute inflammatory pain in humans. Reg Anesth Pain Med. 2001;26(4):322–8.

42. Gray P, Williams B, Cramond T. Successful use of gabapentin in acute pain management following burn injury: a case series. Pain Med. 2008;9(3):371–6.

43. Gustorff B, Hoechtl K, Sycha T, Felouzis E, Lehr S, Kress HG. The effects of remifentanil and gabapentin on hyperalgesia in a new extended inflammatory skin pain model in healthy volunteers. Anesth Analg. 2004;98(2):401–7.

44. Wibbenmeyer L, Eid A, Liao J, Heard J, Horsfield A, Kral L, et al. Gabapentin is ineffective as an analgesic adjunct in the immediate postburn period. J Burn Care Res. 2014;35(2):136–42.

45. Guay DR. Pregabalin in neuropathic pain: a more "pharmaceutically elegant" gabapentin? Am J Geriatr Pharmacother. 2005;3(4):274–87.

46. Wong L, Turner L. Treatment of post-burn neuropathic pain: evaluation of pregablin. Burns. 2010;36(6):769–72.

47. Jones LM, Uribe AA, Coffey R, Puente EG, Abdel-Rasoul M, Murphy CV, et al. Pregabalin in the reduction of pain and opioid consumption after burn injuries: a preliminary, randomized, double-blind, placebo-controlled study. Medicine. 2019;98(18):e15343.

48. Kaul I, Amin A, Rosenberg M, Rosenberg L, Meyer WJ III. Use of gabapentin and pregabalin for pruritus and neuropathic pain associated with major burn injury: a retrospective chart review. Burns. 2018;44(2):414–22.

49. Holbech JV, Jung A, Jonsson T, Wanning M, Bredahl C, Bach FW. Combination treatment of neuropathic pain: Danish expert recommendations based on a Delphi process. J Pain Res. 2017;10:1467.

50. Goutos I, Clarke M, Upson C, Richardson PM, Ghosh SJ. Review of therapeutic agents for burns pruritus and protocols for management in adult and paediatric patients using the GRADE classification. Ind J Plast Surg. 2010;43(Suppl):S51.

51. Edriss A, Mestak J. Management of keloid and hypertrophic scars. Ann Burns Fire Disasters. 2005;18(4):202.

52. Church MK, Church DS. Pharmacology of antihistamines. Indian J Dermatol. 2013;58(3):219.

53. Simons FER. Advances in H1-antihistamines. N Engl J Med. 2004;351(21):2203–17.

54. Vitale M, Fields-Blache C, Luterman A. Severe itching in the patient with burns. J Burn Care Rehabil. 1991;12(4):330–3.
55. Patel T, Yosipovitch G. Therapy of pruritus. Expert Opin Pharmacother. 2010;11(10):1673–82.
56. LaSalle L, Rachelska G, Nedelec B. Naltrexone for the management of post-burn pruritus: a preliminary report. Burns. 2008;34(6):797–802.
57. Jung SI, Seo CH, Jang K, Ham BJ, Choi I-G, Kim J-H, et al. Efficacy of naltrexone in the treatment of chronic refractory itching in burn patients: preliminary report of an open trial. J Burn Care Res. 2009;30(2):257–60.
58. Peer G, Kivity S, Agami O, Fireman E, Silverberg D, Blum M, et al. Randomised crossover trial of naltrexone in uraemic pruritus. Lancet. 1996;348(9041):1552–4.
59. Depetris N, Raineri S, Pantet O, Lavrentieva A. Management of pain, anxiety, agitation and delirium in burn patients: a survey of clinical practice and a review of the current literature. Ann Burns Fire Disasters. 2018;31(2):97.
60. Younger J, Parkitny L, McLain D. The use of low-dose naltrexone (LDN) as a novel anti-inflammatory treatment for chronic pain. Clin Rheumatol. 2014;33(4):451–9.
61. Kim PS, Fishman MA. Low-dose naltrexone for chronic pain: update and systemic review. Curr Pain Headache Rep. 2020;24(10):1–8.
62. Kouwenhoven TA, van de Kerkhof PC, Kamsteeg M. Use of oral antidepressants in patients with chronic pruritus: a systematic review. J Am Acad Dermatol. 2017;77(6):1068–73. e7.
63. Davis MP, Frandsen JL, Walsh D, Andresen S, Taylor S. Mirtazapine for pruritus. J Pain Symptom Manag. 2003;25(3):288–91.
64. Hundley JL, Yosipovitch G. Mirtazapine for reducing nocturnal itch in patients with chronic pruritus: a pilot study. J Am Acad Dermatol. 2004;50(6):889–91.
65. Staender S, Böckenholt B, Schuermeyer-Horst F, Weishaupt C, Heuft G, Luger TA, et al. Treatment of chronic pruritus with the selective serotonin re-uptake inhibitors paroxetine and fluvoxamine: results of an open-labelled, two-arm proof-of-concept study. Acta Derm Venereol. 2009;89(1):45–51.
66. Mendham J. Gabapentin for the treatment of itching produced by burns and wound healing in children: a pilot study. Burns. 2004;30(8):851–3.
67. Yesudian P, Wilson N. Efficacy of gabapentin in the management of pruritus of unknown origin. Arch Dermatol. 2005;141(12):1507–9.
68. Maciel AAW, Cunha PR, Laraia IO, Trevisan F. Efficacy of gabapentin in the improvement of pruritus and quality of life of patients with notalgia paresthetica. An Bras Dermatol. 2014;89(4):570–5.
69. Rayner H, Baharani J, Smith S, Suresh V, Dasgupta I. Uraemic pruritus: relief of itching by gabapentin and pregabalin. Nephron Clin Pract. 2012;122(3–4):75–9.
70. Ahuja RB, Gupta R, Gupta G, Shrivastava P. A comparative analysis of cetirizine, gabapentin and their combination in the relief of post-burn pruritus. Burns. 2011;37(2):203–7.
71. Zachariah JR, Lakshmanarao A, Prabha R, Gupta AK, Paul KM, Lamba S. A prospective study on the role of gabapentin in post-burn pruritus. Eur J Plast Surg. 2012;35(6):425–31.
72. Rogoz K, Andersen HH, Lagerström MC, Kullander K. Multimodal use of calcitonin gene-related peptide and substance P in itch and acute pain uncovered by the elimination of vesicular glutamate transporter 2 from transient receptor potential cation channel subfamily V member 1 neurons. J Neurosci. 2014;34(42):14055–68.
73. Vena GA, Cassano N, Di Leo E, Calogiuri G, Nettis E. Focus on the role of substance P in chronic urticaria. Clin Mol Allerg. 2018;16(1):1–6.
74. Lee J, Jang D, Bae J, Jung H, Park M, Ahn J. Efficacy of pregabalin for the treatment of chronic pruritus of unknown origin, assessed based on electric current perception threshold. Sci Rep. 2020;10(1):1–8.
75. Fehrenbacher JC, Taylor CP, Vasko MR. Pregabalin and gabapentin reduce release of substance P and CGRP from rat spinal tissues only after inflammation or activation of protein kinase C. Pain. 2003;105(1–2):133–41.
76. Gray P, Kirby J, Smith MT, Cabot PJ, Williams B, Doecke J, et al. Pregabalin in severe burn injury pain: a double-blind, randomised placebo-controlled trial. Pain. 2011;152(6):1279–88.
77. Ahuja RB, Gupta GK. A four arm, double blind, randomized and placebo controlled study of pregabalin in the management of post-burn pruritus. Burns. 2013;39(1):24–9.
78. Potenzieri C, Undem BJ. Basic mechanisms of itch. Clin Exp Allergy. 2012;42(1):8–19.
79. Larijani GE, Goldberg ME, Rogers KH. Treatment of opioid-induced pruritus with ondansetron: report of four patients. Pharmacotherapy. 1996;16(5):958–60.
80. Ashmore SD, Jones CH, Newstead CG, Daly MJ, Chrystyn H. Ondansetron therapy for uremic pruritus in hemodialysis patients. Am J Kidney Dis. 2000;35(5):827–31.
81. Koju RB, Gurung BS, Dongol Y. Prophylactic administration of ondansetron in prevention of intrathecal morphine-induced pruritus and post-operative nausea and vomiting in patients undergoing caesarean section. BMC Anesthesiol. 2015;15(1):1–6.

82. Fife D. Practical evaluation and management of atrophic acne scars: tips for the general dermatologist. J Clin Aesthet Dermatol. 2011;4(8):50.

83. Gozali MV, Zhou B. Effective treatments of atrophic acne scars. J Clin Aesthet Dermatol. 2015;8(5):33.

84. Layton A. The use of isotretinoin in acne. Dermatoendocrinol. 2009;1(3):162–9.

85. Layton A, Seukeran D, Cunliffe W. Scarred for life? Dermatology. 1997;195(Suppl. 1):15–21.

86. Rigopoulos D, Larios G, Katsambas AD. The role of isotretinoin in acne therapy: why not as first-line therapy? Facts and controversies. Clin Dermatol. 2010;28(1):24–30.

87. Ganceviciene R, Zouboulis CC. Isotretinoin: state of the art treatment for acne vulgaris. J Dtsch Dermatol Ges. 2010;8:S47–59.

88. Mandekou-Lefaki I, Delli F, Teknetzis A, Euthimiadou R, Karakatsanis G. Low-dose schema of isotretinoin in acne vulgaris. Int J Clin Pharmacol Res. 2003;23(2–3):41–6.

89. Layton A, Dreno B, Gollnick H, Zouboulis C. A review of the European directive for prescribing systemic isotretinoin for acne vulgaris. J Eur Acad Dermatol Venereol. 2006;20(7):773–6.

Physical Therapy

Thomas Koller

Core Messages
- Physiological basics of functional stimulation at the cellular level are the basis for physical therapy.
- Manual dosage needs to be adapted to the wound-healing phase.
- Various forms of physical therapy based on mechanotransduction are available.
- Specific diagnostic and treatment techniques for manual scar therapy are presented.

Introduction

Depending on their size, characteristics, and surface area, the therapy of hypertrophic scars is a special focus during rehabilitation. Promoting mobility, independence, as well as strength and endurance training are often limited or even prevented by fragile scar tissue or tight scar strands.

Applications of physical therapy are based on tissue physiology, wound-healing phases, and empirical-clinical knowledge.

Supplementary Information The online version contains supplementary material available at https://doi.org/10.1007/978-3-031-24137-6_14.

T. Koller (✉)
Musculoskeletal Physiotherapy, Orthopedic and Hand Surgery Rehabilitation, Bellikon, Switzerland
e-mail: thomas.koller@rehabellikon.ch

Fibers and cells that are responsible for high elasticity and mobility are mostly located in the dermis. For this reason, loss or adhesion of this layer leads to massive restrictions (scar contractures). In addition, there are wound-healing processes that lead to physiological restrictions of the scar [1–3].

Fibroblasts react very sensitively to external mechanical stimuli and align collagen fibers (or all fiber types) according to this mechanical force in the extracellular matrix (ECM). If this functional stimulus does not occur in the proliferation phase, for example, because of immobilization, fibroblasts are unable to identify functional alignment and form a mechanically less stable collagen cluster of unspecific collagen type III. If, however, a mechanically adequate stimulus is provided in the proliferation phase, collagen type III will align itself functionally and according to its physiological use. This is of utmost importance for manual scar therapy, since in the remodulation phase the definitive collagen type I always forms in the same direction as the nonspecific collagen type III [4, 5].

Temporary collagen type III does not tolerate acceleration or shear forces. It is mechanically very unstable. Excessive mechanical stimuli tear the temporary structure and inevitably initiate a new inflammatory phase [5].

"Use determines the function"—this is well known. However, the question of which intervention, with which dosage, should be applied in which wound-healing phase and which point in time is not easy to answer. The following sections highlight possible answers based on clinical considerations and empirical experience.

> **Important to Know**
> - Adequately dosed functional stimulation in the proliferation phase is very important for fibroblasts.
> - Fibroblasts use mechanical stimuli to functionally align the temporary collagen type III in the ECM.
> - If the mechanical stimuli in the proliferation phase is set correctly no further reformatting of collagen type I is needed in the remodulation phase. This reduces a weakening of the tissue due to remodeling during the general load build-up in the remodulation phase.

Physiological and Biomechanical Fundamentals for Physical Therapy

Factors that Can Be Influenced Therapeutically in the Case of a Hypertrophic Scar or Scar Surface

In the case of extensive burns, a "pathology of the envelope" must be assumed. The described pathophysiological processes of scar formation result in severe functional limitations and disfigurement, especially in the case of extensive scar surfaces.

The hypertrophic scar is the most common pathological scar after deep dermal defects.

Figure 1 shows the factors that can be influenced by scar therapy. The scar characteristics can be divided into four mechanisms:

1. Increased density
2. Reduced movability
3. Reduced extensibility
4. Tension compensation: formation of scar strands

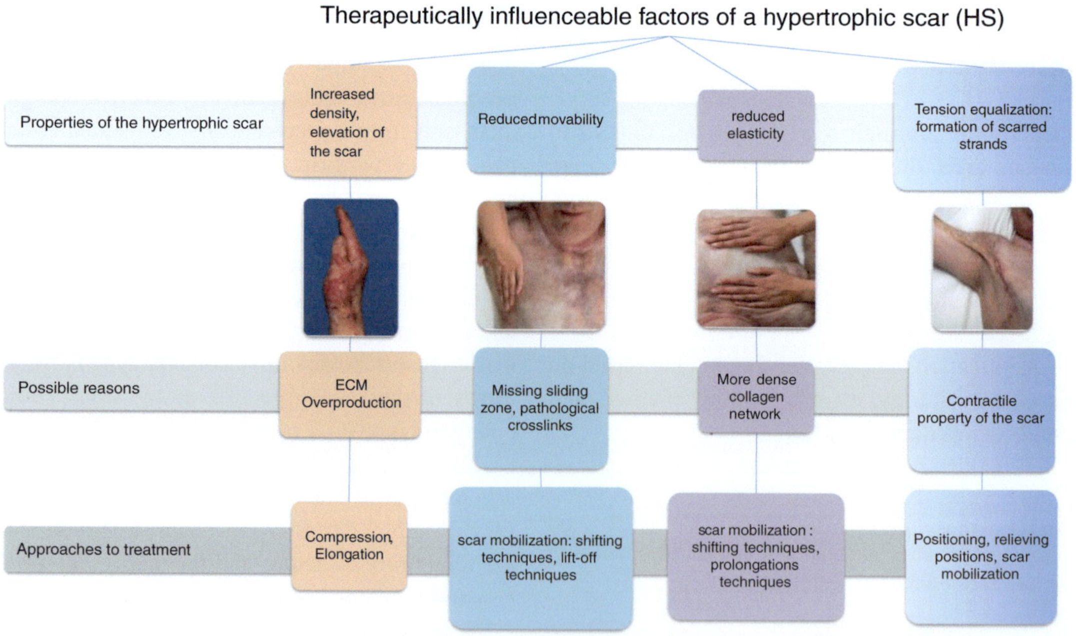

Fig. 1 Overview of factors that can be influenced therapeutically in a hypertrophic scar (four mechanisms) [3, 6–8] (Courtesy of T. Koller)

The mechanical tension in the scar areas and the resulting contractures can develop spontaneously, quickly, and with enormous intensity. The therapist must counteract this tension as much as possible with scar therapy [5, 9]. The aim is to optimally support wound healing by applying functional, physiological stimuli (manual techniques, active exercises, splints, positioning, etc.).

Important to Know
- The hypertrophic scar is the most common form of pathological scarring.
- The cause of hypertrophic scars is not yet fully understood.
- Growth factors (e.g., TGF-Beta 1) play a vital role in scar formation and react to external mechanical forces.
- Some characteristics of the hypertrophic scar can be influenced therapeutically (Fig. 1).

Pain in Deep Dermal Defects

Deep soft tissue injuries (trauma, burns) also destroy pain fibers ($A\delta$ and C-fibers). In general, patient's pain statements are difficult to evaluate, especially in the acute phase and at the beginning of rehabilitation (at the end of the proliferation phase and at the beginning of the remodulation phase). The reasons for this are the generally altered body perception, the partially missing pain fibers in the primary wound area, and the initially high-dose pain medication.

How Do Pain Fibers Differ at the Tissue Level?

The $A\delta$ fiber reacts early and quickly to mechanical influences by reporting strong pulling and pressure. It remains active even in the event of damage.

In contrast, the C-fiber becomes primary in the event of damage (cell wall destruction). It generates the typical pain sensation ("It hurts!"). When cell walls are destroyed, arachidonic acid is released, which is quickly synthesized into prostaglandin.

The C-fiber is very prostaglandin sensitive and reacts by releasing substance P. This process restarts the inflammatory phase with all signs of inflammation (dolor, calor, rubor, tumor, and functio laesa).

It is therefore important to avoid overdosing as much as possible [1, 4–6].

The altered perception of pain also affects cognitive processing in the primary and secondary wound area. Direct and indirect pain transmission can be distinguished here.

Direct Conduction of Pain

As a rule, each area of the skin is mapped in the cortex, which makes it possible to accurately locate a stimulus to the skin. Since the activity of the $A\delta$ fiber in the stressed tissue area (primary wound area) starts early, the body can generate a protective motor response to all stimuli perceived as painful. This prevents renewed cellular damage [1, 5, 6].

Indirect Conduction of Pain

Indirect pain transmission occurs in all kinds of structural injuries. Due to partial destruction of the pain fibers (thermal or bacterial), the primary wound area is temporarily or permanently unable to transmit painful stimuli directly to the cortex. The body therefore compensates these stimuli via the secondary wound area. This is associated with two major disadvantages:

1. The activity of the $A\delta$-fiber in the primary wound area in the inflammatory and proliferation phase is not able to warn of renewed cellular damage. By the time the stimulus set in the primary wound area has mechanically arrived in the secondary wound area, there is already a risk of overdosage in the primary wound area in the form of cell wall damage. This leads to a relapse into the inflammatory phase.

2. In the inflammatory and proliferation phase, the cortical mapping of the primary wound area receives hardly any signals in patients with deep dermal defects. The cortical arrangement of the primary wound area is therefore dependent on indirect information from the secondary wound area. This results in a more difficult differentiated perception with an additional slowed motor and/or verbal protective response. These two disadvantages present therapists with a major challenge.

Thus, pain statements from patients with deep dermal defects are not sufficient to ensure an adequate dosage of the therapeutic intervention. Based on tissue and pain physiology as well as the phases of wound healing, an appropriate functional stimulus can be set using the tactile diagnosis of the first and second connective tissue resistance. This has been empirically well proven [1, 5, 6, 10, 11].

It is the task of the therapist to discuss this pain processing problem in detail with the patient to develop a strategy together. Fear of pain can cause patients to avoid movement. However, it is important that they are again able to distinguish "pulling" (Aδ-fiber) from "hurting" (C-fiber).

> **Caution!**
> - Subjective pain statements by the patient should never be the only criterion for the adequate dosage of therapeutic interventions for deep dermal defects or hypertrophic scars.
> - In addition to the high pain medication in the acute phase and different (emotionally colored) pain perception, the direct or indirect pain conduction is altered.
> - Therefore, objective indicators are required, for example the first and second increases in connective tissue resistance.

Connective Tissue Resistance (R1 and R2)

Basically, it is important to distinguish between the quantity and quality of movement. The quantity of movement is the physically objectively measurable extent of movement. In contrast, the quality of movement includes the flow, dynamics as well as rhythm, and harmony of movement. These are qualities that are subjectively palpable during movement. To be able to assess the quantity and quality of a movement correctly, the therapist first needs theoretical knowledge: What quantity and quality can be expected of a joint or tissue in an uninjured state? In addition, however, extensive practical experience and tactile skills are also required.

As a rule, a healthy joint or tissue always behaves in the same way: within its range of motion, it has a smaller or larger "neutral zone." At the end of the range of motion there is a "physiological space," followed by a "paraphysiological space" (Fig. 2).

The "neutral zone" is usually located in the middle of the range of motion and is characterized by a very small increase in resistance (R1 at the end of "neutral zone"). The "physiological space" begins with the second significant resistance of the connective tissue (R2). The therapist passively mobilizes the tissue to a greater or lesser extent in this area—depending on the intensity of the manual gradation (dosage) and the currently prevailing wound-healing phase. The "paraphysiological space" can only be reached by an impulse mobilization (manipulation). Post-traumatically or postoperatively the anatomical barrier has moved forward. The reason for this is collagen type III, which predominates in the proliferation phase. It is responsible for the integrity of the injured structure and causes the rapid formation of water-soluble crosslinks. Temporary collagen type III does not withstand mechanical shear and acceleration forces very well. Overdosage is therefore quickly possible, especially in the proliferation phase. Microtraumatic injuries trigger new inflammatory phases, which can lead to

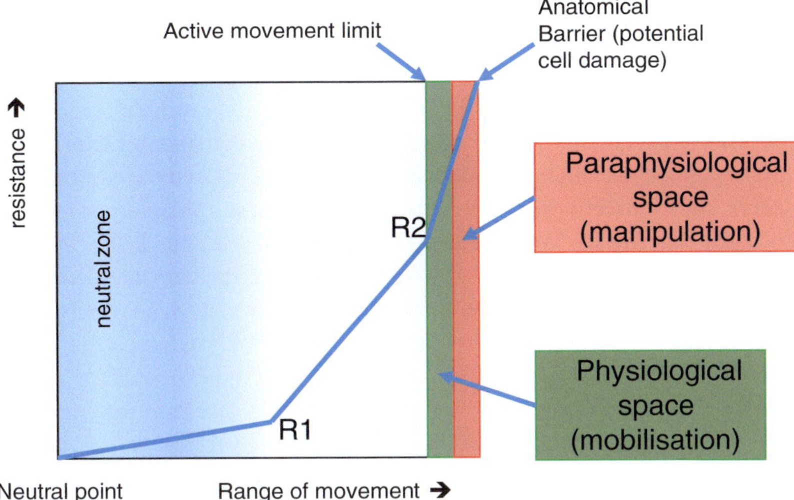

Fig. 2 Behavior of resistance depending on the extent of movement in joints and connective tissue. R1 represents the first and R2 represents the second significant increase in connective tissue resistance. Depending on the intensity of the manual gradation (dosage), therapists treat passively more or less into the physiological space. The paraphysiological space is only achieved by impulse mobilization. If the anatomical barrier is exceeded, cell damage occurs (lesion) which results in an inflammatory reaction. This anatomical barrier is important in posttraumatic and postoperative conditions due to adhesions and water-soluble crosslinks that are moved to the front. Especially in the proliferation phase, this can quickly lead to overdosing. Microtraumatic injuries trigger new inflammatory phases, which result in increased tissue and movement restriction [12] (Courtesy of Own illustration)

increased tissue restriction, and thus restricting movement.

> **Clinical Tip**
>
> - In comparison to healthy skin, the first marked increase in connective tissue resistance usually occurs much faster around a spontaneously healed scar or in an area with surgical coverage.
> - The distance between the first and second marked increase in connective tissue resistance is also usually considerably shorter than in healthy skin.
> - The second marked increase in connective tissue resistance feels hard, stiff, and wooden. The aim is to use therapeutic measures to gradually extend the distance between the first and second marked increase in connective tissue resistance and thus restore the function of the connective tissue.

Mechanical Stimulation

Mechanotransduction

It is known from the literature that the absence of mechanical stimulus is associated with a loss of functional alignment of the fibers. It has also been shown that too much mechanical stress quickly leads to an overdosing (cell damage, renewed inflammatory reaction) [1, 4, 5, 13, 14].

The transmission of mechanical stimuli in the body, for example, by manual techniques, seems to take place in two signaling pathways. Empirically, a "release" in the tissue can often be perceived after only a few minutes. The mechanical stimulus must, therefore, have an effect directly on the tissue, for example, the release of possible pathological crosslinks (water-soluble type) or reactive tonus changes in the connective tissue. The second signaling pathway has been scientifically researched under the term "mechanotransduction." This is the reaction inside the cell to a mechanically applied external stimulus.

If the stimulus is adequate, the cell reacts with a gene transcription and thus influences the cytoskeleton and the ECM and thus the quality of the affected cell [7, 13, 15–19]. The aim of the therapeutically applied manual techniques is therefore not (as previously assumed) to lengthen collagen fibers by stretching but to directly influence cell biological processes by means of adequate stimulation.

What dosage is adequate during the wound-healing phases in relation to functional stimulation at the cellular level? Various aspects are described below:

Bouffard et al. (2008) observed a decrease in TGF-beta 1 concentration and collagen synthesis after tissue injury by 20–30% static tissue stretching for 10 min daily [15].

TGF-beta 1 is a local cytokine that is associated with wound healing and tissue fibrosis. The results of this study suggest that tissue stretching during wound healing leads to a reduction in TGF-beta 1 levels and thus to altered collagen synthesis. This could be an important natural mechanism in limiting excessive scarring [3].

Balestrini and Biliar (2009) were able to demonstrate a positive effect on the extensibility of the extracellular matrix with daily 5% tissue stretching for 24 h. The authors found that a stretching stimulus that was too strong and lasted too long led to increased collagen synthesis and thus to increased tissue restriction. This could only be achieved therapeutically with the help of a splint and well-dosed stimulation [13].

In a review, Andalib et al. (2016) summarized selected studies on mechanotransduction. They also addressed the question of mechanical forces acting on cells. These are given in the former force unit "Dyne" (replaced by the SI unit "Newton" [N] since 1978). The converted data shows that all cells were mechanically stimulated with a force between 0.00002 N and 0.00058 N. In all included studies, a mechanotransduction effect was found [16]. These findings indicate that cells are highly mechanosensitive. Only minimal forces are required for a cell to respond to a mechanical stimulus.

The mechanotransduction process is shown schematically in Fig. 3. The mechanosensors are stimulated by an external mechanical stimulus (here using the example of a fibroblast). These in turn activate "adapter proteins," which are located on the cell nucleus membrane (nuclear membrane). These "adapter proteins" transmit the mechanical stimulus to the cytoskeleton. In this way, they stimulate the skeletal structure. The cell reacts with a gene transcription and passes on correspondingly altered (adapted) processes and products to the extracellular matrix. Thus, a cell response to an external mechanical stimulus takes place [8, 15].

The cytoskeleton of every cell is normally under physiological tension. This tension is in balance with the texture of the ECM and the functional mechanical stimuli in daily life.

In the case of pathological scarring, however, this physiological tension of the cytoskeleton is already increased. This leads to higher sensitivity to mechanical stimuli. Due to the increased collagen deposits and myofibroblast activity, the ECM has a higher tension and stiffness than physiological skin (tissue). This imbalance is responsible for the fact that mechanical stimuli occurring in daily life can already be perceived as overload at the cellular level and lead to an overreaction in the cell. This can end in a pathological fibrosis process.

> **Important to Know**
> - In manual scar therapy, the dosage approach should be selected in such a way that a physiological balance can be restored regarding intra- and extracellular mechanical tension.

Unfortunately, the facts explained so far do not allow a clear conclusion regarding the correct dosage. However, by putting the individual pieces of the puzzle together, it is possible to approach the area of adequate and functional dosage.

It can be assumed that there is a significant difference between the application of a high and

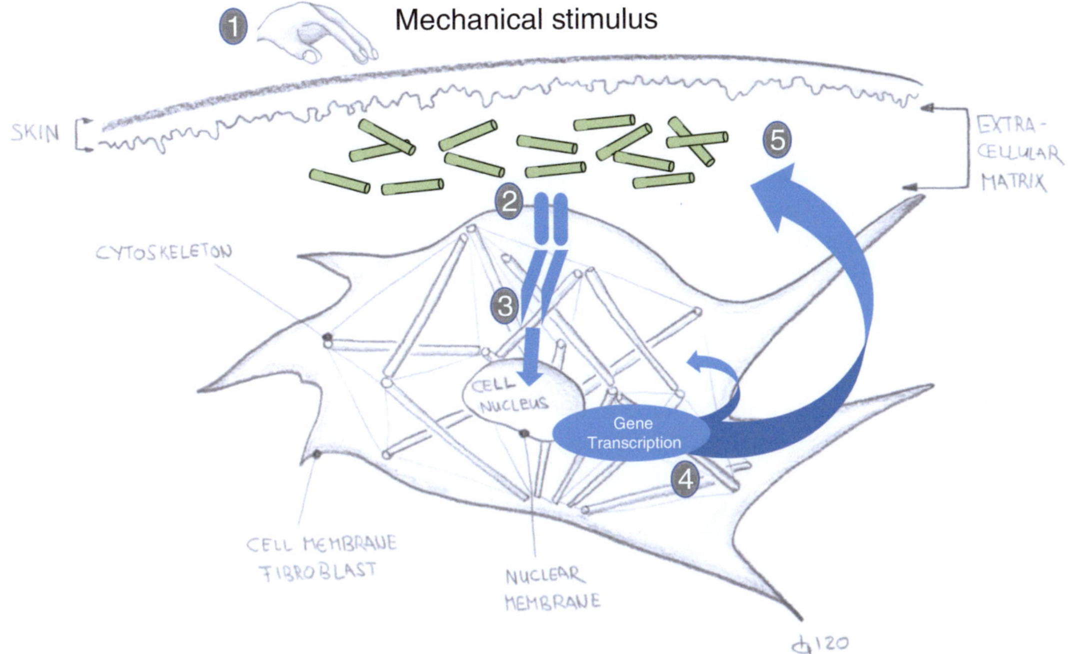

Fig. 3 Schematically depicted mechanotransduction process of the reaction of a fibroblast cell to an external mechanical stimulus [7, 13, 15–19] (Courtesy of T. Koller). (1) A mechanical stimulus is applied by a physiological movement or manual input by hand. (2) Mechanosensors on the cell membrane register the fluid displacement and transmit this signal into the cell. (3) The mechanosensors activate "adapter proteins" which transmit the mechanical stimulus to the cytoskeleton. (4) The cell reacts with a gene transcription and passes on correspondingly altered (adapted) products to the extracellular matrix. (5) Newly functionally aligned collagen networks after an injury or through "new use" due to a new activity

a low dosage. This consideration refers to the active phase of a scar and it is not yet mature state. Therefore, amplitude, duration, and frequency are important parameters that should be considered in connection with the wound-healing phases [15].

Amplitude

Amplitude is defined as the largest excursion of an oscillation or a pendulum from the center position or as the oscillation range. If the mechanical stimulus (the amplitude) is too strong, the reaction of the cell nucleus becomes much less controllable. This can quickly lead to an overreaction of the cell. Due to the persistent inflammatory state, the cell is more sensitive. This leads to the hypothesis that stimuli that are harmless to the physiological skin may already represent an overdose in scars [20].

Since mechanotransductive cell responses are initiated by minimal forces (up to 0.00058 N), functional alignment is already achieved with very gentle manual therapeutic interventions. In the back region, the empirically known marked increases in connective tissue resistance R1 and R2 are 1–2 N for R1 and 2–4 N for R2 [10, 11]. Thus, it can be assumed that manual interventions in the area of R1 probably already provide a sufficiently adequate stimulus for the scar tissue to induce a mechanotransductive response of the cell and thus a functional alignment of the extracellular matrix.

In the proliferation phase, R1 appears to be an important indication for a wound-healing-adapted dosage. In the remodulation phase, a dosage up to R2 is acceptable.

Several years of clinical experience with severely burned patients show that in the proliferation phase manual scar techniques should only be used until the first increase in connective tissue resistance is reached. This is because the tissue is significantly less resilient than comparable connective tissue in the same wound-healing phase [5]. Due to the delayed wound healing, burn scars often have a considerably prolonged proliferation phase. As a result, the transition from R1 to R2 is empirically experienced as smooth (Fig. 4).

In the case of linear (surgical) scars, the clinical situation is more stable. There is no mechanical overdosage if the dosage is increased up to the second connective tissue resistance in the proliferation phase and if it is increased into the second connective tissue resistance in the remodulation phase (Fig. 5).

Koller (2018, 2019) conducted a pilot study on interrater reliability to determine R1 and R2.

The results were promising. Therapists appear to be able to detect the first significant increase in connective tissue resistance with moderate (ICC2 = 0.67) and the second significant increase in connective tissue resistance with good interrater reliability (ICC2 = 0.80). Regarding direct and indirect pain conduction, it can be assumed that C-fiber activity progressively sets in with the second marked increase in connective tissue resistance (R2) and that until R2 mainly the Aδ fibers are active as a "warning signal" of cell damage [10, 11].

Frequency

The frequency describes how fast repetitions within a periodic process follow each other per second. The unit of frequency is Hertz (Hz).

Balestrini and Biliar (2006) found that a cyclical stretch stimulus with 0.2 Hz and moderate

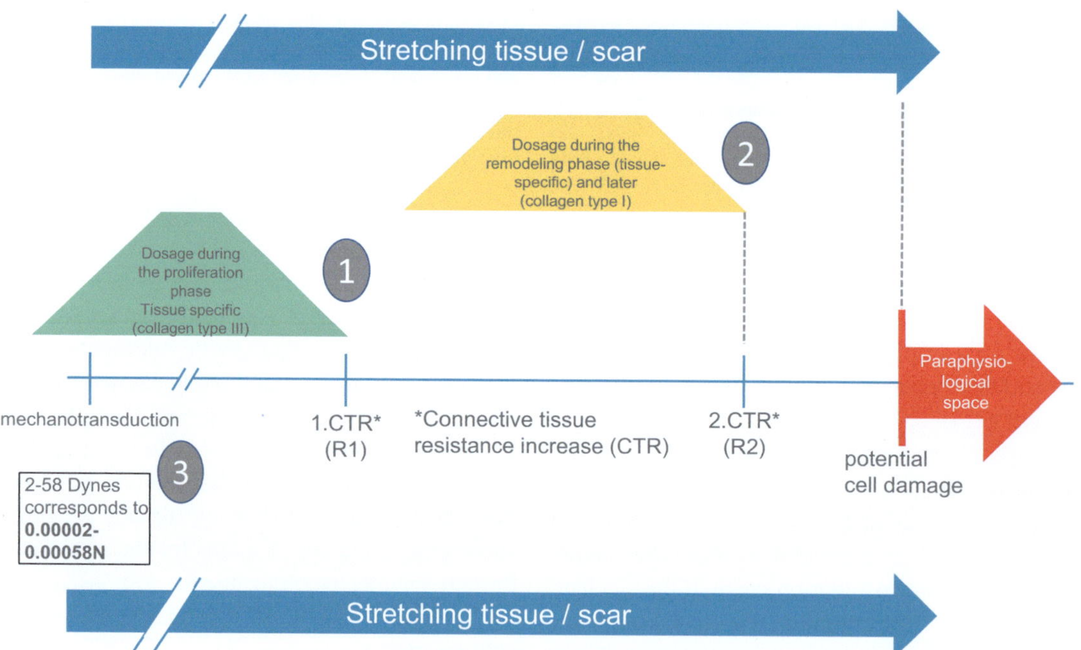

Fig. 4 Summarizing presentation of wound-healing-phase-adapted and tissue-specific dosages in the manual therapy of burn scars (Courtesy of Own presentation). (1) In the proliferation phase, around the first significant increase in connective tissue resistance (amplitude). (2) In the remodulation phase, progressing up to the second remarkable increase in connective tissue resistance (amplitude). (3) R1 and R2 are exemplary. Connective tissue displaceability in the back is within a range of 1–4 N [11] (much higher than the fibroblast needs for mechano-transductive cell response)

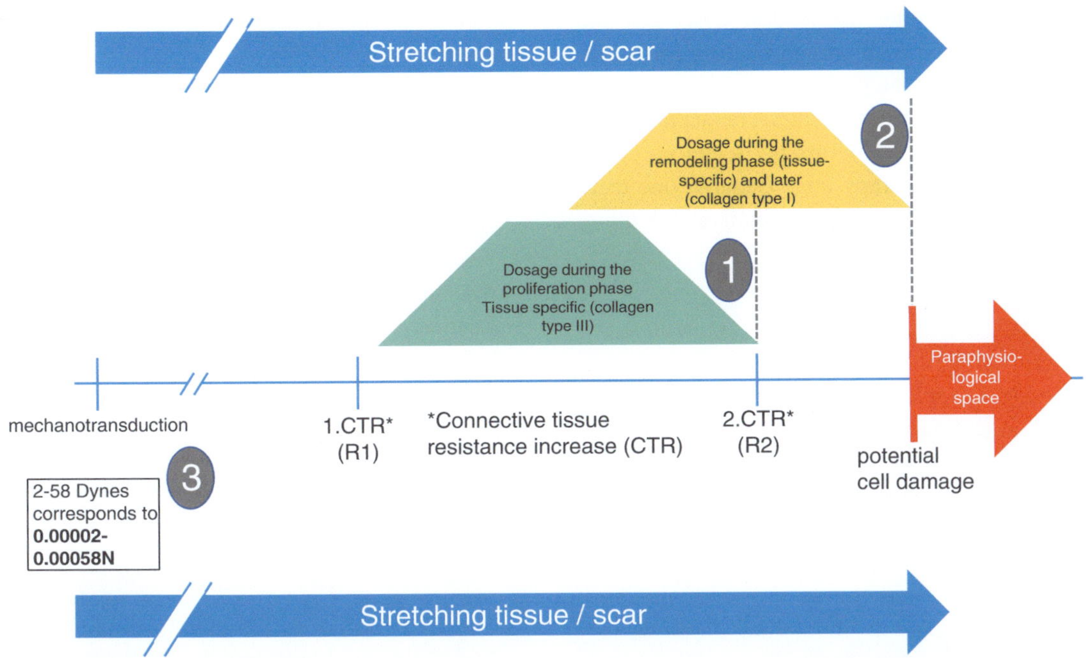

Fig. 5 Summarizing presentation of wound-healing phase adapted and tissue-specific dosages in manual therapy of injured tissue (post-traumatic/postoperative) (Courtesy of Own presentation). (1) In the proliferation phase, progressing up to the second remarkable increase in connective tissue resistance (amplitude). (2) In the remodulation phase, into the second remarkable increase in connective tissue resistance (amplitude). (3) R1 and R2 are exemplary. Connective tissue displaceability on the back is within a range of 1–4 N [11] (much higher than the fibroblast needs for a mechanotransductive cell response)

amplitude stimulates the fibroblasts to produce a more resistant matrix. The tissue density increases, and the fibers are reorganized. Histologically, a significant decrease in thickness was observed. After this stimulus, the tissue was thinner, denser, and better organized [14].

Carano et al. (1996) demonstrated a 200% increase in collagenase production with cyclic stretching on fibroblasts compared to static stretching [21].

Clinically recommendable would therefore be a slight stretching, tailored to the respective wound-healing phase with intermittent oscillation (0.2 Hz) at the end of the respective amplitude. These assumptions correlate with empirical and clinical experience but have not yet been proven in human research.

Duration

How long should a stimulus be applied? This is another fundamental question regarding dosage. Although splints and other stretching techniques are widely used, there are no research results on humans available in the literature. Only effects from animal studies can serve as a basis for clinical considerations and empirical experience.

Bouffard et al. were able to demonstrate good results (reduced TFG-beta 1) with daily 10 min stretching and moderate amplitude (20% stretching) [15]. However, practical experience shows that splint applications over several hours also produce positive effects.

Carano et al. (1996) conducted research on cell cultures of artificial ligaments. They found that a five-minute application time was most effective in terms of wound healing for a previously placed lesion [21].

Empirically, good results are achieved with application times of 1 min per location, three to five times per therapy unit. Usually, one to two therapy units per day are realistic in the clinical setting.

> **Clinical Tip**
> - Recommended dosage **for large-area and deep dermal scars:**
>   - In the *proliferation phase*: around the first marked increase in connective tissue resistance (amplitude)
>   - In the *remodulation phase:* progressively up to the second marked increase in connective tissue resistance (amplitude)
> - Dosage recommendations **for linear scars:**
>   - In the *proliferation phase*: up to the second marked increase in connective tissue resistance (amplitude)
>   - In the *remodulation phase*: progressively into the second marked increase in connective tissue resistance (amplitude)
> - Application duration: In general 1 min per location, three to five times per therapy unit in addition to an oscillating frequency of 0.2 Hz at the end of the respective amplitude

Noninvasive Treatment Options

Scar maturation can have a negative effect on function. Physiological wound contracture leads to increased tension in the tissue and mobility decreases. Therapists try to counteract these negative effects as much as possible to achieve an optimal functional result. The following therapeutic options are based on the mechanotransductor mode of action. They are considered to be

effective and purposeful in terms of regaining function:

- Manual scar therapy
- Compression
- Silicone
- Splints
- Tape (Kinesio®)
- Vacuum massage
- Scar care (with ointments)

> **Important to Know**
> In order to counteract pathological scarring, the following factors must always be considered:
>
> - Avoid increase of blood flow
> - Mechanical forces in adjusted dosage
> - General tension reduction of the tissue
> - Prevent overstrain from daily activities

> **Caution!**
> Sliding on the skin leads to increased shear forces and hyperemia. Excessive external mechanical forces can result in pathological wound healing [8]. The tension can be positively influenced by manual techniques, compression and silicone, splints, tape, and vacuum massage. Behavior that is in line with wound healing is also essential for daily life.

Compression

In everyday clinical practice, textile compression therapy is standard for the prevention and treatment of hypertrophic scars. However, it has not yet been conclusively clarified on which humoral, cellular, or mechanical processes the effect of compression therapy is based [22]. The results of the systematic review and meta-analysis of Ai et al. (2017) show that patients with hypertrophic scarring receiving compression therapy showed significant improvements regarding redness, pigmentation, thickness, and hardness of the scar. In addition, it is known that the application of pressure relieves itching and pain in active hypertrophic scars [23]. Continuous pressure on an active scar causes numerous small vessels to close ischemically. Ischemia leads to increased apoptosis of myofibroblasts during scar maturation causing a reorganization of the extracellular matrix [3]. Compression-induced hypoxia shifts the collagen synthesis toward catabolism [24]. This may lead to the destruction of existing collagen fibers and thus to a lower density of the scar structure. At the same time, the new stimulation (mechanical compression) allows a more functional re-synthesis of collagen. This results in a qualitatively better and functionally more resilient scar tissue [22].

Patients with deep second-degree and third-degree burns as well as with other scars prone to hypertrophy receive customized compression garments [25]. It is recommended to wear compression garments consistently day and night until the end of scar maturation to achieve the most aesthetic scar maturation possible with minimal functional restrictions. A short interruption of the compression therapy is needed to change the compression garment, perform personal hygiene, and care for the scar [22].

The duration of the compression therapy depends on several factors:

- Severity of scars (depth of burn)
- Localization and extension of scars
- Individually different healing reactions
- Acceptance to therapy, patience of the patient and relatives

Empirical values show a period of at least 8–24 months [22].

The following literature-based "three-phase model" of compression has established itself in recent years at the University Hospital Zurich and the Bellikon Rehabilitation Clinic. Flat-knitted products of the Swiss company TTK are used. The terms "comfort" and "strong" refer to the product descriptions by this company.

Phase 1: Early Phase

Patients receive surgical interventions in the acute hospital. As a result, the wound volumes often fluctuate greatly and sometimes the wound areas are still oozing.

Expensive custom-made compression products would not be appropriate in this phase. With tubular bandages (e.g., Eesiban®) and self-adhesive dressings (e.g., CobanTM®), however, a transition from classic wound dressing to compression (10–14 mmHg) can take place early in the healing process. At the same time, early compression can be supplemented by ready-to-wear products. This also improves treatment adherence.

Phase 2: Customized Compression ("Comfort"; Viscose/Elastane)

In this phase, wound healing is largely completed. Patients with extensive wounds are usually transferred to a rehabilitation clinic. People with minor injuries usually receive outpatient follow-up treatment. Now the compression treatment begins with custom-made, soft, comfortable material of compression class II.

Depending on wound healing, a gradual start is also possible. In areas with wounds that are still oozing, materials from the early phase are still used. The custom-made products are used in healed regions.

Phase 3: Customized Compression ("Strong"; Polyamide/Elastane)

Once wound healing is complete, the scar tissue becomes more resilient and pressure sensitivity decreases. The patient is active again and largely independent in daily life. A further individual treatment with more robust material should be aimed for.

They are then more able to tolerate the compression 23 h/24 h. This is a decisive factor for the success of compression therapy [26]. Physiologically healed scars do not necessarily require compression. If patients are involved in therapy decisions, this improves their adherence. If, in addition to the scar problem, lymphatic insufficiency exists, a treatment with compression class III products should be considered.

Custom-made articles should be made of materials that are comfortable to wear and have good haptics. Compression materials that are hard, stiff, or even scratchy are not very well accepted.

Experience shows that compression garments should meet the following requirements [22]:

- Exact reproduction of the skin profile without incisive wrinkling (risk of pressure points)
- Uniform compression with the least possible functional interference
- Few, flat, and flexible seams
- Seams should not be directly on the joints
- Good skin tolerance
- Durable, breathable, and easy to clean.

Colored material can promote acceptance. However, it should be noted that colored materials often have a harder feel due to the higher pigmentation of the material.

The various compression classes (RAL standard) have the following pressure characteristics [27]:

- Compression class I: moderate compression (18.0–21.0 mmHg)
- Compression class II: medium compression (23.0–32.0 mmHg)
- Compression class III: strong compression (34.0–46.0 mmHg)

The unit of measurement [mmHg; millimeters of mercury] is used to specify the static pressure. Measuring instruments for compression therapy are offered by TT Meditrade (Denmark), for example, Kikuhime®.

Silicone

Since 1981, silicone has been used in the treatment of deep dermal defects and hypertrophic scars. Today, it is one of the most common methods of scar treatment, although so far there is only weak evidence for this form of therapy to treat existing scars or for prophylaxis. The effect is based on increased hydration of the scar tissue, caused by silicone gel as a water-impermeable membrane. This mode of action corresponds to an occlusion. In addition, this probably leads to reduced blood circulation or angiogenesis and thus to reduced collagen synthesis [28].

Silicone offers a decisive advantage, especially in burn scars: it reduces the mechanical shearing forces in relation to the "external environment" and thus prevents direct friction on the scar surface. However, there is still no definitive evidence of this.

When should silicone be used in scar therapy? The following methods of application have proven themselves in practice:

Silicone patches:

- In case of excessive mechanical tension on the tissue or scar surface
- In case of hypertrophy and excessive keloid formation
- In case of severe itching (mainly because of the hydration properties)

Customized silicone pads:

- In case of undercuts (recesses/indentations in the tissue)
- In case of anatomically complex shapes
- In case of extensive depressions and unevenness

Silicone in the facial area:

- Always in combination with hard shell masks or partial masks.
- Silicone gel is used for small areas.

To clean or aerate the skin/scar and the silicone pad, daily application breaks of no more than 1 h must be adhered to. The silicone gel is applied twice a day to the lesions being treated.

The advantage of this therapy option is its ease of application. Only rarely do side effects such as folliculitis, erosion, or itching occur.

Silicone gel is often used in combination with other procedures or in postoperative scar prophylaxis. Compared to silicone gel patches, it has the additional advantage that it can also be used on highly visible body parts and over joints. The gel can also be used to apply sun protection products or cosmetics. The side effect of maceration, which is often observed when the patches are worn for a longer period, can also be avoided with silicone gel. Silicone of any kind must not be used on open wounds. Experience has shown that failure to observe daily hygiene measures (during the break in application) can lead to skin irritation.

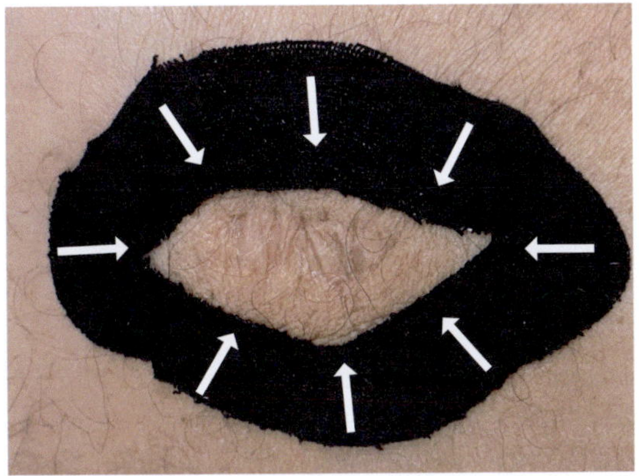

Fig. 6 Tape for mechanical relief of a scar (Figure: Rehabilitation Clinic Bellikon)

Splints

A great advantage of specific, custom-made splints is the duration of application. Splint applications (several times a day in addition to the therapy) make it possible to set a functionally adequate stimulus. Optimal fitting of a splint is often a major challenge at the beginning of rehabilitation and is resource intensive. Due to volume fluctuations resulting from different application techniques of the bandages, potential pressure points are a constant risk, which is why splints must be checked and adjusted regularly. Splints are ideal for the hand, wrists, elbow, ankle, and mouth. The dosage (wearing time, angle, and extent of movement for dynamic splints) must be adapted to the respective wound-healing phase (see Figs. 4 and 5).

Tape

A standard kinesiotape® can be used to relieve scars, wounds, or areas that are subject to excessive mechanical tension. This requires the possibility to apply the tape on physiological skin or already very stable scarred skin. For sensitive skin, skin protection or removal sprays are recommended.

The length of the tape should correspond to the area to be relieved. The therapist cuts the tape lengthwise, and in the middle, fixes the first "anchor" on the tissue and fixes the two branches of the tape "surrounding the scar" (Fig. 6). There should be as much scar tissue as possible between the two legs of the tape. This leads to a visible and noticeable mechanical stress relief.

The tape may remain on the skin for a maximum of 5 days. Further application should only take place after a day's rest. In patients with burn scars, a wearing period of 3 days seems to be optimal [29].

Vacuum Massage

Vacuum massage is a noninvasive mechanical massage technique invented to treat burns and scars. To date, no effects of vacuum massage on thickness and density of human scar tissue have been reported. In the skin endothelial cells, fibroblasts and myofibroblasts embedded in the ECM sense mechanical stimuli (created by vacuum massage) and may promote intracellular processes leading to matrix remodeling. Preliminary results show that the disruption of the epidermis may indicate that vacuum massage could be able to actually breach the skin barrier. The statistically significant changes in the dermal layers could suggest an increased ECM production after vacuum massage [30]. The use of vacuum massage is recommended toward the end of the remodulation phase or outside the classic wound-healing phases.

Strong punctual mechanical vibrations show clinically similar effects; a scientific proof is still missing.

Practical Tips in the Use of Compression Suits and Silicone Inserts

For the orthotist, any large or circular scar area is a challenge. Especially, the concave-shaped areas of the body, such as the palms of the hand or the décolleté area, are not, or only insufficiently, compressed by compression garments. This is where a custom-made silicone insert can help. The second challenge is to put on the compression garment without generating shear to the scar. Excessive shear forces damage the fragile scar surface and inevitably lead to a new inflammatory reaction.

The choice of dressing aids is large, varied, and tolerated very individually by patients. In this chapter, a small selection of dressing aids is used, and illustrated with video sequences (see supplementary material), to explain dressing that is gentle on the tissue and avoids shear forces.

Does Compression Garment Always Compress Equally Well?

Compression garments compress better over straight and convex scar areas than over concave areas of the body. Over concave areas of the body, such as the décolleté, or back area, the scar area to be compressed is often only "spanned" (see Fig. 7a, b). Custom-made silicone pads can be used to compensate these cavities. If the area is very large, full silicone can no longer be used because the specific weight of silicone is very high. For this purpose, either foam materials are ground into shape or silicone foam is cast, and then covered with a thin layer of silicone.

A practical example illustrates the effect of increased compression by a fitted silicone pad. Figure 8a shows a compression class II glove without a silicone pad in the palm of the hand. The spanned cavity can be depressed. If a silicone pad is placed on the concave palm (Fig. 8b, c), there is no longer a cavity and the compression force can act on the scar tissue through the silicone. Fig. 8d, e, shows how effectively a silicone insert can transfer the compression force to the scar tissue.

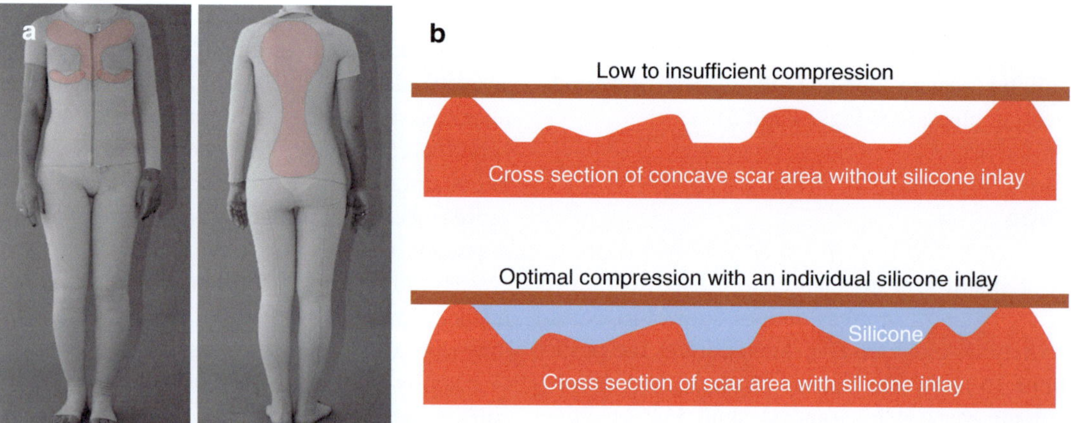

Fig. 7 Insufficient compression of uneven and concave scar areas (Courtesy of Rehaklinik Bellikon). (**a**) Compression is insufficient in the area marked in red. The compression garment "spans" these areas. (**b**) With an individually crafted silicone inlay (for example modeled after a plaster cast), the compression force can be homogeneously distributed over the uneven scar surface

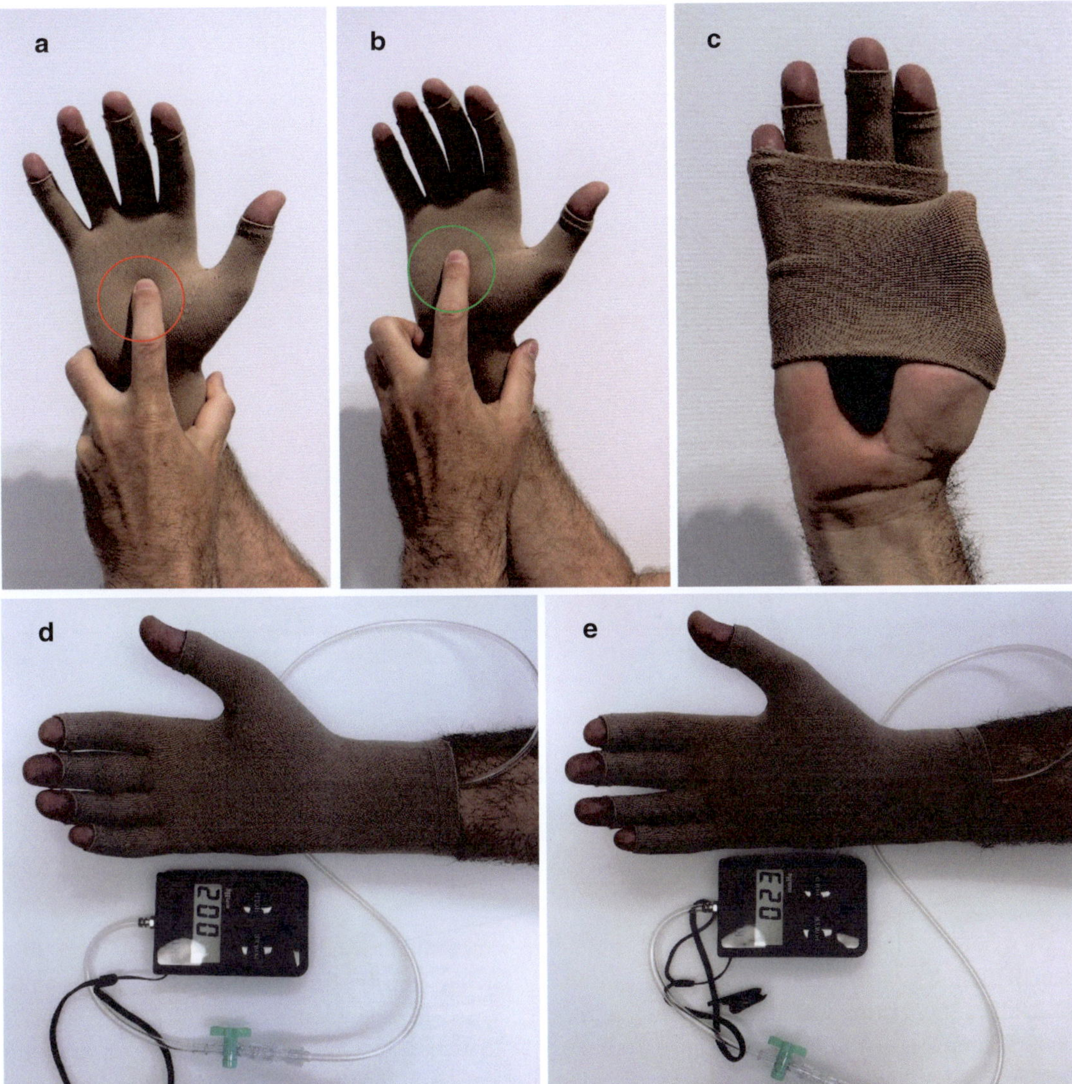

Fig. 8 Effect of silicone inserts on compression forces (Courtesy of Rehaklinik Bellikon). (**a**) Compression class II glove without silicone pad in the palm (red circle).(**b, c**) Compression class II glove with silicone pad in the palm (green circle). (**d**) Pressure measurement [2 mmHg] in the palm of the hand without silicone padding. (**e**) Pressure measurement [23 mmHg] in the palm of the hand with silicone padding. The unit of measurement [mmHg; millimeters of mercury] is used to indicate the static pressure. Measuring instruments for compression therapy are offered by the company TT Meditrade (Denmark), for example Kikuhime®

> **Caution!**
> Compression garments may exert insufficient to no compression on concave and uneven scar surfaces. Custom-made silicone inserts help transfer force to scar tissue.

Compliance as a Basic Prerequisite

The basic prerequisite for effective compression therapy is the patient's consent and willingness to wear the compression garment for 23 h daily. This usually continues until the scar has fully matured (up to 2 years). To achieve this ambitious goal, the individual needs (tolerance level) of the patient must always be considered. If a

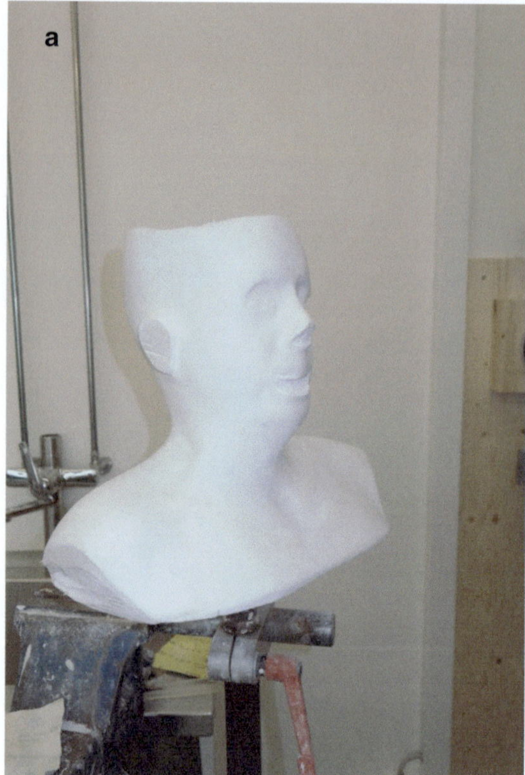

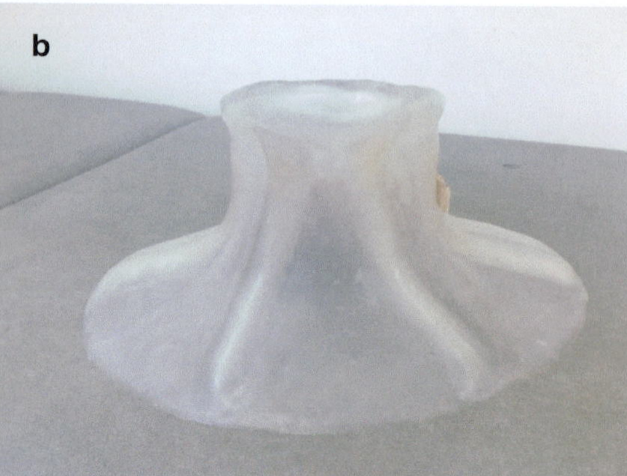

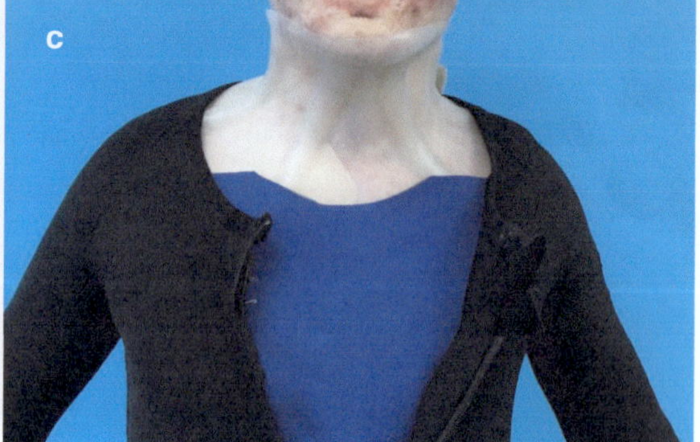

Fig. 9 Silicone collar with light compression (Courtesy of Rehaklinik Bellikon). (**a**) Fabricated plaster model (positive) based on a plaster cast. (**b**) Silicone collar with form-giving silicone reinforcements. (**c**) Patient with silicone collar and compression garment

patient does not agree with the aid, it will not be used. Often, less is more! If a patient with extensive full-body scarring would have to wear a full-body compression suit but is unwilling to do so, perhaps individual parts in severely affected areas can be a compromise solution.

Following technical prerequisites can increase the patient's compliance:

– Proper suture placement: sutures should not pass directly over joints. If this cannot be avoided, they should be placed in such a way that there is as little friction as possible during movement. For example, at the knee medial and lateral to the knee joint. This also applies to zippers.

– Adapted knitting technique: Especially around the joints, a different knitting technique (similar like kneecaps) can significantly reduce mechanical shear forces. This will in turn result in less scar irritation and better compliance on the patient's part.

– Silicone instead of compression: If no compression is tolerated (for example in the neck area), just an individually shaped silicone collar can also achieve a good effect. The compression force is missing here, but the hydrating and micro-massaging properties of the silicone also have a positive effect on the function and quality of the scar tissue (Fig. 9).

Dressing Aids That Avoid Shear Force and Are Gentle on the Tissue

Arion Easy-Slide® Donning Aids

These donning aids are suitable for compression stockings with open toe or hand tip. They can

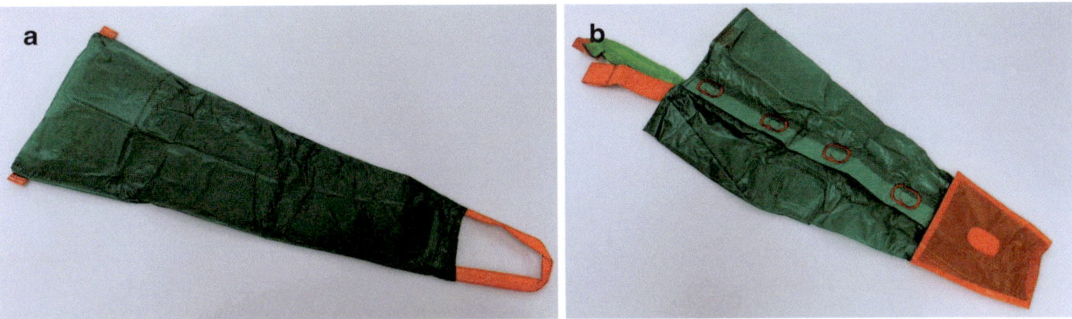

Fig. 10 Donning aid Arion Easy-Slide® for open foot and hand tips (**a**) and for closed foot and hand tips (**b**) (Courtesy of Rehaklinik Bellikon)

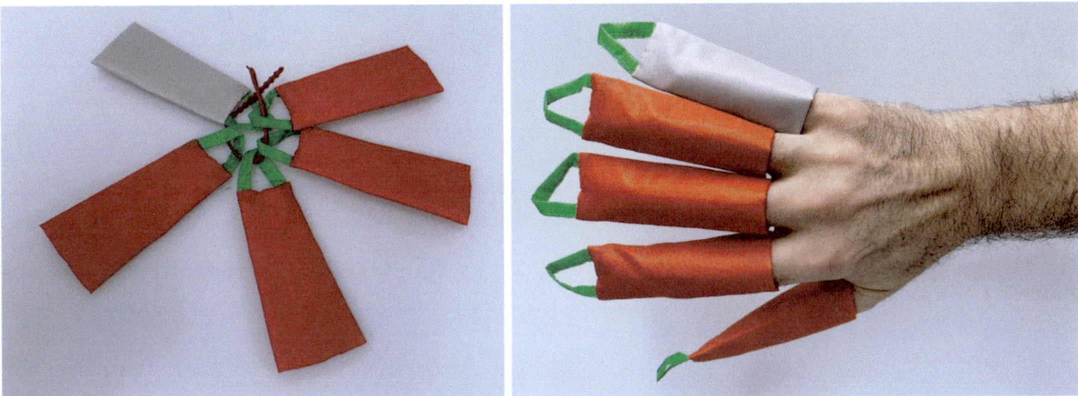

Fig. 11 Arion Dactyna® donning aid for open finger cots or gloves (Courtesy of Rehaklinik Bellikon)

also be used to put on silicone-coated compression stockings without putting too much strain on the fabric and skin. A special Easy-Slide® version is also available for closed-toe compression stockings (Fig. 10a, b). The correct donning procedure is shown in Video 1.

The Arion Dactyna® donning aid is suitable for donning finger cots or entire gloves (Fig. 11). Here, too, the compression material can be applied over the fingers in a way that is very gentle on the tissue (Video 2).

Medi Butler® Dressing Aids

These donning aids are particularly suitable for patients who have little hand strength (Fig. 12). The leg can be pressed into the compression stocking relatively easily. The ribbed stocking then also rolls over the extremity in a way that is gentle on the tissue (Video 3). In addition, rubber gloves can be used to help a little.

DOFF N'DONNER® (DND) Donning Aid

DOFF N'DONNER® is a revolutionary donning aid that is very soft and allows the compression stocking to roll over the limb particularly easily (Fig. 13). It is suitable for both open and closed compression stockings.

The donning technique requires some practice at the beginning (Video 4).

Clinical Tip

Perfectly fitting compression garments with correctly positioned seams or zippers and silicone pads are of no use at all if they are not worn regularly!

Acceptance is always very individual and must be clarified in advance with the patient.

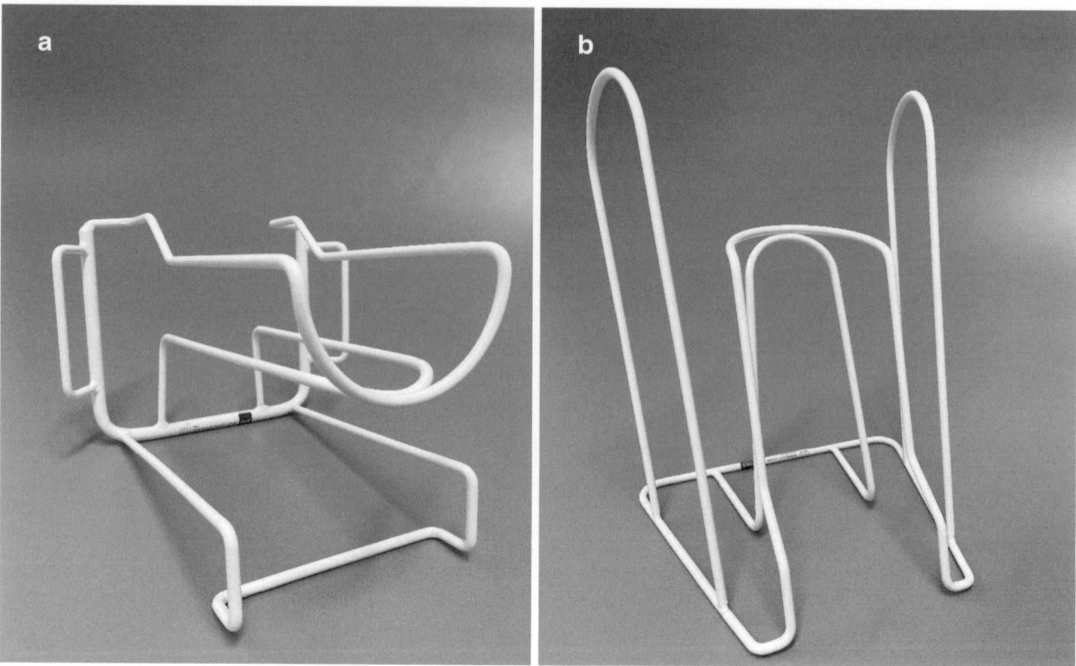

Fig. 12 Dressing aids for arms/gloves "medi Butler®" (**a**) and for legs "medi Lang-Griff Butler®" (**b**) (Courtesy of Rehaklinik Bellikon)

Scar Care

Scar care is of great importance for patients with burns, sometimes even for the rest of their lives. Depending on the depth of the burn, the natural moisture regulation of the skin is reduced or no longer present. This requires care with cream or, in some cases, with silicone pads. Silicone pads are particularly recommended in areas with high mechanical tension such as scar strands, very hypertrophic scars, scars that are difficult to move, over joints, and in circular scar areas.

In general, there is weak to no evidence regarding the effectiveness of scar-specific care products. However, daily, and consistent application of cream to the scar is clinically very relevant. Fewer open areas due to mechanical influences, an increase in mobility, less itching, and less painful scar areas can be observed as clinical effects.

This is done by consistently applying cream or by using silicone pads. When choosing a cream, it is important to ensure that the proportions of lipids and urea are sufficiently high. An oil-in-water base mix works as a good carrier for this.

The lipid additive in creams is supposed to prevent the scar surface from drying out with a thin lipid film, smooth the rough surface, and make the scar more elastic and resistant. Urea has the advantage that it can attract and bind water in the tissue. In this way, the substance allegedly ensures a balanced and high moisture content in the skin or scar and thus also has a positive effect on itching.

It is not possible to explicitly recommend a specific cream; rather, attention should be paid to the proportions of the ingredients "lipid" and "urea." Clinically, good experiences have been made with the following products (list not exhaustive):

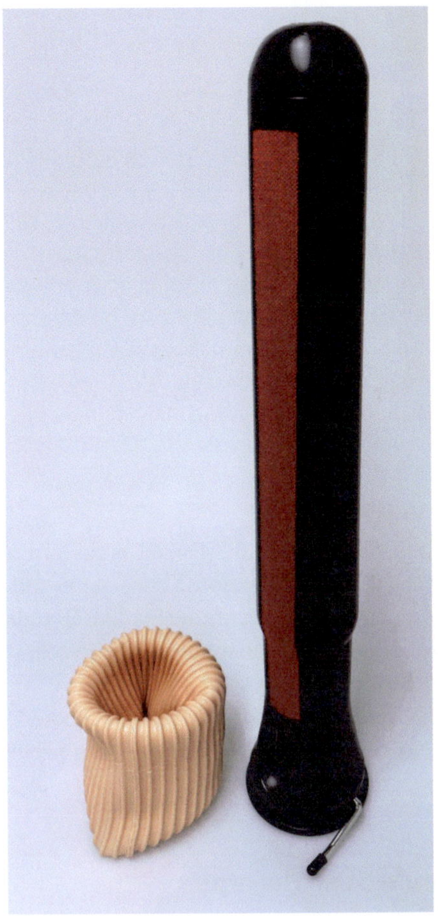

Fig. 13 DOFF N'DONNER® donning aid for arms and legs (Courtesy of Rehaklinik Bellikon)

– NutrientCream (NCR®) (lipid content 40%)
– Excipial® U Hydrolotio (lipid content 11%, urea content 2%)
– Excipial® U Lipolotio (lipid content 36%, urea content 4%)
– Bepanthen® (depending on the product up to 22% lipid content and 5% dexpanthenol)

Bepanthen® also contains the active ingredient "dexpanthenol." The most important function of dexpanthenol is wound healing of the skin, especially the epidermis. Applied to the skin as a water–oil emulsion, the active ingredient is quickly absorbed by the skin. There it is converted to pantothenic acid, which is necessary for the development of coenzyme A. Coenzyme A supports the formation of new cells and increases their biosynthesis capacity [31, 32]. In addition, dexpanthenol increases the skin's ability to retain moisture, which nourishes the skin and improves its elasticity [33]. Furthermore, dexpanthenol also has an antipruritic and anti-inflammatory effect [31, 33, 34].

Another approach is creams with the ingredient "Extractum Cepae." This active ingredient derived from onions is said to have an antiproliferative, antiphlogistic, tissue loosening, and smoothing effect on scar tissue. Systematic reviews on the benefit of "Extractum Cepae" for the prevention or therapy of hypertrophic scars and keloids do not exist; the available evidence from clinically controlled studies is limited. Clinically, no relevant effect could be found when applied to several patients. Side effects such as itching and reddened areas after applying a cream with the active ingredient "Extractum Cepae" predominated in these cases.

Application

Bepanthen® is recommended in the early phase. This cream can already be applied to crusted wounds. Its additional ingredient "dexpanthenol" has been shown to positively support wound healing.

NCR® is also a good cream for the early phase. It should only be applied to closed wounds without scabs. It is suitable for areas that are repeatedly dry and under great mechanical tension. It has a very greasy consistency and is therefore somewhat tedious to apply.

Later on, it is increasingly possible to switch to Excipial® U Lipolotio and Excipial® U Hydrolotio. Due to its lower fat content, Excipial® U Hydrolotio can be applied with ease. For more exposed areas, it is recommended to use the more lipid-rich Excipial® U Lipolotio.

Basically, the skin must be creamed as often as possible so that it does not show any dry patches. The frequency varies depending on the product used. It is often necessary to treat certain areas with an oilier product than other areas. Clinically, in the early phase, 2–3 times a day is recommended, later 1–2 times a day.

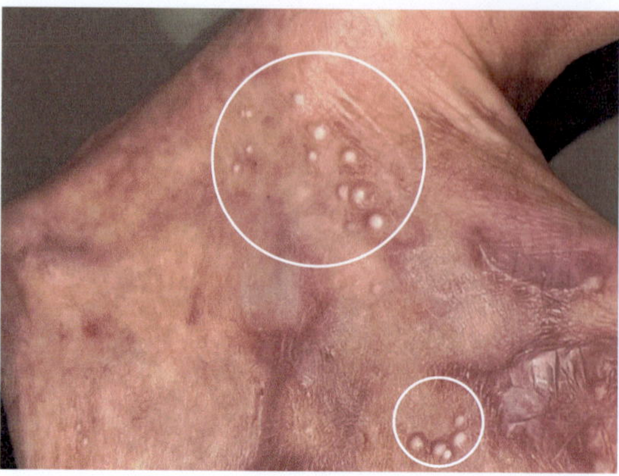

Fig. 14 Scar surface after applying oily cream for too long with clogged sebaceous glands (light dots) (Figure: Property of the Bellikon Rehabilitation Clinic)

Caution!

If a cream containing too much oil is used for too long, the skin pores become clogged and small sebaceous inclusions form, which can be seen as light spots (Fig. 14).

The remedy is to change to a less oily product and to shower regularly (if the wound situation allows this). The sebaceous inclusions are reversible. However, it takes months for the body to break them down again.

Important to Know
- **Goal:** NO dry patches and no sebaceous inclusions.
- **Lifelong care:** It is important to find a product that suits the patient and that they can and will use regularly. Strong fragrances are not recommended!
- **Combination with silicone:** Care should be taken that there is no cream under the silicone. This means: Clean the silicone after wearing it and let it dry, apply cream to the skin and let it dry as well, then apply the silicone again a few hours later. As a rule, areas with silicone pads should only be treated with cream once a day.
- **Costs:** The costs for the creams are not fully covered by all insurance companies. It is essential to clarify what is paid for by the respective insurance (also country-specific); otherwise there is a risk of immense costs for the patient. If possible, switch to a product paid for by the insurance company in the inpatient setting so that the patient can be discharged well prepared for the outpatient setting.

Sun Protection

As long as the scar or scarred areas are active (increased vascularization), consistent sun protection is strongly recommended. UV radiation can lead to hyperpigmentation, so the scars must be consistently covered or creamed!

After scar maturation, the scar should continue to be protected with at least sun protection factor 50.

Manual Scar Therapy

Manual scar therapy is not clearly defined in the literature. Terms such as "scar massage" or "soft tissue techniques" are also used. The manual scar techniques described in the following belong to the category of "Soft Tissue Techniques" and are gentler, more specific, and easier to dose.

Basically, the anamnestic procedure is identical to that for patients with physiotherapy or occupational therapy indications. The evaluation only includes a few additional questions and examinations of the skin tissue.

Acquisition Findings

Anamnesis: Additional scar-specific questions

- Ask about itching: How often? At what time of day? Where?

- Intensity of itching? Coping strategies?
- Painful scars? Pulling scars?
- Scar areas, scar strands, and wounds?
- Which scars/scar strands restrict which function most?
- Which scars/scar strands are aesthetically the most disturbing?
- Is compression clothing available? Is it applied?
- Are any aids available, e.g., splints?
- What is the frequency and duration of application?
- Are compatibility and useability given? Are there any problems?
- Are other aids necessary?

Objective examination: Additional examinations for scars

- *Inspection of the scars:* The patient must be undressed so that hypertrophic areas, scar strands, open wounds, etc. can be identified.
- *Evaluation criteria:* Color, surface, open areas, mechanically stressed areas, and scar strands.
- *General active range of motion*: Assessment at the activity level from a functional point of view.
- *Recognize compensation strategies with:* "Hand to mouth," "Tilt upper body forward," "Adjust the longitudinal axis of the body to be neutral in sitting and standing position," "Dressing," "Gripping," "Walking," "Stairclimbing," etc.
- *Passive range of motion:* What structure limits the motion?

  Where in the tissue do mechanical tensions arise? Where is the first or second significant increase in connective tissue resistance?

Specific Tests According to Jaudoin

As a rule, patients should not have any fresh cream applied before all specific testing or manual scar treatment. Otherwise the therapist's hand will slip over the skin. As a result, neither a specific diagnosis nor a treatment is possible. In addition, the application of shear forces is a contraindication in all phases of wound healing.

Capillary Refill Test (CRT)

The Capillary Refill Test makes it possible to determine the wound-healing phase in which the scar is currently in. This is decisive for the later dosage of the techniques (collagen type III or I). Inflammatory mechanisms lead to an enlargement of the capillaries in the periphery. The time required for revascularization is inversely proportional to the inflammatory factors still active in the tissue [35]. Scientific evidence on the Capillary Refill Test is not yet available.

Procedure: Apply pressure to the scar for about 3 s, release and stop the time until the color has completely adapted to the surrounding tissue color:

- Revascularization <3 s— >high inflammatory state of the tissue
- Revascularization >3 s— >inflammatory processes subside

Shifting Test (Displaceability)

With the shifting test, the mobility of the tissue in different directions can be measured. In physiological tissue, the greatest displacement is between the subcutis and fascia (or, depending on the location, in relation to the periosteum) [1].

Procedure: Place the hand flat on the tissue and let it sink in well.

Then slowly move the tissue in each direction until the first or second marked increase in connective tissue resistance is reached. The therapist documents the restricted directions in steps of thirds:

- Freely movable
- 1/3 restricted = slight restriction
- 2/3 restricted = medium restriction
- 3/3 restricted = no movement possible

The displaceability is tested on all functionally relevant scars in cranial-caudal and medial-lateral directions. It is important to focus on the entire scar and to test all areas.

Example: Scar strand in the axilla. The tissue on the thorax must be movable cranially. This is the basic prerequisite for adequate shoulder function.

Lift-Off Test

This test measures the displaceability of the tissues relative to each other as well as the density of the tissue. The decrease in density can be achieved by compression through controlled ischemia (apoptosis of myofibroblasts) [3].

Procedure: Let thumb and index finger slowly "sink" into the tissue. To prevent pinching, the therapist initiates a supination movement of the forearm. Now a skin fold develops between the fingers, which must be assessed. To ensure objectivity, the therapist measures the approximation of the thumb to the index finger [in cm]. Depending on the region of the body, place the fingers 1–3 cm apart at the beginning and measure the distance again after the skin fold has formed.

Extension Test

This test measures how far point A can be moved from point B. The therapist tests at the beginning and end of the scar strand as well as *on the* scar strand itself. In addition, measurements are taken in neutral position and at the end of the movement (limited by the scar strand). Only tissue in the same wound-healing phase should be between the hands. Open or mechanically fragile areas between point A and point B are not allowed.

Procedure: "sink" into the tissue with both hands and then move the hands apart until the first or second marked increase in connective tissue resistance is reached. Usual range: for extremities and thorax at least one hand width, on the neck, face, and fingers at least one finger width. Documentation is once again possible in thirds:

- Freely movable
- 1/3 restricted = slight restriction
- 2/3 restricted = medium restriction
- 3/3 restricted = no movement possible

Treatment Techniques

The following treatment techniques were developed by the therapists Godeau, Jaudoin, and Guillot [35–37]. The procedure described here corresponds to current evidence [5]:

This applies to all treatment techniques:

- No sliding over the skin (friction/shear forces).
- Do not use creams.
- Avoid open wounds.
- Techniques are not painful, patient tolerates pulling.
- Dosage: Depending on the phase of wound healing, note the first and second increase of connective tissue resistance and the type of scar (see Figs. 4 and 5).

Shifting Technique

"Sliding" (without sliding on the skin): make contact with the skin, "sink in," slowly move the tissue until resistance is felt (can also be done circular). Notice tissue resistance (adhesions) and then intensify movement in the functional direction. Continued movement in the tissue is prevented by recessing or delimiting, i.e., fixates the fragile or unaffected area with one hand, with the other he mobilizes the scar (Fig. 15; Video 5).

Shifting Technique at the Wound Margin

One hand holds the scar tissue in place; the other hand gently moves the unaffected tissue in a circular motion. In this manner, the therapist tries to influence the margin of the wound. The procedure can also be performed the other way round: hold the unaffected tissue and gently move the scar tissue in a circular motion (Fig. 16; Video 6).

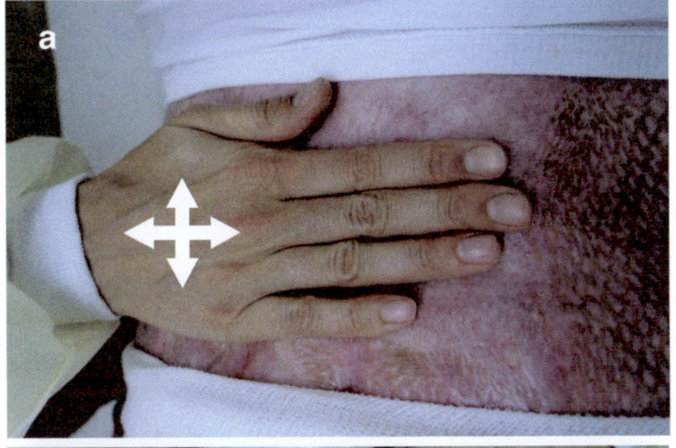

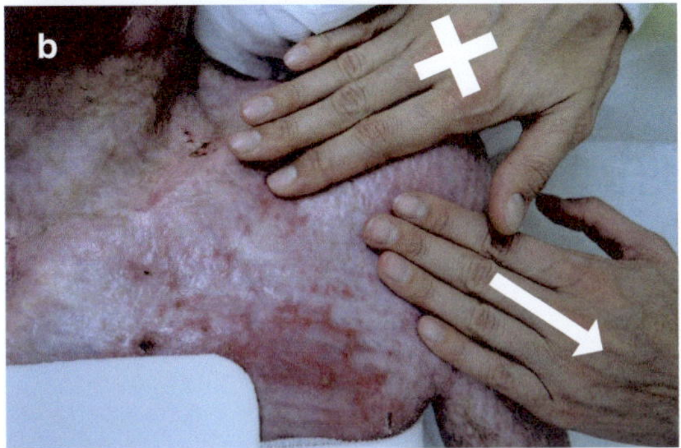

Fig. 15 Shifting technique (**a**) and shifting technique with stop (**b**) (Courtesy of Rehabilitation Clinic Bellikon)

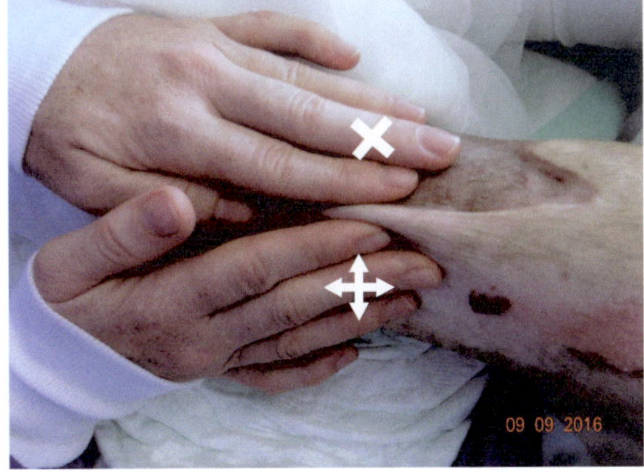

Fig. 16 Displacement technique at the wound margin. Fix the upper hand and move the lower hand. (Figure: University Hospital Zurich)

Lift-Off Technique

Proliferation phase: Gently "sink" into the tissue with thumb and forefinger, lift off the skin fold via a slight supination of the forearm, and hold it (Fig. 17; Video 7).

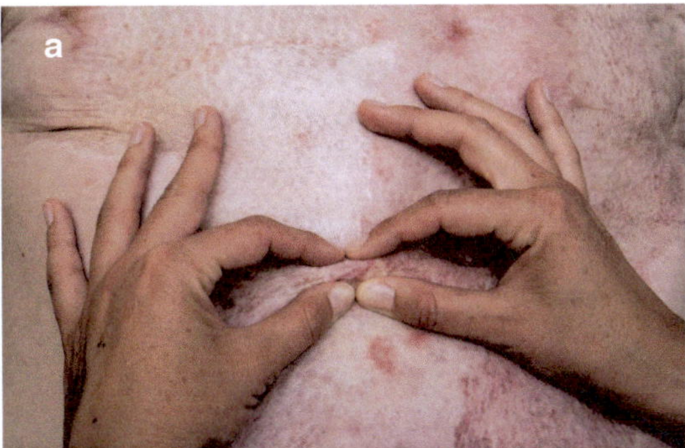

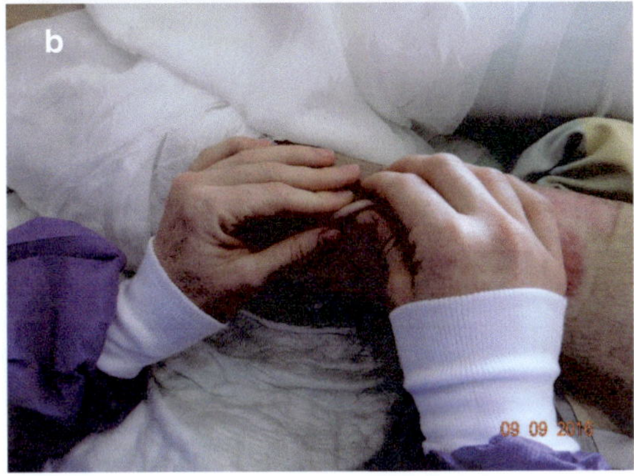

Fig. 17 Form skin fold (**a**); in the remodulation phase, form skin fold and move within (**b**) (Courtesy of University Hospital Zurich)

From the *remodulation phase* onwards, the skin fold can be moved gently within itself (without slipping over the skin). This technique can also be applied directly on a scar strand.

Extension Technique

In order to achieve an extension of the tissue, extension techniques are used in the area of the scar strand as well as in the area before and after. Two techniques can be distinguished.

The two-point technique is suitable for plane and convex scar surfaces (e.g., thorax, extremities, MCP joints, ventral knee, etc.). The three-point technique is used for concave scar surfaces (e.g., axilla, neck, elbow bend, first commissure, etc.). The scar tissue between the hands must be in the same wound-healing phase. Open areas must be left out.

Two-Point Technique

Place both hands on the tissue, "sink in," then gently pull outwards (point A moves away from point B) (Fig. 18; Video 8).

Three-Point Technique

The three-point technique is basically identical to the two-point technique.

The therapist places the hands in such a way that he can place a fixed point (third point) between points A and B with his index finger (Fig. 19; Video 9). This prevents the tissue in the concavity that is under tension from lifting off.

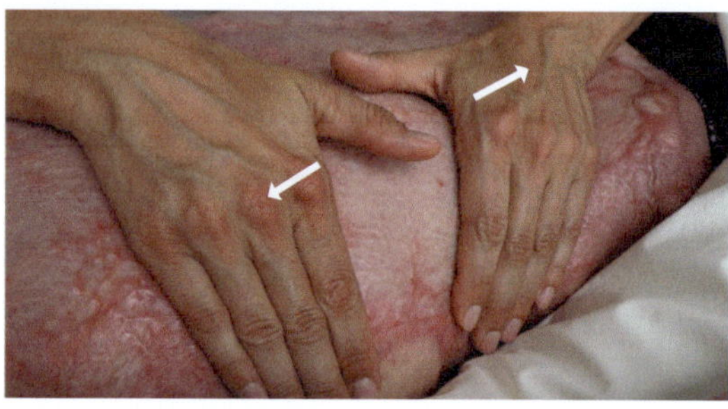

Fig. 18 Two-point extension technique for convex surfaces. (Figure: Bellikon Rehabilitation Clinic)

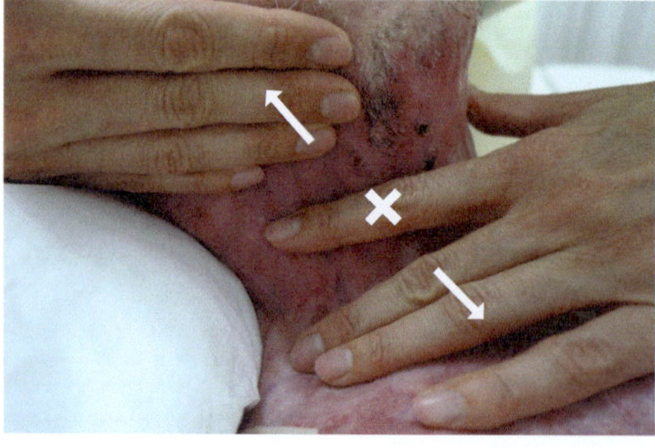

Fig. 19 Three-point extension technique for concave surfaces with fixed point in the center. (Figure: Bellikon Rehabilitation Clinic)

Clinical Tip

- A specific scar assessment precedes the appropriate treatment techniques. The aim is to determine the current phase of wound healing, the quality of the scar or scar surface, potential limitations, and general mobility. This information forms the basis for manual scar therapy and individual therapeutic measures.
- It is particularly important to start with an adequately dosed manual scar therapy at the beginning of the proliferation phase. This ensures functional alignment at the tissue level and is crucial for the best possible maintenance of function later.
- The treatment of large, deep dermal scars requires a lot of time and specific knowledge about pathophysiological processes during wound healing or scar formation.

Conclusion

To be able to initiate the correct processes at the cellular level, adequate manual dosing is a basic requirement. Overloading the tissue inevitably leads to cellular damage and triggers a new inflammatory reaction with all cardinal symptoms. Understrain, on the other hand, leads to the formation of crosslinks and reduced elasticity and resilience.

In the follow-up treatment of deep dermal defects and hypertrophic scars, additional parameters must be considered. Compression, silicone, vacuum massage, tape, and splint therapy offer valuable support here.

References

1. Van den Berg F. Das Bindegewebe des Bewegungsapparates verstehen und beeinflussen. Stuttgart: Thieme; 2011.
2. Bayat A. Skin scarring. BMJ. 2003;326(7380):88–92.
3. Tomasek J, Gabbiani G, Hinz C, Chaponnier C, Brown R. Myofibroblasts and mechano: regulation of connective tissue remodeling. Nat Rev Mol Cell Biol. 2002;3(5):349–63.
4. Koller T. Physiologische Grundlagen manueller Mobilisation von Narben und Bindegewebe und Dosierung bei großflächig brandverletzten Patienten. Manuelle Therapie. 2016;20:239–43.
5. Koller T. Physiotherapeutische Werkzeuge zur funktionellen Mobilisation von Narben und Bindegewebe sowie Dosierung bei großflächigen Narbenplatten. Manuelle Therapie. 2017;21:237–43.
6. Butler D, Mosley D, Lorimer G. Schmerzen verstehen. Berlin/Heidelberg: Springer; 2009.
7. Khan K, Scott A. Mechanotherapy: how physical therapists' prescription of exercise promotes tissue repair. Br J Sports Med. 2009;43(4):247–52.
8. Langevin H, Bouffard N, Fox J, Palmer B, Wu J, Iatridis J, Barnes W, Badger G, Howe K. Fibroblast cytoskeletal remodeling contributes to connective tissue tension. J Cell Physiol. 2011;226(5):1166–75.
9. Jaudoin D, Mathieu Y, Weber S, Ponthus C, Bruel H, Petit V, Chun E, Gauthier J, Galaup F, Kints A. Physiothérapie de la cicatrice après une brûlure grave (unveröffentlichtes Weiterbildungsskript). 2010.
10. Koller T. Manualtherapeutische Bestimmung des Bindegewebewiderstands bei Narben und Narbenplatten. Manuelle Therapie. 2018;21:81–7.
11. Koller T. Intertesterreliabilität und Kriteriumsvalidität bei der Bestimmung der Haut-und Bindegewebswiderstände (BGW) im physiologischen Gewebe—eine Pilotstudie. Manuelle Therapie. 2019;23:1–19.
12. Maitland G. Manipulation der Wirbelsäule. Berlin: Springer; 2008.
13. Balestrini J, Biliar K. Magnitude and duration of stretch modulate fibroblast remodeling. J Biomech Eng. 2009;131:051005–1. https://doi.org/10.1115/1.3049527.
14. Balestrini J, Billiar K. Equibiaxial cyclic stretch stimulates fibroblasts to rapidly remodel fibrin. J Biomech. 2006;39(16):2983–90.
15. Bouffard N, Kenneth R, Cutroneao G, Badger J, White S, Buttoph T, Ehrlich H, Stevens-Tuttle D, Langevin H. Tissue stretch decreases soluble TFG B1 and type-1 procollagen in mouse subcutaneous connective tissue: evidence from ex vivo and in vivo models. J Cell Physiol. 2008;214(2):389–95.
16. Andalib M, Dzenis Y, Donahue H, Lim J. Biomimetic substrate control of cellular mechanotransduction. Biomater Res. 2016;20:11. https://doi.org/10.1186/s40824-016-0059-1.
17. Eckes B, Nitsch R. Cell-matrix interactions in dermal repair and scarring. Fibrogenes Tissue Repair. 2010;3:4. https://doi.org/10.1186/1755-1536-3-4.
18. Li-Tsang C, Feng B, Huang L, Liu X, Shu B, Chan Y, Cheung K. A histological study on the effect of pressure therapy on the activities of myofibroblasts and keratinocytes in hypertrophic scar tissues after burn. Burns. 2015;41(5):1008–16.
19. Huang C, Holfeld J, Schaden W, Orgill D, Ogawa R. Mechanotherapy: revisiting physical therapy and recruiting mechanobiology for a new era in medicine. Trends Mol Med. 2013;19(9):555–64.
20. Moortgat P. Physikalische Narbenbehandlung. Berlin: Scar Academy DACH; 2017.
21. Carano A, Siciliani G. Effects of continuous and intermittent forces on human fibroblasts in vitro. Eur J Orthod. 1996;18(1):19–26.
22. Lehnhardt M, Hartmann B, Reichert B, editors. Verbrennungschirurgie. Berlin/Heidelberg: Springer; 2016.
23. Ai J, Liu J, Pei S, Sheng-Duo P, Liu Y, De-Sheng L, Hong-Min L, Pei B. The effectiveness of pressure therapy (15–25 mmHg) for hypertrophic burn scars: a systematic review and meta-analysis. Sci Rep. 2017;7:40185.
24. Sergiou M, Ott S, Farmer S. Comprehensive rehabilitation of the burn patient. In: Hernorn D, editor. Total burn care. Philadelphia: Saunders Elsevier; 2007. p. 620–51.
25. Künzi W, Wedler V. Wegweiser Verbrennungen. In: Beurteilung und Behandlung von Verbrennungen bei Erwachsenen. Montagnola: IBSA, Institut Biochimique; 2003.
26. Meier P. Versorgungsmöglichkeiten durch Kompression. Kongressvortrag, vol. 03. Leipzig: OT-World; 2016.
27. Scheer R. Clinical innovation: compression garments for managing lymphoedema. Wounds Int. 2017;8(2):34–8.
28. Flak E. Wirksamkeit einer neuen topischen Silikonzubereitung in einer verdickten Narbenentstehung und einer überschiessenden Narbenbildung bei Patienten mit frisch geschlossenen Verbrennungswunden. Dissertation, Ruhruniversität Bochum. 2010.
29. Moortgat, P. et al. (2015): Tension reducing taping as a mechanotherapy for hypertrophic burn scars—a proof of concept. Annals of Burns and Fire Disasters—vol XXVIII—Supplement EBA. 2015.
30. Meirte J, Moortgat P, Anthonissen M, Maertens K, Lafaire C, De Cuyper L, Hubens G, Van Daele U. Short-term effects of vacuum massage on epidermal and dermal thickness and density in burn scars: an experimental study. Burns Trauma. 2016;4:27.
31. Dermatologie: Entzündungsprozesse mit Dexpanthenol behandeln. In: Deutsche Apothekerzeitung. Nr. 51, 17. Dezember 2000, S. 66 (deutsche-apotheker-zeitung.de [abgerufen am 1. Oktober 2021]).

32. Stozkowska W, Piekoś R. Investigation of some topical formulations containing dexpanthenol. Acta Pol Pharm. 2004;61:433–7.

33. Ebner F, Heller A, Rippke F, Tausch I. Topical use of dexpanthenol in skin disorders. Am J Clin Dermatol. 2002;3(6):427–33. PMID 12113650

34. Proksch E, Nissen HP. Dexpanthenol enhances skin barrier repair and reduces inflammation after sodium lauryl sulphate-induced irritation. J Dermatol Treat. 2002;13:173–8. PMID 19753737

35. Gavroy J, Poveda K, Oversteyns B, Plantier W, Roug D, Griffe C, Teot L. Interet du test de viropression dans le suivi des cicatrices de brulures a partir de 50 observations. Ann medit Burns Club. 1995;VIII:1.

36. Godeau J. Massage dermo-épidermique sur séquelles cicatricielles de brûlures. Les Annales. 2005;5(40):37–9.

37. Guillot M. Principes généraux de rééducation fonctionnelle du brûlé. Les brûlures. Paris: Elsevier; 2010. p. 233–49.

Management of Hypertrophic Scars in Pediatric Burn Patients

Alen Palackic, Robert P. Duggan, Camila Franco-Mesa, and Ludwik K. Branski

Introduction

Wound healing is a complex, physiologic ballet that requires precise convergence of numerous cellular and humoral cascades in harmony [1]. Physiologic requirements and demands change as we age [1, 2]. Thus, it should be no surprise that children and adults differ in notable aspects when considering wound healing [3]. Even within the pediatric population, healing and scar physiology have certain peculiarities [1]. Factors such as the inflammatory response, characteristics of extracellular components, and the environment surrounding the injured tissue are essential to understand the scarring discrepancies between these patient populations [4, 5].

A. Palackic · L. K. Branski (✉)
Department of Surgery, University of Texas Medical Branch, Galveston, TX, USA

Division of Plastic, Aesthetic and Reconstructive Surgery, Department of Surgery, Medical University of Graz, Graz, Austria
e-mail: alpalack@utmb.edu; lubransk@utmb.edu

R. P. Duggan · C. Franco-Mesa
Department of Surgery, University of Texas Medical Branch, Galveston, TX, USA
e-mail: rpduggan@utmb.edu; camfranc@utmb.edu

Pathophysiology

We will detail the differences in scarring exhibited by each pediatric age group. For general information, see the respective chapter(s).

Fetal

During the fetal period, skin wounds heal without scar formation [6]. Although the mechanism responsible for this is still unclear, several theories have been described [3, 6]. At 8 weeks of gestation, skin cells exist as a single layer, but by 24 weeks, the epidermis is indistinguishable from that of a newborn. The dermis, however, is thin and is progressively filling with extracellular matrix components [6]. There is a lack of inflammatory response attributed to a markedly decreased macrophage migration. Without the major influx of these cells, the healing process is carried out in a noninflammatory environment. Growth factors expressed in the fetal period are also different from adults. Lower levels of TGF-β 1, TGF-β 2, and platelet-derived growth factor (PDGF) accompanied by elevated levels of TGF-β 3 have been described. Ferguson et al. confirmed that mimicking these growth factor ratios outside the fetal period improved the quality of resulting scars. The fetal environment contains high levels of adhesion molecules and selective growth factors in a hyaluronic acid-rich amniotic fluid [6]. These conditions provide an amplified noninflammatory setting that allows scarless or minimum scarring. As gestational age increases, so does the inflammatory response, and the resulting scars become more visible [4, 6].

Neonates and Infants (−12 Months)

Neonatal and infant skin have unique properties attributed to their transition period [2]. The decreased inflammatory response seen in the fetal period persists in a less dramatic state throughout the neonatal stage and, to an even lesser degree, into infancy. As a result, scarring is only barely noticeable under most conditions during this time. Wounds tend to close quickly due to the accelerated granulation tissue formation rate and extracellular matrix deposition. Topical absorption is exaggerated at these ages due to an immature stratum corneum. These patients are more vulnerable when exposed to irritating environmental substances such as adhesives, feces, urine, tape, and continuous pressure [2].

Toddlers and Children (1–12 Years)

The scarring process in this age group tends to be quite unpredictable. After age two, the inflammatory response begins to strengthen and only intensifies with age [3]. Pajulo et al. reported an elevated concentration of interleukin 6 (IL-6) and metalloproteinase 9 (MMP-9) associated with increased neutrophil infiltration in early stage wounds (Pajulo). In the acute phase, the extracellular matrix modification is related to the intensity of the proinflammatory response [7]. Children have a rapid healing phase with a robust remodeling phase. This combination can result in hypertrophic scarring or keloid formation [3]. Thus, children are more prone to develop hypertrophic scarring, to the point that it is not an uncommon result for wounds sustained in this age group. In burned children less than 5 years of age, a 50% hypertrophic scarring rate was reported by Spurr et al. in 1990 [8]. Lawrence et al. would evaluate the prevalence of hypertro-

phic scarring after burn injury in 2012, reporting a rate of 32–75% [9]. Risk factors for pathologic scarring included darker skin, female gender, neck and upper extremity injury, more severe burns, prolonged healing time, and surgical interventions [9]. Ten years later, and despite advances in treatment, pathologic scarring is still frequent, with a 30–90% incidence of keloids or hypertrophic scars, according to Barone et al. [10] Mechanism of injury and quality of treatment also impact scar formation [3]. Traumatic wounds, such as burns, often have protracted healing times, increasing the risk for hypertrophic scarring [11]. Injuries closed under high degrees of tension experience an increased influx of inflammatory mediators, promoting pathologic scar formation [3, 12].

Adolescence (12–18 Years)

As age increases, so does the possibility of excessive wound healing [5]. In other words, adolescent skin has a greater capacity to scar than younger counterparts. Cytokine response during this period is quite different; TGF-β 1, TGF-β 2, and interleukins 6 and 8 are noticeably increased. Hyaluronic acid is decreased, and collagen type I is present to a greater extent than collagen III [5, 6]. By adolescence and early adulthood, the scarring process can be divided into the well-known three stages of inflammation, proliferation, and remodeling [13]. Overall, the adolescent wound healing mechanisms are virtually the same as those in young adults [3, 5, 6].

Nonsurgical Approaches

The best treatment for hypertrophic scarring is prevention. Optimal management of the initial wound environment decreases mortality and will lessen the burden of hypertrophic scarring as the wound heals and as the patient ages. Whether or not hypertrophic scarring occurs is dramatically influenced by the duration of wound healing. Wounds that heal in under 21 days are markedly less likely to become hypertrophic, whereas those wounds taking longer than 25 days to heal are at risk [14]. Prompt debridement and wound coverage promote timely wound healing and, in turn, decrease the reconstructive burden later in life. Attention to wound tension at the time of closure will foster more rapid and organized healing. Avoiding local or systemic factors that impair wound healing, such as wound infection or corticosteroid usage, will speed wound closure and diminish future pathological scarring [15, 16].

Compression Garments

Persistent physical compression of burn scars has been reported and recommended since the 1970s [17, 18]. Dr. Duane L. Larson and his team at the Galveston Shriners Hospital for Children observed that scars under thermoplastic splints used in preventing contractures were soft and smooth and rarely became hypertrophic. Later, in conjunction with plastic surgeon Ted Huang at the neighboring University of Texas Medical Branch, it was reported that a pressure of at least 15 mmHg applied continuously for at least 6 months was required to cause the changes that were being observed clinically [18]. No single pathway for the efficacy of compression garments has been elucidated. External compression has been shown to affect the scar extracellular matrix, making it more rigid. This rigidity then stimulates increases in mechanoreceptor number and increases in apoptotic signaling. Local hypoxia due to compression also is thought to play a role in decreasing collagen overproduction [19, 20]. Clinical reports and series would be published over the decades exhibiting the efficacy of compression bandages and other garments [21–25]. Results were encouraging, but randomized studies were lacking [26].

Chang et al. conducted a trial randomizing burn patients to compression garment therapy versus no compression garments. Their early findings in 122 patients were contrary to the widespread trend of the time, finding no benefit in compression garments [27]. Future randomized studies did, however, indicate that compression therapy improved scar quality [28, 29].

Investigation into optimal degree and duration of compression has occurred since its initial popularization [29–31]. Engrav et al. enrolled patients aged 7–65 over 12 years to be randomized to low- or normal-pressure garments applied over forearm burns. Patients were instructed to wear their garments for 23 hours a day, removing only to bathe, and were taught the proper application of the garment by their manufacturer. Wide pressure ranges in both the low (mean 6.4 mmHg) and normal (mean 25 mmHg) groups were present, highlighting the difficulty of applying a consistent and prescribed pressure "dose" for the treatment of hypertrophic scars. Their rigorous study design and follow-up confirmed the efficacy of compression garments and highlighted the difficulty of applying controlled compression over tissue for the duration required to modify scars. Importantly, they strongly recommend the use of compression garments in children and adolescents. In the same year, Candy et al. reported the results of a trial randomizing adult burn patients to normal (10–15 mmHg) versus high (20–25 mmHg) compression. All patients demonstrated improved scar thickness at 5 months, but high-pressure scars, those under at least 20 mmHg of pressure, improved more consistently. Controlling pressure application again was noted to be difficult, with pressure loss being more significant in the high compression group [30].

Additional randomized clinical trials are needed to prove the efficacy of pressure therapy more definitively. However, the current body of evidence supports their use as first-line therapy to prevent hypertrophic burn scars. Compression garments may be fashioned out of numerous materials with or without splints, and a multidisciplinary approach involving occupational and physical therapists is necessary to fashion ergonomic devices. Certain body areas are more receptive to compression therapy. Areas of flexion in the limbs likely receive less consistent pressure for the duration of treatment. As such, the overlying scar is less affected. The ideal duration of wear for maximal benefit has yet to be determined. Clinical trials begin with daily wear after reepithelization has occurred and advise at least 6 months of therapy. However, recent trials have shown that at this time, there is little difference between compression, silicone, or no therapy at all [32].

Any intervention over most of a day will have compliance issues. Loose pressure garments may be more comfortable for daily wear but provide little long-term benefit. More restrictive garments that provide over 40 mmHg of compression may seem appealing, offering a higher dose of pressure while patients are compliant. However, these pressures risk paresthesias and can decrease overall compliance. Restrictive garments may also be uncomfortable in warmer and humid climates, and compression and moisture may macerate the underlying skin and foster dermatologic reactions. In young patients who cannot dress themselves, caregivers may struggle with fitting garments daily. As children rapidly grow, garments may become too restrictive, and replacements may be needed, an unforeseen cost that ultimately promotes discontinuation. Adolescents may be reluctant to wear compression garments in social situations. In children, particularly those prone to hypertrophic scarring or with a family history of pathogenic scarring, compression therapy is a cost-effective treatment for hypertrophic scarring. Treatment can be initiated once wounds have re-epithelized and will likely occur for at least 12 months. Caregivers and patients should be counseled on the importance of daily wear, and replacement garments should be readily available as the child ages.

Silicone

Silicone was first described as a treatment for burn scars in the 1980s [33]. At that time, potential mechanisms of action had yet to be described. Like compression therapy, there is no single unifying pathway that accounts for silicone's efficacy. Silicone products have been described as mediating their scar-modulating effects through altering tissue oxygenation, scar polarization, increased temperature, decreased tension, and direct effects of the silicone molecule itself. The most plausible mechanism involved silicone's ability to create an occluded and hydrated environment. This environment decreases fibroblast activity and diminishes scarring. Furthermore, a hydrated and occluded environment may decrease nociceptor activity in the scar and decrease neurogenic inflammation driving hypertrophic scarring [19, 34]. Silicone sheeting may also reduce tension by transmitting forces to the edge of the sheet, away from the forming scar.

Despite widespread use, the evidence supporting silicone is less robust than desired, and findings are conflicting [31, 35, 36]. Many silicone products are available in diverse applications ranging from silicone sheets to sprays and foams applied to scars. No one product is clearly more efficacious than others, and the ideal duration of therapy has not been established [32]. In a randomized trial with intraindividual comparisons, Steinstraesser et al. compared the addition of silicone sheeting versus silicone spray to pressure therapy. At 18 months, their results did not suggest any additive benefit due to either silicone product when compared to compression therapy alone [35]. Wiseman et al. randomized patients 18 and under to silicone gel, pressure therapy, or combined therapy; at 6 months of therapy, the silicone-only patients had significantly thinner scars than the combined therapy group. Still, no other differences in scar quality were found between groups [32]. Inherent in the study design is the practice of compression therapy and silicone products in the pediatric population despite the lack of high-level evidence for either product or their use in conjunction.

Caregivers and patients may have fewer compliance issues with silicone products than with pressure garments. Sheets and strips may be placed directly over scarred areas rather than compressing entire limbs. More self-conscious wearers may find silicone products to draw less attention than compression garments. Most products tend to be single-use, and costs may accumulate over the recommended therapy duration. Patients may develop folliculitis or other dermatological reactions secondary to the occlusive nature of the dressings. Both are widely recommended and well-tolerated despite lacking high-level evidence for either compression garments or silicone products [37]. Further investigations are needed to determine the optimal timing for initiation of therapy and the duration of wear to achieve maximal benefit.

Scar Massage

Scar massage is employed globally to manage not only hypertrophic scars but also well-healing traumatic or surgical scars [37–39]. Its reported benefits include alterations to the scar appearance and quality, including increased pliability and decreased scar thickness. Essential patient quality of life improvements related to their scar has been reported as well, including decreased pruritis and decreased hypersensitivity and pain [38, 40–44]. A systematic review by Ault et al. analyzed scar massage in hypertrophic burn scarring [38]. Only two reviewed studies focused on pediatric populations [43, 44]. Morien et al. prospectively enrolled pediatric burn survivors to receive scar massage by trained therapists once a day for 20–25 min. Patients were over 2 years postburn with well-matured scars. In their small series of eight patients, range of motion throughout the scarred area improved within 3–5 sessions [43]. Patiño et al. randomized 30 pediatric patients to receive 10 min of massage by their primary caregiver for 3 months or to receive no massage. At the conclusion of the study, the massage intervention failed to show improvements in scar quality; however, pruritis was improved [44].

Unlike silicone or compression therapy, scar massage may have no associated costs for patients. Furthermore, it can be performed by the patient themselves once properly instructed and by caregivers. The potential psychosocial benefit of scar massage, including decreased depression and anxiety, is enough to recommend this relatively benign intervention for the pediatric population. Future investigations into the idea techniques and their implementation will help provide more evidence-based recommendations to parents and caregivers.

Injections of Corticosteroids

The intralesional injection with corticosteroids into the hypertrophic scar is another nonsurgical approach commonly applied in pediatric burn patients. Intralesional injections have long been shown to reduce scar height, volume, pain, and pruritis and improve pliability [16, 45]. Triamcinolone acetonide is the most used corticosteroid for pathological scarring in pediatric patients postburn. On a cellular level, injections work to inhibit collagen production; suppress inflammation; attenuate the proliferation of fibroblasts and keratinocytes; limit oxygen and nutrient delivery; and halt the migration and phagocytosis by immunoregulatory cells [41, 46]. In pediatric patients, the intralesional injection may be accompanied by pain and discomfort, which can be minimized when combined with topical lidocaine cream prior to injection. In pediatric burn patients, corticosteroids can be combined with other preventive therapies, including silicone gel therapy, pulsed dye laser treatment, and cryotherapy [45, 47]. Corticosteroid injections can be done several times; however, there should be at least a 2-month interval between two injections as overloading the scar with steroids can result in epidermal thinning and the appearance of telangiectasia.

Autologous Fat Transfer (AFT)

AFT or also widely known as fat lipofilling may be beneficial as an adjuvant treatment option for postburn scarring in children [48]. The adipose-derived stem cells have a variety of regenerative and metabolic properties and growth factors involved in the remodeling process, promoting rapid revascularization and a decrease in fibrosis [49]. Using the Coleman technique, fat adipose-derived stem cells can be harvested and reinjected at 2–4 week intervals until healing [48]. Applying the same technique, reinjections may also be performed at a 12 weeks interval after healing [50]. AFT may also alleviate pruritis and neuropathic pain associated with hypertrophic scars. Despite these positive findings, more research is needed to determine the efficacy of AFT and its combination with other treatment options such as laser therapy in this population [51, 52].

Laser and Surgical Approaches

Laser and Light Therapy

There have been significant advancements in laser and light therapy technology in recent decades. These therapies are now used with conventional surgical options or exclusively to avoid more invasive procedures [53]. Compared to the previously described nonsurgical treatment options, a core advantage of lasers is the improvement of the scar in a few sessions, rather than the gradual improvement only after months or years of therapy. Different lasers have been utilized in pathological and nonpathological burn scars, including the 585–595 nm pulsed dye laser, the 585 nm short-pulsed dye laser, the Er:Yag laser, and the ablative and non-ablative fractional CO_2 laser [54]. Briefly, laser therapies are based on selective thermolysis, which permits the targeted application of energy into tissues with minimal damage to surrounding areas. Lasers emit different wavelengths of light targeting different chromophores, compounds within the body, such as melanin, hemoglobin, and water. Energy in the form of photons excites the target chromophore and ultimately leads to selective tissue damage [55]. Numerous studies have shown scar size and quality improvement following laser therapy sessions [56]. Furthermore, it has been shown that laser therapy improves erythema, texture, contracture, neuropathic pain, function, and overall quality of life [57–60]. However, most of these findings have been shown in the adult burn population; the literature on laser use in pediatric patients is scarce. Nevertheless, there are studies reporting their experiences with laser therapy, showing improvement in scar quality in pediatric burn patients.

Two commercially available lasers are most widely reported in the literature [61]. The first is the 585 nm short-pulsed dye laser (Syneron Candela VBeam Perfecta, Wayland, MA), whose target chromophore is hemoglobin. Destruction of hemoglobin-containing tissues leads to necrosis in capillaries and the reduction of scar erythema, and improvements in pliability and pruritus [62]. Next is the fractional carbon dioxide laser (The UltraPulse® Lumenis) which is an ablative fractional resurfacing (AFR) machine with different setting options; ActiveFXTM (lowest energy and highest density) and DeepFXTM (balance between energy and density). These two settings are commonly applied for superficial and deep treatments, respectively. In contrast to the pulsed dye laser, an ablative fractional laser improves the scar's height, volume, thickness, and overall texture [56, 60, 61]. Both mechanisms can be used to treat hypertrophic scars. In a retrospective review, Zuccaro et al. report that using a pulsed dye laser in conjunction with an ablative fractional carbon dioxide laser significantly improved scar pigmentation, vascularity, pliability, and height. Also significant was the finding that the two lasers could be safely combined in a single case [62]. A recent prospective cohort study by Patel et al. would confirm the efficacy of carbon dioxide laser in pediatric burn survivors. The authors suggested that laser treatment of scars provides an excellent alternative to more invasive therapies and a more immediate alternative to more conservative scar treatments [54]. The treatment with ablative fractional laser can be combined with reconstructive surgical techniques, which has become a popular and efficacious treatment approach [59]. However, once a scar is fully matured, treatment with laser therapy alone is not a replacement for surgical reconstruction, which will be discussed in the following section.

In the pediatric population, it is crucial to individualize the use of lasers and consider each scar as its own clinical problem to optimize results. Once a wound is healed, the treatment team should consider laser treatment in the early phase to prevent scar contracture and increase other treatments' responses using the ActiveFXTM CO_2 laser. At our institution, Shriners Children's Texas, recently matured scars with red or raised appearance are commonly treated with intense pulsed light (IPL). These patients also may benefit from the intralesional corticosteroid injections, typically with Kenalog 10 mg or 40 mg (Bristol Myers Squibb, New York City, New York, USA). Scars with intense pruritis are also considered for IPL therapy or fat grafting. While benefits may be apparent after a single session, scars typically require multiple rounds of laser therapy before a treatment plateau is reached. The scar should be allowed to heal between treatments, 6–8 weeks, so the response to treatment can begin to be observed and documented. More extensive scars will require more sessions than limited ones. Depending on the scar quality and symptoms, ActiveFXTM and DeepFXTM fractional CO_2 laser can be applied in one single session for superficial and deep treatment, respectively. This approach is primarily applied in thicker scars with erythema and pruritis. Every session should be performed under intravenous sedation to reduce discomfort and pain. Regarding pain management, additional intradermal injections or regional nerve blocks can be utilized in pediatric patients, which has also been reported in the literature [63].

Surgical Scar Revision

Although there have been advancements in conservative treatment approaches, surgical treatment remains integral in the management of excessive scarring postburn. No two scars are the same, and every case needs to be considered individually to match the surgical plan with the patient's complaints and goals. The timing of scar revision surgeries should be considered carefully, and children should be monitored throughout their growth and development. The scar tissue does not grow as fast as the child during the growth period, leading to asymmetric growth and motor impairment. Therefore, it is crucial to anticipate the need for potential scar surgery prior to the development of permanent sequelae. Furthermore, surgeries should be considered at least 1 year after healing to allow for scar maturation.

If surgery is required, our approach generally follows the reconstructive ladder, carefully considering where laser or corticosteroid-based therapies may be employed as a complement. Patients presenting to our clinic have a detailed surgical plan in place, including areas of possible surgical intervention and laser therapy, including previous laser settings and treatment response. Still, patients and caregivers guide our approach; care is taken to address the most pressing complaints first, whether or not they were part of the surgical plan beforehand.

Local tissue rearrangements are a workhorse for burn reconstruction. The most common and valuable techniques for contracture release include various forms of Z-, W-, V-Y, or Y-V-plasty, which every reconstructive burn surgeon should master. These techniques elongate tissue along a contracture, camouflage scar tissue in favor of cosmesis, and release tension, resulting in decreased inflammation and hypertrophic scarring [64]. Based on the hypertrophic scar location, local flaps can be utilized in various forms. Hypertrophic scars of the face are commonly released with multiple Z-plasty in combination with ablative CO_2 laser treatment. Local V-Y advancement flaps release the commissures around the mouth. In the hand, small scarring bands and mild forms of scarring in the palm can be released by Z-plasty. Within the web spaces, the jumping man Z-plasty, STAR-plasty, or Y-V flaps have been established as valuable techniques for scar release, as they create concavity and length [65]. In the region of the nose, the nasal turndown flap, consisting of the dorsal surface of the nose and made up of skin graft and scar, has been established as a useful surgical technique [66].

Depending on the severity of contracture and location, skin grafts may be needed to introduce unscarred tissue where local tissue rearrangement is insufficient. For the reconstruction of eyelids, we always use a full-thickness skin graft for the lower lid and a thick split-thickness skin graft (STSG) for the upper lids. In the axillary and popliteal regions, we frequently use fasciocutaneous transposition flaps. To prevent contracture in these regions, split-thick skin grafts may be needed adjacent to transposition flaps. The neck is the most challenging area to treat in terms of contractures. A simple, one-stage application of STSG almost always results in a later contracture. Other approaches involve bioartificial skin substitutes (e.g., Integra) combined with STSG. Although they offer an excellent cosmetic result, contracture recurrence still occurs in 50% of cases [67]. The NovoSorb Biodegradable Temporising Matrix (BTM), a synthetic polyurethane dermal matrix, plus STSG, potentially better prevents contracture recurrence; however, more evidence is needed to recommend this approach definitively. In our experience, a possible approach to prevent contractures is a two-stage approach with the French/McCauley technique with surgical release plus Cadaver skin, followed by second-stage grafting with thick STSG from the back. Scalp alopecia is also a very commonly treated condition postburn. Here, we use tissue expansion to increase the surface area of the hair-bearing scalp gradually. Later, the expander is removed, and scarred tissue is excised, with the area of alopecia now being covered by the expanded scalp. Tissue expansion in the pediatric burn population continues to be a safe and effective reconstructive option.

Conclusion

The best treatment for hypertrophic scarring is prevention. Optimal management of the initial wound environment decreases mortality and will lessen the burden of hypertrophic scarring as the wound heals and as the patient ages. The current approach is to reduce pathological scar formation with early acute surgical intervention and various nonsurgical modalities, in combination with scar revision. It is crucial to monitor and follow up children with excessive scars during their growth period. In recent years, there has been advancement in the technology of lasers, and their popularity has grown; however, follow-up studies and randomized controlled trials are lacking. Up to date, there is no absolute standard of care, and well-designed randomized controlled trials and innovations are needed to find the "holy grail" in the treatment of pathological scarring in pediatric burn patients.

References

1. Gantwerker EA, Hom DB. Skin: histology and physiology of wound healing. Facial Plast Surg Clin North Am. 2011;19(3):441–53. https://doi.org/10.1016/j.fsc.2011.06.009.
2. Steen EH, Wang X, Boochoon KS, et al. Wound healing and wound Care in Neonates: current therapies and novel options. Adv Skin Wound Care. 2020;33(6):294–300. https://doi.org/10.1097/01.ASW.0000661804.09496.8c.
3. Sanchez J, Antonicelli F, Tuton D, Mazouz Dorval S, François C. Particularités de la cicatrisation de l'enfant [specificities in children wound healing]. Ann Chir Plast Esthet. 2016;61(5):341–7. https://doi.org/10.1016/j.anplas.2016.05.001.
4. Huhn EA, Jannowitz C, Boos H, et al. Fetale wundheilung. Aktueller stand und neue perspektiven [fetal wound healing: current status and new perspectives]. Chirurg. 2004;75(5):498–507. https://doi.org/10.1007/s00104-004-0878-9.
5. Wang PH, Huang BS, Horng HC, Yeh CC, Chen YJ. Wound healing. J Chin Med Assoc. 2018;81(2):94–101. https://doi.org/10.1016/j.jcma.2017.11.002.
6. Ferguson MW, O'Kane S. Scar-free healing: from embryonic mechanisms to adult therapeutic intervention. Philos Trans R Soc Lond Ser B Biol Sci. 2004;359(1445):839–50. https://doi.org/10.1098/rstb.2004.1475.
7. Pajulo OT, Pulkki KJ, Alanen MS, et al. Correlation between interleukin-6 and matrix metalloproteinase-9 in early wound healing in children. Wound Repair Regen. 1999;7(6):453–7. https://doi.org/10.1046/j.1524-475x.1999.00453.x.
8. Spurr ED, Shakespeare PG. Incidence of hypertrophic scarring in burn-injured children. Burns. 1990;16(3):179–81. https://doi.org/10.1016/0305-4179(90)90034-t.
9. Lawrence JW, Mason ST, Schomer K, Klein MB. Epidemiology and impact of scarring after burn injury: a systematic review of the literature. J Burn Care Res. 2012;33(1):136–46. https://doi.org/10.1097/BCR.0b013e3182374452.
10. Barone N, Safran T, Vorstenbosch J, Davison PG, Cugno S, Murphy AM. Current advances in hypertrophic scar and keloid management. Semin Plast Surg. 2021;35(3):145–52. https://doi.org/10.1055/s-0041-1731461.
11. Xu QL, Song JH. Zhonghua Shao Shang Za Zhi. 2018;34(8):509–12. https://doi.org/10.3760/cma.j.issn.1009-2587.2018.08.005.

12. Son D, Harijan A. Overview of surgical scar prevention and management. J Korean Med Sci. 2014;29(6):751–7. https://doi.org/10.3346/jkms.2014.29.6.751.

13. Broughton G 2nd, Janis JE, Attinger CE. Wound healing: an overview. Plast Reconstr Surg. 2006;117(7 Suppl):1e. https://doi.org/10.1097/01.prs.0000222562.60260.f9.

14. Deitch EA, Wheelahan TM, Rose MP, Clothier J, Cotter J. Hypertrophic burn scars: analysis of variables. J Trauma. 1983;23(10):895–8.

15. Cubison TC, Pape SA, Parkhouse N. Evidence for the link between healing time and the development of hypertrophic scars (HTS) in paediatric burns due to scald injury. Burns. 2006;32(8):992–9. https://doi.org/10.1016/j.burns.2006.02.007.

16. Ogawa R. The most current algorithms for the treatment and prevention of hypertrophic scars and keloids. Plast Reconstr Surg. 2010;125(2):557–68. https://doi.org/10.1097/PRS.0b013e3181c82dd5.

17. Larson DL, Abston S, Evans EB, Dobrkovsky M, Linares HA. Techniques for decreasing scar formation and contractures in the burned patient. J Trauma Inj Infect Crit Care. 1971;11(10):807–23. https://doi.org/10.1097/00005373-197110000-00001.

18. Linares HA, Larson DL, Willis-Galstaun BA. Historical notes on the use of pressure in the treatment of hypertrophic scars or keloids. Burns. 1993;19(1):17–21. https://doi.org/10.1016/0305-4179(93)90095-P.

19. Yagmur C, Akaishi S, Ogawa R, Guneren E. Mechanical receptor–related mechanisms in scar management: a review and hypothesis. Plast Reconstr Surg. 2010;126(2):426–34. https://doi.org/10.1097/PRS.0b013e3181df715d.

20. Li-Tsang CWP, Feng B, Huang L, et al. A histological study on the effect of pressure therapy on the activities of myofibroblasts and keratinocytes in hypertrophic scar tissues after burn. Burns. 2015;41(5):1008–16. https://doi.org/10.1016/j.burns.2014.11.017.

21. Baur PS, Larson DL, Sloan DF, Barratt GF. An in situ procedure for the biopsy of pressure-wrapped hypertrophic scars. J Invest Dermatol. 1977;68(6):385–8. https://doi.org/10.1111/1523-1747.ep12496949.

22. Tolhurst DE. Hypertrophic scarring prevented by pressure: a case report. Br J Plast Surg. 1977;30(3):218–9.

23. Garcia-Velasco M, Ley R, Mutch D, Surkes N, Williams HB. Compression treatment of hypertrophic scars in burned children. Can J Surg. 1978;21(5):450–2.

24. Judge JC, May SR, DeClement FA. Control of hypertrophic scarring in burn patients using tubular support bandages. J Burn Care Rehabil. 1984;5(3):221–4. https://doi.org/10.1097/00004630-198405000-00007.

25. Rose MP, Deitch EA. The clinical use of a tubular compression bandage, Tubigrip, for burn-scar therapy: a critical analysis. Burns. 1985;12(1):58–64. https://doi.org/10.1016/0305-4179(85)90184-6.

26. Anzarut A, Olson J, Singh P, Rowe BH, Tredget EE. The effectiveness of pressure garment therapy for the prevention of abnormal scarring after burn injury: a meta-analysis. J Plast Reconstr Aesthet Surg. 2009;62(1):77–84. https://doi.org/10.1016/j.bjps.2007.10.052.

27. Chang P, Laubenthal KN, Lewis RW, Rosenquist MD, Lindley-Smith P, Kealey GP. Prospective, randomized study of the efficacy of pressure garment therapy in patients with burns. J Burn Care Rehabil. 1995;16(5):473–5. https://doi.org/10.1097/00004630-199509000-00002.

28. Van den Kerckhove E, Stappaerts K, Fieuws S, et al. The assessment of erythema and thickness on burn related scars during pressure garment therapy as a preventive measure for hypertrophic scarring. Burns. 2005;31(6):696–702. https://doi.org/10.1016/j.burns.2005.04.014.

29. Engrav LH, Heimbach DM, Rivara FP, et al. 12-year within-wound study of the effectiveness of custom pressure garment therapy. Burns. 2010;36(7):975–83. https://doi.org/10.1016/j.burns.2010.04.014.

30. Candy LHY, Cecilia L-TWP, Ping ZY. Effect of different pressure magnitudes on hypertrophic scar in a Chinese population. Burns. 2010;36(8):1234–41. https://doi.org/10.1016/j.burns.2010.05.008.

31. Friedstat JS, Hultman CS. Hypertrophic burn scar management. Ann Plast Surg. 2014;72(6):S198–201. https://doi.org/10.1097/SAP.0000000000000103.

32. Wiseman J, Ware RS, Simons M, et al. Effectiveness of topical silicone gel and pressure garment therapy for burn scar prevention and management in children: a randomized controlled trial. Clin Rehabil. 2020;34(1):120–31. https://doi.org/10.1177/0269215519877516.

33. Perkins K, Davey RB, Wallis KA. Silicone gel: a new treatment for burn scars and contractures. Burns. 1983;9(3):201–4. https://doi.org/10.1016/0305-4179(83)90039-6.

34. Mustoe TA. Evolution of silicone therapy and mechanism of action in scar management. Aesthet Plast Surg. 2008;32(1):82–92. https://doi.org/10.1007/s00266-007-9030-9.

35. Steinstraesser L, Flak E, Witte B, et al. Pressure garment therapy alone and in combination with silicone for the prevention of hypertrophic scarring. Plast Reconstr Surg. 2011;128(4):306e–13e. https://doi.org/10.1097/PRS.0b013e3182268c69.

36. Anthonissen M, Daly D, Janssens T, Van den Kerckhove E. The effects of conservative treatments on burn scars: a systematic review. Burns. 2016;42(3):508–18. https://doi.org/10.1016/j.burns.2015.12.006.

37. Liuzzi F, Chadwick S, Shah M. Paediatric postburn scar management in the UK: a national survey. Burns. 2015;41(2):252–6. https://doi.org/10.1016/j.burns.2014.10.017.

38. Ault P, Plaza A, Paratz J. Scar massage for hypertrophic burns scarring—a systematic review. Burns. 2018;44(1):24–38. https://doi.org/10.1016/j.burns.2017.05.006.

39. Holavanahalli RK, Helm PA, Parry IS, Dolezal CA, Greenhalgh DG. Select practices in management and

rehabilitation of burns: a survey report. J Burn Care Res. 2011;32(2):210–23. https://doi.org/10.1097/BCR.0b013e31820aadd5.

40. Roques C. Massage applied to scars. Wound Repair Regen. 2002;10(2):126–8. https://doi.org/10.1046/j.1524-475X.2002.02107.x.

41. Finnerty CC, Jeschke MG, Branski LK, Barret JP, Dziewulski P, Herndon DN. Hypertrophic scarring: the greatest unmet challenge after burn injury. Lancet. 2016;388(10052):1427–36. https://doi.org/10.1016/S0140-6736(16)31406-4.

42. Krakowski AC, Totri CR, Donelan MB, Shumaker PR. Scar management in the pediatric and adolescent populations. Pediatrics. 2016;137(2):e20142065. https://doi.org/10.1542/peds.2014-2065.

43. Morien A, Garrison D, Smith NK. Range of motion improves after massage in children with burns: a pilot study. J Bodyw Mov Ther. 2008;12(1):67–71. https://doi.org/10.1016/j.jbmt.2007.05.003.

44. Patiño O, Novick C, Merlo A, Benaim F. Massage in hypertrophic scars. J Burn Care Rehabil. 1999;20(3):268–71. discussion 267.

45. Atiyeh BS. Nonsurgical management of hypertrophic scars: evidence-based therapies, standard practices, and emerging methods. Aesthet Plast Surg. 2007;31(5):468–94. https://doi.org/10.1007/s00266-006-0253-y.

46. Krusche T, Worret WI. Mechanical properties of keloids in vivo during treatment with intralesional triamcinolone acetonide. Arch Dermatol Res. 1995;287(3–4):289–93. https://doi.org/10.1007/BF01105081.

47. Arno AI, Gauglitz GG, Barret JP, Jeschke MG. Up-to-date approach to manage keloids and hypertrophic scars: a useful guide. Burns. 2014;40(7):1255–66. https://doi.org/10.1016/j.burns.2014.02.011.

48. Piccolo NS, Piccolo MS, Piccolo MT. Fat grafting for treatment of burns, burn scars, and other difficult wounds. Clin Plast Surg. 2015;42(2):263–83. https://doi.org/10.1016/j.cps.2014.12.009.

49. Sultan SM, Barr JS, Butala P, et al. Fat grafting accelerates revascularisation and decreases fibrosis following thermal injury. J Plast Reconstr Aesthet Surg. 2012;65(2):219–27. https://doi.org/10.1016/j.bjps.2011.08.046.

50. Coleman SR. Long-term survival of fat transplants: controlled demonstrations. Aesthet Plast Surg. 1995;19(5):421–5. https://doi.org/10.1007/BF00453875.

51. Huang SH, Wu SH, Chang KP, et al. Alleviation of neuropathic scar pain using autologous fat grafting. Ann Plast Surg. 2015;74(Suppl 2):S99–S104. https://doi.org/10.1097/SAP.0000000000000462.

52. Huang SH, Wu SH, Lee SS, et al. Fat grafting in burn scar alleviates neuropathic pain via anti-inflammation effect in scar and spinal cord. PLoS One. 2015;10(9):e0137563. Published 2015 Sep 14. https://doi.org/10.1371/journal.pone.0137563.

53. Fisher M. Pediatric burn reconstruction: focus on evidence. Clin Plast Surg. 2017;44(4):865–73. https://doi.org/10.1016/j.cps.2017.05.018.

54. Patel SP, Nguyen HV, Mannschreck D, Redett RJ, Puttgen KB, Stewart FD. Fractional CO2 laser treatment outcomes for pediatric hypertrophic burn scars. J Burn Care Res. 2019;40(4):386–91. https://doi.org/10.1093/jbcr/irz046.

55. Patil UA, Dhami LD. Overview of lasers. Indian J Plast Surg. 2008;41(Suppl):S101–13.

56. Donelan MB, Parrett BM, Sheridan RL. Pulsed dye laser therapy and z-plasty for facial burn scars: the alternative to excision. Ann Plast Surg. 2008;60(5):480–6. https://doi.org/10.1097/SAP.0b013e31816fcad5.

57. Klifto KM, Asif M, Hultman CS. Laser management of hypertrophic burn scars: a comprehensive review. Burns Trauma. 2020;8:tkz002Published 2020 Jan 16. https://doi.org/10.1093/burnst/tkz002.

58. Issler-Fisher AC, Fisher OM, Smialkowski AO, et al. Ablative fractional CO2 laser for burn scar reconstruction: an extensive subjective and objective short-term outcome analysis of a prospective treatment cohort. Burns. 2017;43(3):573–82. https://doi.org/10.1016/j.b.

59. Issler-Fisher AC, Waibel JS, Donelan MB. Laser modulation of hypertrophic scars: technique and practice. Clin Plast Surg. 2017;44(4):757–66. https://doi.org/10.1016/j.cps.2017.05.007.

60. Hultman CS, Friedstat JS, Edkins RE, Cairns BA, Meyer AA. Laser resurfacing and remodeling of hypertrophic burn scars: the results of a large, prospective, before-after cohort study, with long-term follow-up [published correction appears in Ann Surg]. Ann Surg. 2015;260(3):519–32.

61. Anderson RR, Donelan MB, Hivnor C, et al. Laser treatment of traumatic scars with an emphasis on ablative fractional laser resurfacing: consensus report. JAMA Dermatol. 2014;150(2):187–93. https://doi.org/10.1001/jamadermatol.2013.7761.

62. Zuccaro J, Muser I, Singh M, Yu J, Kelly C, Fish J. Laser therapy for pediatric burn scars: focusing on a combined treatment approach. J Burn Care Res. 2018;39(3):457–62. https://doi.org/10.1093/jbcr/irx008.

63. Cantatore JL, Kriegel DA. Laser surgery: an approach to the pediatric patient. J Am Acad Dermatol. 2004;50(2):165–88. https://doi.org/10.1016/j.jaad.2003.08.004.

64. Hundeshagen G, Zapata-Sirvent R, Goverman J, Branski LK. Tissue rearrangements: the power of the Z-Plasty. Clin Plast Surg. 2017;44(4):805–12. https://doi.org/10.1016/j.cps.2017.05.011.

65. Sorkin M, Cholok D, Levi B. Scar Management of the Burned Hand. Hand Clin. 2017;33(2):305–15. https://doi.org/10.1016/j.hcl.2016.12.009.

66. Taylor HO, Carty M, Driscoll D, Lewis M, Donelan MB. Nasal reconstruction after severe facial burns using a local turndown flap. Ann Plast Surg. 2009;62(2):175–9. https://doi.org/10.1097/SAP.0b013e31817d87ed.

67. Hunt JA, Moisidis E, Haertsch P. Initial experience of Integra in the treatment of post-burn anterior cervical neck contracture. Br J Plast Surg. 2000;53(8):652–8. https://doi.org/10.1054/bjps.2000.3436.

Part IV

Scar Rehabilitation

Medical Tattooing for Aesthetic Optimisation

Thomas Rappl, Mario Barth, Dominique Bossavy, Paul Wurzer, Lars-Peter Kamolz, and Sebastian P. Nischwitz

Introduction

Skin grafting, different kinds of local and free flaps and other various techniques serve essential requirements as well as functional improvement in plastic and reconstructive surgery. Nevertheless, the aesthetic outcome sometimes leaves something to be desired, and surgical or other therapeutic means cannot further ameliorate a situation or are not wanted. Hypertrophic scarring, colour mismatch, superficial irregularities of the grafted skin, loss of elasticity and dermal thickness, hair loss, contour irregularities, etc. might impair a perfect postoperative outcome and patient's satisfaction. Not only traumatic/surgical sequelae, sometimes also a "natural flaw" is of highly disturbing character to a patient, leaving even the most-adapted surgeons without an idea on how to improve the situation surgically. Local flaps, skin grafts and areola sharing are the most frequent techniques for nipple areola complex (NAC) reconstruction in reconstructive breast surgery. We find the technique of contralateral areola-skin sharing to be the ideal choice for patients who were reconstructed with autologous tissue. Colour match and circumferential areola border can be created extremely similar to the contralateral side. Nevertheless, the sharp edges usually remain a telltale sign even in the best surgical outcomes. In such cases, medical tattooing can bring perfection to an already good-looking skin graft, i.e. by camouflaging the sharp edges of the skin graft.

After skin-sparing mastectomy, the remaining skin is often too thin to perform local flaps or even skin grafting. The risk of penetrating the skin and subsequent extrusion of the mammaprosthesis is high. In these cases, medical tattooing can offer a variety of benefits, for example as an enhancement of contour symmetry and to restore colour mismatch [1].

Medical tattooing also offers various benefits in burn patients like enhancement of symmetry in

T. Rappl (✉) · P. Wurzer · S. P. Nischwitz
Research Unit for Tissue Regeneration, Repair and Reconstruction, Division of Plastic, Aesthetic and Reconstructive Surgery, Department of Surgery, Medical University of Graz, Graz, Austria
e-mail: Thomas.rappl@medunigraz.at;
paul.wurzer@medunigraz.at;
Sebastian.nischwitz@medunigraz.at

M. Barth
Mario Barth Starlighttattoo, South Las Vegas, NV, USA
e-mail: mb@starlighttattoo.com

D. Bossavy
Dominique Bossavy, Beverly Hills, CA, USA
e-mail: dominique@dominiquebossavy.com

L.-P. Kamolz
Research Unit for Tissue Regeneration, Repair and Reconstruction, Division of Plastic, Aesthetic and Reconstructive Surgery, Department of Surgery, Medical University of Graz, Graz, Austria

COREMED—Cooperative Centre for Regenerative Medicine, JOANNEUM RESEARCH Forschungsgesellschaft mbH, Graz, Austria
e-mail: lars.kamolz@medunigraz.at

facial contours or scar camouflaging. Overall, medical tattooing offers a range of treatments including:

- Enhancement of contour symmetry (lips, brows, eyelids, etc.).
- Restoration of the appearance of hair loss due to alopecia (includes restoration of eyebrows, eyelash definition, simulation of scalp hair).
- The diminishment of the appearance of scar tissue due to skin trauma, including burns.
- Vitiligo colour restoration [2].
- Complete reconstruction of the NAC using 3D tattooing.

Technique

Medical tattooing after burn injuries represents a perfect option when reconstructions using skin grafts are followed by pigment mismatch, hair loss and contour deformities. Nowadays, this tattoo technique is mostly performed by a specialised tattoo artist to improve colour match and contour deformities using colours like carbon black, titanium dioxide, etc. The ink is injected by an electric tattoo machine armed with single or multiple needles. Figure 1 shows the process of medical tattooing in vivo.

Burned skin shows a cooler temperature than healthy skin, and pigment appears differently through the scar tissue depending on the degree of the burn. This must be taken into consideration when choosing the right colour mixture. The medical tattooing process, performed under aseptic/sterile conditions, inserts pigment into the dermis, which requires the use of an electric tattoo machine. The ink is inserted using disposable single or a group of needles that are soldered on a bar attached to an oscillating unit. The needles are driven in and out of the skin 80–150 times per second. Needle speed and frequency are crucial when performing medical tattooing treatments to suit the different structures and tolerance of the skin. Needle selection is a critical consideration for any treatment. Smaller needles can penetrate the skin better if there is obvious scar tissue. However, some scar tissue can also be fragile as the structure of the skin is unstable, and this would warrant using a larger needle causing less trauma to the skin [3]. Initially, in order to work through scar tissue smaller needle groupings have to be selected; the smaller the needle the crisper the result. The finer the line, the less noticeable the tattooing will appear. Larger needle grouping gives softer results, for the blending in of the full colour [3]. Different inks are composed of different ingredients, like inorganic materials (titanium dioxide, iron oxide, carbon black, azo dyes, acridine, quinolone, phthalocyanine and naphthol), and organic materials—dyes made from ash and other mixtures. Modern tattooing inks are carbon-based pigments. The pigments used in the field of medical tattooing must be produced under extremely tight guidelines to ensure they are of the highest industry standard and quality.

Through the injection, pigment is dispersed throughout a homogenised layer through the epidermis and upper dermis. The immune system activates phagocytes as a reaction on foreign material. During the healing process, the damaged skin and surface pigment flake away. Following the needling process, collagen growth is induced by granulation tissue formation in the dermal layer. The pigment is captured within the

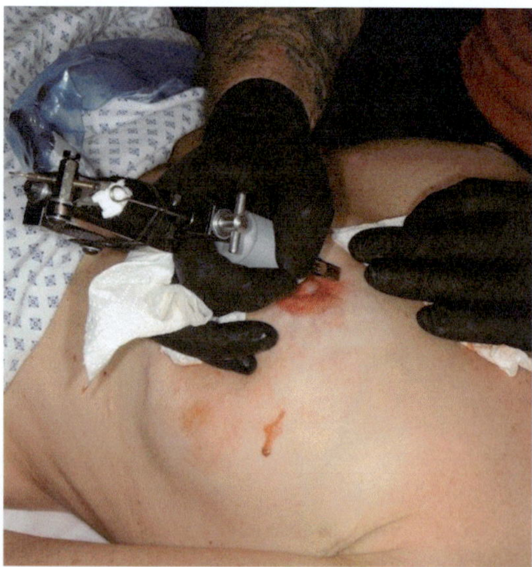

Fig. 1 The process of performing a medical tattooing of the NAC on the left side after the NAC was lost in a prior procedure

fibroblasts, which are concentrated in the dermis/epidermis junction. The pigment stays stable over several years, with a potential migration into the deeper dermis after decades.

After surgical art has reached its limits, medical tattooing opens up the field for possible improvement. Besides covering the whole scared or skin-grafted area with a work of art tattoo, camouflaging the colour mismatch has proven to enhance colour as well as skin texture due to the positive effect of multiple skin-puncture inducing a skin-regenerative processes following the dermal needling. Clinical findings have proven the upregulation of elastin and collagen production following multiple needling. Care has to be taken to find a matching colour in between tanned and pale skin. The procedure has an immediate effect. It has to be taken into account that the colour becomes lighter after a few weeks and that tattoos may fade out with time [4]. Therefore, the revision could be done using the same technique. Generally, a review is not needed for another 12–18 months following a cover-up.

Facial contouring: Hair-baring areas in the face after scarification or skin grafting often look like patches. On one hand, improvement of the colour might be taken in account; on the other hand, tattooing can simulate hair by introducing the pigment into the dermis using a single needle into the dermis similarly to the natural hair pattern. Creating eyebrows using multiple needles is another option to reconstruct eyebrows on hair-bearing supraorbital scarring. Sometimes it is difficult to recreate facial lines and contours exactly by surgery. Especially lip contours and borders between white and red lip might be impossible to reconstruct sufficiently. In these cases, medical tattooing can help to create a perfect line and contour.

NAC reconstruction: Tattooing the nipple in a 3D way provides the visual illusion of real nipple [5]. Indications for NAC tattooing are quite liberal and favoured in patients with thin skin (e.g. radiation). Many women also do not want further surgery but prefer to have a subjectively "complete breast" [6]; for these patients NAC tattooing is also a great solution. To underline the importance of medical tattooing in NAC reconstruction many analyses have been performed [7–11]. In most

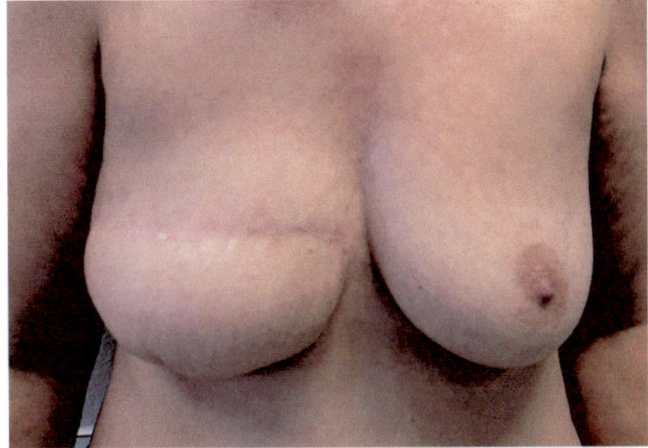
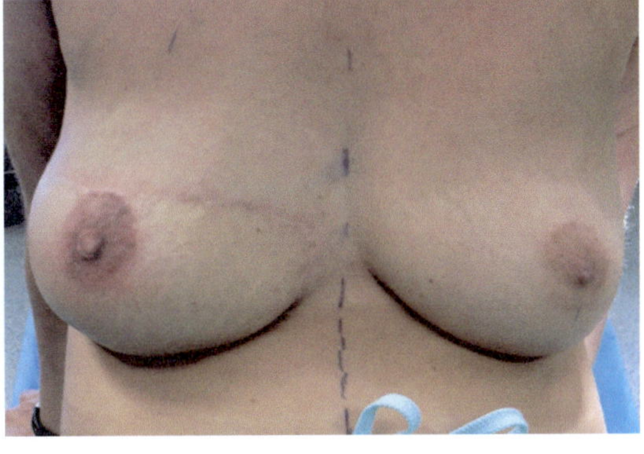

Fig. 2 Pre (up) and post (below) medical tattooing of the NAC after breast reconstruction

studies, a great patient satisfaction could be achieved with close to no adverse events. Especially when having undergone an implant-based reconstruction, the worst-case scenario is to lose the implant due to further complications in NAC reconstruction. The only downsides reported are the lacking projection and the fading over time. However, the latter can easily be countered by a touch-up tattooing session once the colour fades. In general, the aesthetic outcome of reconstructed NACs is lower compared to tattooed NACs. By tattooing, NACs can look more similar to original NACs because of the possibility of creating a fading effect on the edges, which simulates a more natural look than skin grafts or otherwise reconstructed solutions. NAC tattooing however can also be used in addition to a surgical solution: in capable hands, the benefits of both procedures can be combined [12, 13].

NAC tattoos should be performed by a tattoo artist who is skilled in 3D tattoos to receive a 3D effect of the nipple. Colours like carbon black, titanium dioxide, glycerine and isopropyl alcohol are applied using an electric tattoo machine. Figure 2 shows the result of a NAC tattooing after breast reconstruction using a free flap.

Reconstructive Cases

To treat scared lips, a fine 1#needle configuration with a light wash of skin tone has to be applied with emphasis on constricted scar from graft perimeters. Also, the change in lip commissure-to-commissure distance at rest and when smiling has to be taken into account to achieve an improvement after the treatment.

The two presented cases (Figs. 3 and 4) show a very tight scar tissue meaning that the medical tattooing procedure had to be done very slowly using a fine needle, to avoid tissue laceration, and bouncing back of the needle. The pigment was implanted into the skin with a pointillism method. This technique was very successful in

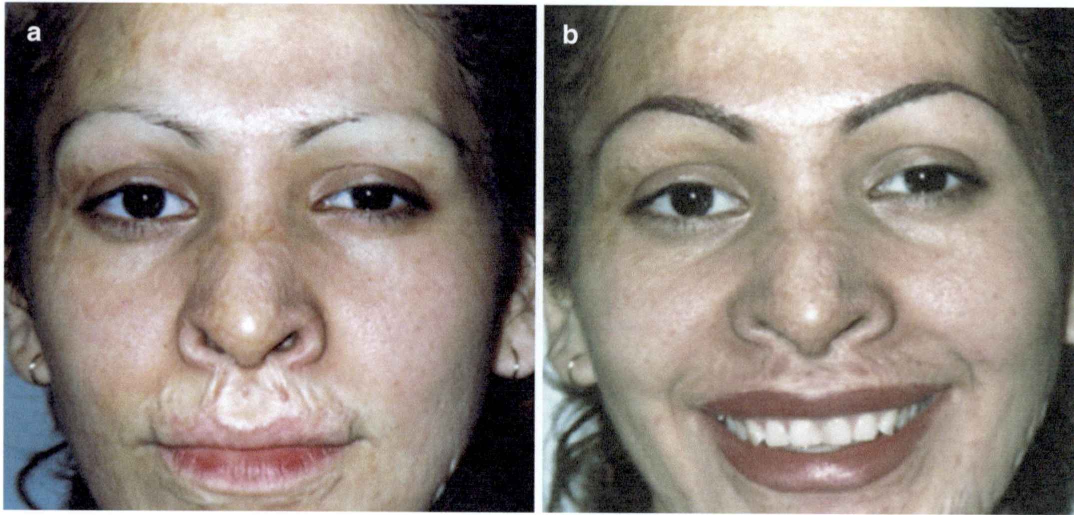

Fig. 3 Pre (**a**) and post (**b**) medical tattooing of the lips and eyebrows. Pics. courtesy Dominique Bossavy

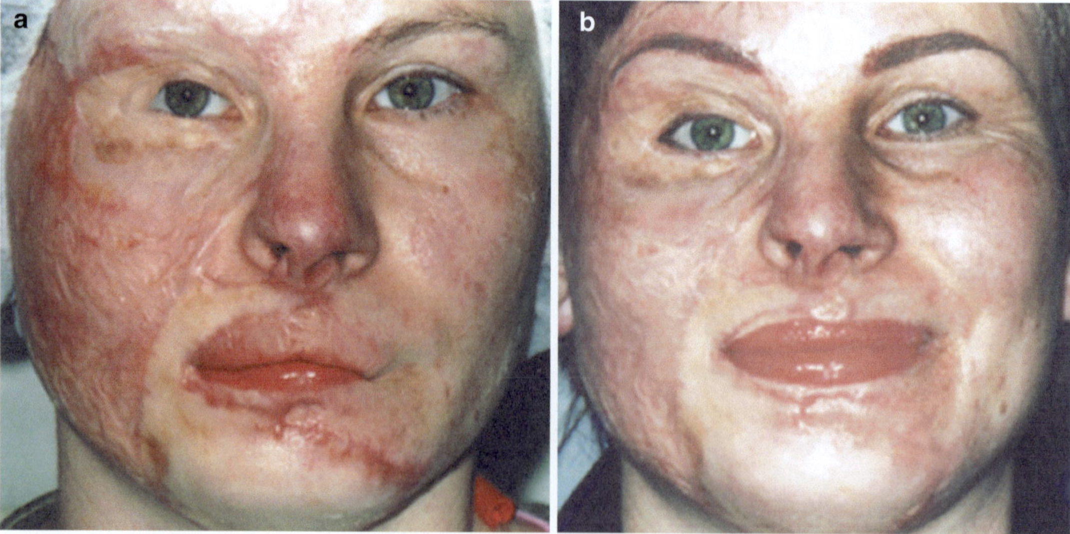

Fig. 4 Pre (**a**) and post (**b**) medical tattooing of the lips, around the eyes and eyebrows

breaking down and loosening the tight scar tissue due to the penetration. Eight different shades of pigment were used on this patient to match the patient's skin colour and to minimise the permanent redness. This resulted in a significant overall release and increased elasticity, translating to a 75% reduction of scleral show as well as more mobility in the lips. The process was applied three times. Usually, during the fourth session, the canthus area was restored to create the illusion of a normal eye corner and restored eyebrows. Finally, on the fifth visit, after successful release of constriction, the lips' shape and contour were designed.

Risks and Complications

Improper sterilisation of tattooing needles and tattoo ink in public tattoo parlours can cause a wide range of diseases and skin reactions [14–16].

Infection

Pyodermal infections can include temporary inflammation at the sites of needle punctures, superficial infections such as impetigo and ecthyma, and deeper infections such as cellulitis, erysipelas and furunculosis. Other transmissible infections include hepatitis, syphilis, leprosy, tuberculosis cutis, rubella, chancroid, tetanus and molluscum contagiosum. An outbreak of infection with *Mycobacterium chelonae* from premixed tattoo ink has also been reported [17]. Hepatitis C has been shown in epidemiologic studies to be transmissible via nonsterile needles. Human immunodeficiency virus is also theoretically transmissible this way, but this is difficult to confirm because the virus has a long incubation period.

Cutaneous Reactions

Skin reactions to tattooing include aseptic inflammation and acquired sensitivity to tattoo dyes, especially red dyes, but also to chromium in green dyes, cadmium in yellow dyes, and cobalt in blue dyes [16]. The reaction can manifest as either allergic contact dermatitis or photoallergic dermatitis. Cutaneous conditions that localise in tattooed areas include vaccinia, verruca vulgaris, herpes simplex, herpes zoster, psoriasis, lichen planus, keratosis follicularis (Darier disease), chronic discoid lupus erythematosus and keratoacanthoma.

Other possible conditions include keloid, sarcoidal granuloma, erythema multiforme, localised scleroderma and lymphadenopathy [14–16].

Burns During Magnetic Resonance Imaging (Rare Complications)

The metallic ferric acid pigments used in tattoos can conduct heat on the skin during magnetic resonance imaging [18], resulting in traumatic burns. This has also been reported to occur with tattoos with nonferrous pigments [2]. Patients should be asked before this procedure if they have tattooing so that this complication can be avoided.

Conclusion

Case series showed that a combination of reconstructive surgery and medical tattooing is a promising collaboration to improve aesthetic outcome and patient satisfaction in reconstructive surgery. Colour temperature must be taken into consideration when choosing the right colour mixture. The medical tattooing process, performed under aseptic/sterile conditions, inserts pigment into the dermis, which requires the use of an electric tattoo machine. Needle speed and frequency are crucial when performing medical tattooing treatments to suit the different structure and tolerance of the skin. Furthermore, needle selection is a critical consideration for any treatment. Smaller needles can penetrate the skin better if there is obvious scar tissue.

The intradermal injection leads to a dispersion of the colour in the upper dermis and epidermis, allowing visual appearance of reconstructed NAC, hair, skin appendages or facial contours.

One main consideration is to match an adequate skin tone between light and tanned skin, since the tattoo itself does not tan when exposed to sunlight. The pigment usually stays stable over time with a tendency to fade after years, as can be seen in regular tattoos. This effect usually is countered by a revision of the tattooing using the same technique once the fading is obvious.

Medical tattooing can serve to improve appearance and symmetry, which in turn helps diminish the visual effects and promotes an improved feeling of self-esteem. Patients reported a confidence boost and a sense of liberation, with a regained sense of normality, and a sense to have gotten back what had been taken away by oftentimes traumatic circumstances. The benefit of medical tattooing is undeniably a valuable application, to bridge the gap between surgery and the aftermath of scar disfigurements. Furthermore, medical tattooing has proven to be a safe and predictable technique which maximises patient's satisfaction and improves the postoperative outcome.

References

1. Tsur H, Kaplan HY. Camouflaging hairless areas on male face by artistic tattoo. Plast Reconstr Surg. 1993;92(2):357–60.
2. Franiel T, Schmidt S, Klingebiel R. First-degree burns on MRI due to nonferrous tattoos. AJR Am J Roentgenol. 2006;187:W556.
3. Betts K. Medical tattooing. Aestheticsjournal.com. 2016.
4. Conway H, Mckinney P, Climo M. Permanent camouflage of vascular nevi of the face by intradermal injection of insoluble pigments (tattooing): experience over twenty years with 1022 areas. Plast Reconstr Surg. 1967;40:457.
5. Halvorson EG, Cormican M, West ME, Myers V. Three-dimensional nipple-areola tattooing: a new technique with superior results. Plast Reconstr Surg. 2014;133(5):1073–5. https://doi.org/10.1097/PRS.0000000000000144.
6. Weissler EH, Schnur JB, Lamelas AM, Cornejo M, Horesh E, Taub PJ. The necessity of the nipple: redefining completeness in breast reconstruction. Ann Plast Surg. 2017;78(6):646–50. https://doi.org/10.1097/SAP.0000000000000943.
7. Liliav B, Loeb J, Hassid VJ, Antony AK. Single-stage nipple-areolar complex reconstruction technique, outcomes, and patient satisfaction. Ann Plast Surg. 2014;73(5):492–7. https://doi.org/10.1097/SAP.0b013e318276dac0.
8. Cha HG, Kwon JG, Kim EK, Lee HJ. Tattoo-only nipple-areola complex reconstruction: another option for plastic surgeons. J Plast Reconstr Aesthet Surg. 2020;73(4):696–702. https://doi.org/10.1016/j.bjps.2019.11.011.
9. Goh SC, Martin NA, Pandya AN, Cutress RI. Patient satisfaction following nipple-areolar complex reconstruction and tattooing. J Plast Reconstr Aesthet Surg. 2011;64(3):360–3. https://doi.org/10.1016/j.bjps.2010.05.010.
10. Uhlmann NR, Martins MM, Piato S. 3D areola dermopigmentation (nipple-areola complex). Breast J. 2019;25(6):1214–21. https://doi.org/10.1111/tbj.13427.
11. El-Ali K, Dalal M, Kat CC. Tattooing of the nipple-areola complex: review of outcome in 40 patients. J Plast Reconstr Aesthet Surg. 2006;59(10):1052–7. https://doi.org/10.1016/j.bjps.2006.01.036.
12. Sowa Y, Kodama T, Hori T, Numajiri T. A medical tattooing technique for enhancing the three-dimensional appearance of the nipple-areola complex after flap-based nipple reconstruction. Aesthetic Plast Surg. 2021;45(6):2631–6. https://doi.org/10.1007/s00266-021-02471-5.
13. Cha HG, Kwon JG, Kim EK. Simultaneous nipple-areola complex reconstruction technique: combination nipple sharing and tattooing. Aesthetic Plast Surg. 2019;43(1):76–82. https://doi.org/10.1007/s00266-018-1247-2.
14. Sperry K. Tattoos and tattooing. Part II: gross pathology, histopathology, medical complications, and applications. Am J Forensic Med Pathol. 1992;13:7–17.
15. Ci J. Tattoo-associated dermatoses: a case report and review of the literature. Dermatol Surg. 2002;28:962–5.
16. Kaur RR, Kirby W, Maibach H. Cutaneous allergic reactions to tattoo ink. J Cosmet Dermatol. 2009;8:295–300.
17. Kennedy BS, Bedard B, Younge M, et al. Outbreak of Mycobacterium chelonae infection associated with tattoo ink. N Engl J Med. 2012;367:1020–4. https://doi.org/10.1056/NEJMoa1205114.
18. Price RR. The AAPM/RSNA physics tutorial for residents. MR imaging safety considerations. Radiological Society of North America. Radiographics. 1999;19:1641–51.

Treatment and Rehabilitation of the Patient with a Scar

Lisa Martin and Fiona Wood

Core Messages

- Patients experience constant disruptions to daily living on a physical, emotional and social level.
- By understanding the potential difficulties experienced by people with scars, health care practitioners gain context and empathy, and this puts them in stronger position to understand rehabilitation strategies.
- By non-judgemental listening, the MDT team can facilitate effective reintegration and rehabilitation that align with patients' values.
- Rehabilitation should be patient-centric, with goals aligning with overarching, value-driven aims.
- Every effort should be made to put some control into the hands of the patient which can improve feelings of self-efficacy.
- Reaching milestones, especially return to work, is important.
- Partner, family and social support are central to a good recovery.

L. Martin (✉)
Burn Injury Research Unit, University of Western Australia, Crawley, WA, Australia

Fiona Wood Foundation, Murdoch, WA, Australia
e-mail: lisa.martin3@health.wa.gov.au

F. Wood
Burn Injury Research Unit, University of Western Australia, Crawley, WA, Australia

Fiona Wood Foundation, Murdoch, WA, Australia

Burn Service of Western Australia, Fiona Stanley Hospital, MNH (B) Main Hospital, Level 4, Burns Unit, Murdoch, WA, Australia
e-mail: Fiona.wood@health.wa.gov.au

Introduction

A multidisciplinary, timely and holistic approach to scar care is necessary as the physical, psychological and social components of scarring are inseparable. There are physical challenges, such as itch, pain, discomfort, heat intolerance and restriction of movement. Challenges can be psychological, such as managing emotions, managing relationships and managing stigma, and can be social, such as appearance concerns, avoidance of engagement and social isolation.

Health care practitioners (HCPs) who treat patients with scars must seek to understand the interactions between the physical, psychological and social impacts to deliver holistic care. This is an important concept for the treating medical team because influences on one component can affect other components. For example, poor mobility and a decrease in participation in fitness activities (reduction in physical function) can lower mood in otherwise healthy people (reduction in psychological function), let alone those recovering from illness or injury [1]. This can then reduce interaction with previously attended social groups, in this case, sporting groups (reduction in social function), and may also diminish belief in the self to perform previously performed activities (further reduction in psychological function). In this way, the influences of the three domains of biological, psychological and social impacts fluctuate and their contribution to the current health situation is dynamic [2]. Thus, opportunities to improve recovery grow because an intervention in one area may influence the others and therefore improve overall well-being.

In addition, HCPs need to understand the actual lived experience of the patient who wears the scars. The impact on their quality of life, their perceptions of the scarring and their priorities for treatment are key to the choices made for reconstructive surgery, scar management and other treatment options. Patients' opinions about required surgery and treatment are likely to differ from HCPs for both adult and paediatric patients, and establishing a patient-centric model of care is important [3–5].

> **Caution!**
> Patients' opinions about required surgery and treatment are likely to differ from health care practitioners for both adult and paediatric patients, and establishing a patient-centric model of care is important.

Any scar can impact daily life, whether from injury, illness, surgery, self-harm, acne or stretch marks. Scars can be fine line, widespread, atrophic, contracted or raised. Medical advances have influenced the scars that are seen in clinical practice. Laparoscopic surgical techniques have replaced open surgery in many areas of clinical practice, thus reducing the size of the resultant scars. In burn care, there has been a long focus on early intervention to reduce scarring [6] and time to healing has been identified as an important factor [7, 8]. However, improvements in burn care have led to burn survival from very large body surface area burns, resulting in bigger burn scars for some survivors [9], and thus more scarring [10, 11].

Despite the fact that scars arise from multiple aetiologies, much of the published research focuses on burn scarring, an area that is supported by a significant body of peer-reviewed evidence. Scars from burn injuries cover more of the skin surface and are more likely to be present in multiple bodily locations. In addition, burn scarring is more likely to have physical symptoms, especially pain and itch [9, 12]. Other fields of research into the impact of scars focus on surgical scars that are in visible body locations, such as thyroid surgery [13–15], scars that have other related psychosocial impacts, such as those that result from mastectomy [16], and scars associated with high levels of stigma such as those from non-suicidal self-injury [17, 18]. Scars can be impactful whether large or small, hidden or visible, or hypertrophic, atrophic, or keloid. Some people overcome challenges better than others despite similar severity, bodily location and functional limitations of the scar [19]. Practitioners need to understand the lived experience of scarring from the perspective of the patient in order to understand how to deliver useful support for reintegration to the family, the workplace and the community. By understanding the potential difficulties experienced by people with scars, HCPs gain context and empathy, and this puts them in a stronger position to understand rehabilitation strategies.

First, this chapter will explain the impact of scarring, from the 'big picture' of increased health risks for the population of people who live with a scar to the individualised lived experience of people who wear their scars for life [20–25]. Second, the chapter will discuss how the clinician and the health care team can facilitate effective reintegration and rehabilitation through their daily practice, choice of treatments and approach to care.

Scar Impact

The Big Picture

Longitudinal studies indicate that posttraumatic stress disorder (PTSD) after burn has been reported in up to 45% of patients [26, 27]. For burn injury, a diagnosis of mental health disorder does not account for the many patients who experience sub-clinical degrees of stress, anxiety or depression which is normal after burn [28]. A similar incidence of emotional problems has been reported after mastectomy [16]. The associations between PTSD and the skin are complex and reciprocal, with the psychological effects of scarring resulting in PTSD, and PTSD exacerbating skin disorders because of greater systemic inflammation and dense sympathetic nervous innervation of the skin [29].

> **Important to Know**
> The associations between PTSD and the skin is complex and reciprocal, with the psychological effects of scarring resulting in PTSD, and PTSD exacerbating skin disorders because of greater systemic inflammation and dense sympathetic nervous innervation of the skin.

Epidemiological data demonstrated that first-time mental health admissions in the 5-year period following burn were three to seven times higher in patients who have had an unintentional burn compared to an uninjured control group. Mental health admission classifications included mood and anxiety disorders, psychotic disorders and alcohol or drug-related disorders. This cohort included more than 10,000 burn admissions with 96% of patients with a burn less than 20% TBSA followed for up to 30 years postburn [30]. This supports other evidence that suggests that burn severity is not a predictor of longer-term psychopathology postburn [31]. Postburn psychosocial research has focused on psychopathology and quality of life [19] with attention on correcting problems and deficits, and regular clinical practice accepts the absence of a mental disorder as an acceptable goal.

Secondary traumatic events can drive the initial acute stress response from the scar-inducing event to augment negative long-term impacts. Posttraumatic stress responses are likely to be greater if there have been other unrelated psycho-

logical stressors or psychological disorders [32] or adverse childhood experiences [33].

> **Caution!**
> Secondary traumatic events can drive the initial acute stress response from the scar-inducing event to augment negative long-term impacts. Posttraumatic stress responses are likely to be greater if there have been other unrelated past psychological stressors.

Understanding the Lived Experience of Scarring

A true understanding of the lived experience of scarring can be difficult to achieve without personal experience, but it is important to gain some understanding of the reality of the challenges of living with a scar. To understand what the experience of scarring is like we need to visit qualitative accounts and analysis, and back this up with quantitative data on symptom prevalence.

Physical symptoms of the scar occur regardless of scar type. Tightness, pain, throbbing and discomfort can be continually present affecting daily life and activities. Feelings of tightness and pulling restrict the ability to move in normal ways whilst attending to the simplest of tasks, depending on the bodily location of the scar [20]. For example, those with scars from mastectomy have pain and adherence problems that reduce arm movement and adversely affect sleep, leisure activities, sports, work and home duties [21]. For those with burn scarring to the lower limbs, bending down or walking downhill can be difficult, or for facial scars with microstomia, using cutlery, or for hand burns, turning a page [22]. Long-term pain in digits impacts dexterity, and learning to compensate for loss of hand function due to scarring or loss of digits is challenging [9]. Pain and sensitivity across scarred fingers have been reported to prohibit bag carrying when shopping, difficulties in hygiene practices such as brushing teeth, and difficulties with driving. The inability to wear shoes led to long-term use of slippers and flip-flops, increasing social isolation for one burn survivor who would not leave their home unless necessary many years after the injury [23].

Other physical sensations may be constantly present such as burning or stinging sensations, sensitivity to touch or sensations that feel like an electric shock. This may present suddenly, graphically described by a burn survivor as having knives stuck into him and being punched at the same time [20]. Sensitivity can be exacerbated by contact with clothing, or temperature extremes. For example, getting into a hot shower can exacerbate both sensitivity [9] and itch [22]. Sensitivity to temperature and the lack of ability to regulate temperature through sweating are important consequences of scarring that can have unforeseen consequences. This can alter choice of employment, such as the inability to work in a commercial kitchen or for jobs that are based outdoors. It can restrict the choice of travel destination or holiday activity [22] or simply the mode of travel, not wanting to travel by plane for fear of being stuck in a confined space and unable to seek cool fresh air [24]. It can alter choice of fitness activity because of perceived heat intolerance during exercise or choice of leisure activity, for example the patient who was unable to use their season ticket to watch their favourite team play because he was unable to sit in the hot sun [23]. Consequently, work–life balance can be significantly altered for years following the event or injury that resulted in the scar [23, 24].

Itch is a significant problem that has been reported in up to 62% of burn scars and 56% of non-burn scars [9] and described as 'really unbearable', 'tormenting' to experience and 'annoying' because it will not stop. Itch can affect sleep, leading to further problems with mood and ability to function. Patients are unable to scratch the itch because of tenderness and risk of breakdown due to scar fragility [20]. Itch is associated with poor mental health [34, 35]. The presence of itch may affect the choice of activity, for instance swimming might be avoided because of increased itch [22]. Scar fragility and fear of breakdown also impact activity choice and reduce

options for the type of physical activity engaged in because of increased protective behaviours.

Thus, physical symptoms are often constant; they affect multiple aspects of daily life and inhibit routine aspects of daily living such as movement, eating and drinking. They restrict the types of physical activities that are available to the person, and they interrupt sleep at night. The biggest issues, as identified by burn patients during the first 12 months after their injury, were identified as reduced range of motion, pain, poor sleep, itch and fatigue [36]. Daily life is difficult [25] and people become resigned to accept limited physical outcomes [23]. The physical symptoms are a constant reminder of the scar and the associated event.

> **Important to Know**
> Physical symptoms are often constant; they affect multiple aspects of daily life and inhibit routine aspects of daily living such as movement, eating and drinking.

The emotional effects of living with a scar are varied and complex. Emotional issues include feelings of vulnerability, guilt, blame and shame, intrusive thoughts and flashbacks, self-consciousness, sadness and anger [19, 26, 37]. Looking at scars for the first time can be very confronting [38]. Following mastectomy, one woman reported she had felt unprepared for what to expect, she felt as though she had been butchered and cried uncontrollably. She felt unable to show her husband the scars, and her mother suggested she could hide the scars under a dressing [16]. Cold weather may be welcomed as it gives the opportunity to cover up with clothing, but can hinder physical comfort as pain and stiffness increase [21]. Hiding scars is a common reaction with all types of scarring [20].

Most patients think their scars are unsightly and are unhappy with the way they look. The emotional response is not simply a reaction to their objective self-assessment of the scar appearance in the present moment but reflects the fact that the scars act as a constant visual reminder of their cause, and scar-related experiences that have occurred since. For example, a 20-year-old male with a hypertrophic facial scar was laughed at by his friends, who told him that he deserved it [20].

> **Important to Know**
> Emotional issues include feelings of vulnerability, guilt, blame and shame, intrusive thoughts and flashbacks, self-consciousness, sadness and anger.

In a social context, people may feel stigmatised by the scars, fearing judgement [9, 20, 39]. People report feeling ugly, embarrassed, humiliated, self-conscious and did not feel they were normal. They are particularly anxious about the reactions of other people [22, 40]. They were concerned that other people might think they were criminals, had engaged in self-harm behaviours, or that they were weak-willed, weird or on drugs [20]. Socially, all aspects of engagement with others can be difficult. The attempt to hide scars from other people to avoid unwanted attention and questioning occurs; this might include camouflage with make-up, over dressing or changes in gesticulation, posture and general body language. People fear rejection and initial eye contact may be avoided in case the other person does not want to engage, or that they would engage too much and ask unwanted questions. Trying to maintain eye contact can be difficult if the other person becomes 'fixated' on the scar [20]. This is supported by quantitative research using eye-tracking monitors that demonstrated that observers of images of people who had thyroidectomy neck scars direct their attention towards the neck rather than the face [14]. People talk about 'putting on a brave face to the world' [40] or 'putting on a brave face to the kids' [9].

> **Important to Know**
> Remember that there might be hidden emotions not revealed to you as recovery is a 'double track' of stress and resilience and patients often put on a 'brave face'.

Unwanted questions are found to be inevitable, and in time people learnt to close conversations rapidly. Questions from strangers, or those asked in a hostile manner or asked in transient situations, for example the supermarket, were met with little need to explain. Questions from friends, when asked with underlying care and concern, would be answered more fully, especially if the social interaction was likely to be more prolonged, such as at a dinner party. In these circumstances, there were more feelings of obligation to explain and tell the story, sometimes to the point of telling the story before being asked to pre-empt the questions that were felt to be inevitable. A quantitative study that assessed all-cause scarring state that 56% of patients found that their scars had affected their confidence, and for the subgroup of burn patients that 45% had gained unwanted attention [9]. Appearance concerns and co-existing PTSD symptoms are particularly problematic, as re-experiencing occurs when asked about the scars or the event [40].

All of these issues led to a reluctance to leave the house unless it was necessary, and to increased social isolation. They felt less sociable, wanted to be alone and actively avoided situations such as public transport or shopping where they could be stared at by strangers [23]. People report a new understanding of friendship, of 'finding out who their friends are' as some of their friends disappeared and their friendship group narrowed to long-term, trusted people they could confide in. They pretend they are 'ok' so that they don't lose more friends [24, 41]. For those who do leave the house and who pursue leisure activities, their choice of activity is described as distressing if scars are exposed, such as swimming or surfing. Scars are felt to be ugly and people with scars do not want to get changed into a swimming costume at a beach or a pool [9, 20, 24]. There was a sense of sadness in accepting the need for change [25].

> **Important to Know**
> Socially, people may feel stigmatised by the scars, fearing judgement. People report feeling ugly, embarrassed, humiliated, self-conscious and did not feel they were normal.

Body Image

A review of body image concerns after burn reports mixed results when comparing satisfaction with appearance between a burn scar group and another reference group or a normative population [42]. However, there were some consistent findings that body image is worse at the time of discharge in women after a burn, with no mediation from burn severity (as measured by TBSA). However, TBSA did negatively affect improvement over time for women compared to men, especially for patients with facial burn scars. Generally, body image is worse with higher TBSA, longer length of stay, the presence of facial burn scars and for those whose scars persist over time [42]. Body image difficulties may peak at 6 months postburn, with small improvements by 12 months [43]. Overall, it seems that negative impacts on body image, sexuality and relationship persist in the first year following burn injury despite physical and functional recovery [44]. There is some evidence to suggest that preburn body image will affect postburn body image, with those who put more importance into their appearance before the burn more adversely affected afterwards [45]. Body image issues are associated with symptoms of depression in the postburn period whilst the patient is undergoing reconstructive surgery, especially in women [46], a worrying finding as depression is a barrier to burn recovery [47]. Good social support can be protective against body image concerns if partners still find them attractive and seek intimacy, and family and friends do not focus on their scars. This helps them to know that others recognise that they are still the same person inside despite their altered appearance, often mirroring how they feel [48]. This aids acceptance, which is important in recovery [49].

Intimate relationships can be fraught with anxiety, whether scarring is visible or easily hidden with clothing [45]. A 22-year-old woman found that disclosing a burn experience to a potential new partner when chatting casually in a bar caused them to change their attitude and back off [40]. However, it has been recently reported that burn survivors are as sexually active and are as often in romantic relationships, as a normative comparison group, unrelated to TBSA or bodily location of the burn scar [50].

There is less evidence of the effects on scarring on children, whereby study participants are often recruited from convenience samples, such as burn camps. This creates a selection bias in the reporting of the impacts of scarring on children with scars because that which is reported in the literature are for children who have received more intervention, more social support, and who have been encouraged to use approach-focused coping strategies. In addition, comparison groups may not be ideal, where a cohort of Australian patients was compared to a US normative control [42]. However, body image concerns peak in late teen/early adulthood making this group vulnerable to mental health issues, as is reflected in the epidemiological data [51]. Hence, the social consequences of scarring affect relationships at intimate levels, friendship levels and community levels [40, 52, 53].

Understanding the Lived Experience of Recovery

There are ways in which the patients' perception of recovery may differ from the perception of the medical team. Patients see recovery as a process not a destination. This process is a non-linear journey, a roller coaster with twists and turns.

This journey is seen as being personal and individual, and setbacks are considered to be a normal part of this. The process is stressful, and setbacks have to be worked through. These are not seen to be failures but are part of the process. The patient needs to be part of the process, specifically with the need to engage in decisions made. Every effort should be made to put some control into the hands of the patient which can improve feelings of self-efficacy [54]. Recovery is reported more than cessation of self-harm in the case of non-suicidal self-injury scars and involves the development of resilience [17]. Self-efficacy and self-determination are important factors for good postburn recovery [25, 55].

Often, the lived experience of burn injury supports the concept of patients experiencing a 'double track' of recovery. This is when posttraumatic stress symptoms occur alongside posttraumatic growth experiences. Posttraumatic growth (PTG) refers to the psychological growth that results from the reappraisal of life and an adjustment of worldview. It is 'growth' because development occurs beyond pre-trauma levels and is true for those who have survived burn. It is not the opposite of posttraumatic stress but means that psychologically there are positive and negative aspects that run together. Stress precedes growth, is thought to be necessary to trigger growth and growth may act as a buffer to stress. PTG involves a reframed worldview that seeks acceptance and meaning, identifies values, is future focused and seeks new ways to thrive [41, 47, 55–58].

It takes time to make any sense out of the life changes that occur after burn, and it feels as though it is simply about putting one step in front of another, with some determination to overcome the limitations of the injury [23]. Early in recovery patients make subconscious assessments of pain and function and later purposefully evaluate their strength, movement and appearance [25]. There is conflicting evidence about the influence of total burn surface area (TBSA) on PTG after burn [58, 59]. Females reported higher PTG scores [58] and PTG and positive reframing does not occur in the presence of depression [25, 47]. Humour is important, but must come from self-reflection and new insights, and is a form of reframing. Hope for the

future and acceptance of the circumstances are key to good recovery [23–25].

> **Important to Know**
> Burn survivors can feel pressured to put on a front of positivity. This might result in a public and a private side of managing the challenges of scarring.

Patients often use downward comparisons to improve how they feel about their own scars [25]. They might express gratitude that the area of the scar is not bigger, that their scar is not on their face or hands or that they have been burnt as adults not children [24, 60]. However, this comes with a warning to the HCP, family or anyone other than the patient—this is not something you can tell them! Being told they were 'lucky' that the scars are not worse can be distressing and invalidating and can make some people feel they are being selfish or self-indulgent [48]. Burn survivors can feel pressured to put on a front of positivity [48]. This might present as a public and a private side of managing the challenges of scarring and its cause. For example, they may also outwardly downplay body image concerns, whilst simultaneously internalising feelings of body dissatisfaction [61]. It is important for HCPs to bear this in mind when managing patients who do well; what you see on the surface might hide deeper issues.

The management of scars is challenging for patients. Pressure garments are reported to be uncomfortable, cause friction on sensitive skin, are hot to wear, and cause increased itch. These unwanted sensations only resolve when the garment is removed. Garments take time to put on, take off and maintain, and the physical restriction of the garments can reduce range of motion and can make activities of daily living difficult [62]. In addition, garments can make some people feel conspicuous when in public and this can be a barrier to adherence [63]. Other patients adapt to wearing the garments and feel that they can be useful to hide the scars giving protection and security with an 'emotional barrier' [5].

Moving towards a new normal is important, and close involvement of family, accepting their new appearance as normal and empowerment through self-care are important for patients who are emerging from the 'trauma bubble'. The milestone of return to work was found to be especially important with burn survivors 'rethinking' how that might happen [64].

Scar-Focused Reintegration in Clinical Practice

Measuring Quality of Life and Impact of Scarring

Measures that assess the physical and psychosocial aspects of scarring are addressed in the chapter about Scar Assessment. The clear understanding of what is being assessed and by whom is essential in tracking the scar evolution and its impact on the individual. These assessments provide an opportunity to track the effectiveness of the interventions and can guide the treatment plan. For example, understanding which scar symptoms cause emotional triggers for individual patients can enable targeted treatment of those symptoms to help reduce the constant reminders.

There are specific measures that assess the experience of living with scarring on quality of life [65]. These include the Brisbane Burn Scar Impact Scale (BBSIP) [12], the Burn-Specific Health Scale Brief (BSHS-B) [66] and the Burns Outcome Questionnaire (BOQ) [67]. In addition, the Satisfaction with Appearance Scale (SWAP) was devised using some questions from the BSHS-B and was designed to measure subjective satisfaction with appearance, social and behavioural impacts of the scar [68]. These in-depth measures of quality of life can give insight into individual issues as well as pooling quantitative data which can identify predictors of risk, highlighting those in most need of therapeutic inter-

vention and identifying appropriate timing of intervention.

Use of Language: Victim vs. Survivor

Please note that the word 'victim' has not been used in this chapter. We want patients to move away from the belief that they are a 'victim' to thoughts of survivorship. The word 'victim' suggests passivity and lack of agency, implying powerlessness. The word 'survivor' suggests determination, adaptation and resilience. This is true regardless of the cause of scarring, whether a non-intentional or intentional injury, or the result of a medical procedure. In addition, when there is a concurrent cancer diagnosis, the word 'survivor' is far from perfect because it implies that the danger has passed. Following trauma, this can be helpful, but following a cancer diagnosis and successful treatment, recurrence is possible and therefore the danger might not have passed [69].

> **Important to Know**
> Using the word 'survivor' suggests determination, adaptation and resilience. Using the word 'victim' suggests passivity and lack of agency, implying powerlessness.

Communication of the Multidisciplinary Team

The team of HCPs treating the patient needs to be aligned in their messaging and language with regular review and clear documentation of the journey. The united approach of the team must be firmly based on individual patient needs, so non-judgmental listening is key. Honesty is important to build trust, and it is important to keep in mind realistic outcomes for the individual patient. On the other hand, we do not want to give self-limiting beliefs by telling a patient that something is not achievable.

> **Clinical Tip**
> Non-judgemental listening is key. Honesty is important to build trust, and it is important to keep in mind realistic outcomes for the individual patient.

There are a number of key messages that patients need to hear from the treating team. Firstly, it is necessary to encourage self-belief and self-efficacy. Patients need to believe that they have the strength and resilience to get through this time period, and just because something seems impossible today does not mean that it will be impossible tomorrow, or next week or next year. It is simply that they can't do it yet. The burn experience might already have taught them that they are stronger than they thought, and reflecting on this can be a useful reminder to patients. Most importantly, patients need to have some control over what is happening to them and to make choices about their care and treatment where possible. Secondly, it is important to help the patient understand that recovery is a roller-coaster ride, and sometimes taking one step back is normal. As well as acknowledging this fact, if patients are discouraged with their progress, make their goals more short-term and achievable. Hope and determination can be facilitated by feeding back progress to the patient, reminding them of how far they have come and the hurdles they have conquered to date. Thirdly, it is important to communicate the hope that there will be improvements into the future with a focus on the importance of explaining trajectory of scar progression and therapeutic opportunities.

> **Clinical Tip**
>
> Encourage self-belief and self-efficacy. Patients need to believe that they have the strength and resilience to get through this.

In summary, the team needs to use an open and honest, patient centric, approach that encourages self-belief, self-compassion and determination in order to motivate patients towards better recovery.

Goal Setting

The process of recovery requires the engagement of the patient, not just the patient being the recipient of the administrations of the treating team. The perceptions of need for scar management may differ between the patients' viewpoints and the HCPs' viewpoints [3]. Identifying the patient's individual values is important, and assessment can start by identifying desired activities that are prevented by the scar, either functionally or psychosocially. Setting value-driven goals and encouraging meaningful engagement for recovery is a priority that needs to be addressed along the clinical journey.

> **Clinical Tip**
> Long-term value-driven aims need to be identified, and short-term rehabilitation goals should be set that are specific, measurable, achievable, realistic, and timely.
>
> Return to normal activities and meaningful activities is an important goal for patients. It is important to have realistic discussions with respect to the return to previous roles and responsibilities. For the HCP, it is necessary to identify the patient's values and to align recovery goals to these. For example, if the patient previously enjoyed playing golf or baseball, then goals related to ensuring range of motion in the shoulders, or hand grip, become meaningful and motivational aims for the patient. The long-term aim needs to be identified, and then short-term rehabilitation goals should be set that align with this and that are specific, measurable, achievable, realistic, and timely ('SMART goals') [70].

In the context of goal setting the importance of milestones needs to be recognised, such as the return home from hospital, return to work, return to driving and return to other activities that are personally important to the patient. We want patients to realise their own personal strengths and to mark their goals against their current priorities. At each stage, we need to recognise that control needs to be handed to the patient with recognition that behavioural disengagement may indicate the need for increased input.

> **Important to Know**
> The milestone of return to work was found to be especially important with burn survivors 'rethinking' how that might happen. Work-life balance can be significantly altered for years following the event or injury that resulted in the scar.

The Importance of Addressing the Physical Symptoms of Scarring

Pain is a significant factor in scar management beginning at the time of the injury or incision. The establishment of a pain management plan tailored to the individual is ideal. At the outset, the use of general anaesthetic for extensive dressing changes and local anaesthetics prior to interventions can reduce the long-term impact of pain. A combination of pharmacological strategies with narcotics, simple analgesia and anti-inflammatory agents combine to reduce acute pain. Poorly managed pain at the onset is associated with the development of chronic pain syndrome associated with the scarred body site.

Furthermore, itch is a debilitating symptom impacting on every aspect of the individual's life specifically linked with pain and driving sleep disturbance. Sleep quality is an area in need of discussion and understanding the individual's circumstance and opportunities to help, for example cool shower and hydration prior to sleep and regular sleep patterns.

> **Clinical Tip**
> Addressing these physical symptoms will have a positive impact on psychosocial functioning
>
> - Pain
> - Itch
> - Discomfort
> - Altered sensation
> - Heat intolerance
> - Restriction of movement
> - Sleep hygiene

Ongoing pain and itch, or sleep disturbance related to scarring, require an assessment of medical history and an examination to develop a management plan. A multidisciplinary approach linked with allied health practitioners can facilitate the multi-faceted approach, including strategies such as massage, stretching and pressure techniques that will influence the physical aspects of the scar, highlighting the importance of maintaining connection with all the services, discussed in depth in the respective chapters.

Encouraging Compliance with Therapy

Maintaining engagement with the multidisciplinary team is important for compliance with treatment. Reasons for disengagement need to be assessed; it might be that the patient perceives that they have reached their recovery goals and they think, rightly or wrongly, that there are no further treatments that may help. However, it is important to remember that behavioural disengagement can indicate that a patient is using avoidance coping styles [71].

Although scar outcome is individual in terms of ultimate appearance and acceptability to the

> **Caution!**
>
> A 'red flag' for poor recovery can include behavioural disengagement, which may present as non-compliance with care, missed appointments and disengagement with the treating team.

patient it is important to explain to patients the usual trajectory of scarring, so that they understand what they might expect in the long term. As well as understanding these long-term scar outcomes, it is helpful to then focus on the short-term scar management steps that will help to get them there.

Health care practitioners need patients to be intrinsically motivated; in other words, patients must want to comply with therapy because they can understand the benefits therein. Intrinsic motivation is associated with greater determination, improved mood and well-being and better outcomes. If behaviours are externally controlled, so that patients feel they have to comply, challenges can feel more difficult to overcome. As behaviour becomes more integrated, future challenges are more easily overcome [72].

Priorities for patients are to achieve good scar outcomes for appearance and function, and this will help to drive treatment compliance, especially for pressure garments. There are factors that can result in non-adherence with pressure garments. Occupational therapists and other members of the multidisciplinary team need to educate patients and their families about what to expect with pressure garment therapy. Patients want to have prior warning about potential sensory problems such as itch, discomfort, friction and heat. In addition, education about pressure garment regimens helps with future planning and realistic expectations. If there is a choice of fabric, colour or design for their individual situation, the patient should be involved in this to allow a sense of control [63]. Describing how garments are thought to act on the scar and the benefits on scar outcome may help motivate the patient to comply with treatment. In addition, although itch might increase, the garments can protect against

breakdown from scratching and can protect fragile scars. Sun protection is important, and it is important to explain that garments are not protective to UV rays, and that sunscreen needs to be used for protection against further damage, such as skin cancer [73]. There is some evidence to suggest that scar massage might have short-term benefits for itch and pain and also improve scar vascularity, pliability and height. In addition, it might have a positive effect on mood by reducing depression and anxiety [74]. Long-term goals are important and it is important to provide future hope for patients by explaining that there are further treatments that can improve scar outcome, such as ablative, fractional, CO_2 laser to improve pain, itch and dermal architecture, contracture restrictions and range of motion [75–77].

As previously indicated the physical and psychosocial aspects of scarring are intimately linked, and the understanding that physiotherapy and occupational therapy have significant roles in the management of scarring is important. The therapeutic opportunities are detailed and discussed in the respective chapters. Physical functional rehabilitation, with stretches, positioning and driving range of movement, specific scar management with massage, pressure garments and topical therapies are a core part of recovery. In addition, the focus on return to work and normal activities is essential for a successful rehabilitation.

Psychological Screening and Referral Strategies

It is essential to manage the patient's emotions with empathy and early assessment is pivotal, exploring for indicators which would drive referral to psychology and psychiatric services. Coping strategies used after trauma can be adaptive or maladaptive. Problem-focused coping methods are useful if the intervention can change the outcome, and emotion-focused coping methods are useful when the outcome is fixed and requires acceptance [78]. Some types of coping avoid engagement with the problem, and these are less useful for adaptation. These might include self-distraction or denial and can be appropriate strategies in the immediate aftermath of the injury, but are not helpful in the longer term, and frequent use of these can increase stress and reduce well-being [79].

As previously described in this chapter, your patients may use humour, positive reframing and downward comparison to cope [24]. Finding meaning and purpose may be positive behaviours with some patients using religious or spiritual beliefs to support their recovery journey. Hope is important, and positive reframing is protective against depression, with new insights for the patient helping them to accept the situation and move on with life [25, 41].

> **Caution!**
> Depressive symptoms prevent good recovery and might be worse in the rehabilitation phase. Look out for behavioural disengagement, venting and self-blame which have been associated with injury-related distress and posttraumatic stress disorder.

Remember that there might be hidden emotions not revealed to you as recovery is a 'double track' of stress and resilience and patients often put on a 'brave face'. This means you need to be aware of the 'red flags' that might indicate that a patient needs more professional support. Depressive symptoms prevent good recovery and might be worse in the rehabilitation phase compared to the acute phase after burn [80]. Other signs can be predictive of depression, such as behavioural disengagement, venting and self-blame which are coping strategies that have been associated with injury-related distress [81] and posttraumatic stress disorder [82]. Behavioural disengagement is when the patient appears to have given up trying to manage the problem [83]. Thus, a 'red flag' for poor recovery can include behavioural disengagement, which may present as non-compliance with care, missed appointments and disengagement with the treating team. Self-blame is when a person attaches their cur-

rent circumstances to their own actions [83]. Venting is the expression of negative feelings to find relief [84]. Emotional triggers and flashbacks can be indicative of PTSD and are barriers to recovery [85]. The HCP must be observant of these behaviours and signs for early screening for depression and/or PTSD symptoms for referral to psychological services. Specialist psychological programmes might include social cognitive behavioural therapies or social skills training [86, 87].

> **Clinical Tip**
> Early detection and treatment of depression and PTSD are important, and a quick screen for these during burn recovery can be a rapid and easy indicator for psychological referral.

In summary, early detection and treatment of depression and PTSD are important, and screening for these during burn recovery can be a quick and easy indicator for psychological referral. Reasons for non-compliant patients should be established and patients can be assessed for depression. HCPs can also be observant for venting or self-blame behaviours that indicate poor coping strategies and are barriers to recovery.

Social Screening and Support

Social screening needs to assess the non-medical factors that account for between 30 and 55% of health outcomes, the social determinants of health. The World Health Organization states that 'In countries at all levels of income, health and illness follow a social gradient: the lower the socioeconomic position, the worse the health'. These factors include education level, income and welfare, employment, job (in)security, nutrition, housing, social inclusion, non-discrimination, early childhood development, conflict, and access to good health care [88]. These considerations must be applied to the cultural, environmental, and individual circumstances for the patient. Appropriate involvement of the social work team is required as part of the treating multidisciplinary team at all stages of the recovery journey.

The process of recovery requires support from family, friends, and the wider community, as well as health care professionals. A trusted confidante who has given long-term support is an important source of help and comfort for people with scars [24]. Supportive partners need to give reassurance that they still find them attractive, balanced with recognition that they still see the same person beneath the scars. It is important for the patient to do things with friends and family, and interact with friends, neighbours and strangers. The support of family and close friends will help the person manage other people's reactions and manage social situations [48].

Important to Know

A trusted confidante who has given long-term support is an important source of help and comfort for people with scars.

Supporting the Family

Families of burn survivors have reported feeling powerless, stressed and dejected. They have initially looked forward to the return home of their loved one after discharge, only to find there are difficulties with care at home, lack of sleep for themselves and financial strain. Roles change, and partners may become the new 'hub' of the family network [89]. Families may be under strain, both before and after the patient's discharge. The family can feel more supported by the team if they are included in care and decision-making, and when HCPs communicate directly with them. Education about the patient's needs should be given, and they should be included in routine care activities, such as scar massage and the donning and doffing of pressure garments, to increase confidence. Developing routines can be helpful to family members [64]. Communication between the patient and their families should be

encouraged, as families and partners want to help but don't necessarily know the best way to go about it. They might be confused about how much help to give, and the patient might want different levels of practical support on different days or might feel they are being a burden if they ask for help [24]. Partners and close family members should be encouraged to seek support from their GP or mental health services for psychological support. In addition, if there are burn support groups or local community organisations that support carers, HCPs should make these known to stressed families for further support.

Clinical Tip

Family should be included in care and decision making where possible.

Support from friends, neighbours and the community is often appreciated by both the patient and their family, and some seek support from their faith or from religious organisations [89]. Partners and families should be made aware that it is normal to find the situation difficult, and that they can also seek support via their GP, clinical psychology services or other local supportive organisations.

Dealing with Other People

Learning to deal with other people is an important part of recovery. People with visible scars are very aware of the double takes, stares and glances that come their way, and this can lead to self-consciousness and apprehension. This may result in a fear of rejection, together with the tendency to link the disfigurement to any adverse social experiences, and social skills can decline [87]. These patients might benefit from social skills training. In addition, the inevitable questions need to be addressed, and learning to tell the story in different ways is helpful to recovery. Questions come at unexpected times, in random places, by strangers as well as friends, and learning ways to effectively and politely close a conversation and thus *not* tell the story can be important too. Unexpected questions can trigger unwanted flashbacks of the event or other associated memories and thus having prepared and practiced responses can be helpful to manage these situations [90]. Preparing stories can help recovery, and patients might require professional psychological support to achieve this. Narrative psychology is about subjectively reconstructing the event, and survivors who can do this in a redemptive way can be psychologically healthier in the longer term [91].

> **Important to Know**
> For patients, the inevitable questions need to be addressed and learning to tell the story in different ways is helpful to recovery.

Peer support is often found to be helpful for patients, as talking to other survivors enables reflection and reframing. Other survivors have credibility because they have the lived experience and understand the reality of what lies before someone who is early in their recovery journey. This can bring meaning, hope, reassurance, acceptance and new possibilities for the future [92, 93]. However, for one-to-one support, it is important to match patients well [94] and group support might be more beneficial for some [93]. Not all survivors feel that they need peer support strategies because their personal support system is thought to be good enough and that their recovery trajectory is satisfactory. For those who do receive peer support it is important to ensure the time is right for the patient, with inpatient peer support sometimes being too early [94]. In fact, the need for peer support might be greater many years postburn [95].

Burn survivors sometimes turn to social media and blogging to share their stories. In these online biographies, they retell the event, describe the social support they have received, discuss how they have adapted to a new body image, how they have been treated by others and how they have found a new life course [96]. It is important for people to be able to tell the story behind the scar, and particularly helpful when learning how to deal with the inquisitive and unwanted questions from other people.

Other types of online resources are sought for all types of health advice. Discussion boards and online forums can provide places for people to discuss issues, and unfiltered communication can be analysed. For those with NSSI scars, the reflections were that the scars were part of the identity of the person, how hard they were to accept and that acceptance was a process. For some the visible scars told a story of strength in the face of adversity and survival, but some expressed shame, of not wanting to wear their story on their arms for others to see [18].

Conclusion

The scar worn for life can act as a constant reminder of the traumatic event in an individual's life. The resulting impact can be reduced by focused and comprehensive care with respect to the physical aspects of the scar but there will remain a unique pattern of coping with psychosocial sequelae. Taking the time to listen to the patient's concerns will help drive goal setting and progress throughout the clinical journey. The validation of the patient's unique journey informs the foundation of individualised patient-centric care, giving hope for their future.

References

1. Antunes HK, Leite GS, Lee KS, Barreto AT, Dos Santos RV, de Sá Souza H, Tufik S, de Mello MT, et al. Exercise deprivation increases negative mood in exercise-addicted subjects and modifies their biochemical markers. Physiol Behav. 2016;15:182–90.
2. Jull G. Biopsychosocial model of disease: 40 years on. Which way is the pendulum swinging. Br J Sports Med. 2017;51(16):1187–8.
3. Rea S, Goodwin-Walters A, Wood F. Surgeons and scars: differences between patients and surgeons in the perceived requirement for reconstructive surgery following burn injury. Burns. 2006;32:276–83.
4. Wood A, Clugston S, Rawlins J, Rea S, Edgar D, Wood F. Burn patients, parents and doctors: are we in agreement? Burns. 2012;38:487–92.

5. Jones L, Calvert M, Moiemen N, Deeks J, Bishop J, Kinghorn P, et al. Outcomes important to burn patients during scar management and how they compare to the concepts captured in burn-specific patient reported outcome measures. Burns. 2017;43:1682–92.

6. Engrav L, Heimbach D, Reus J, Harnar T, Marvin J. Early excision and grafting vs. nonoperative treatment of burns of indeterminant depth: a randomized prospective study. J Trauma. 1983;23(11):1001–4.

7. Chipp E, Charles L, Thomas K, Moeimen N, Wilson Y. A prospective study of time to healing and hypertrophic scarring in paediatric burns: every day counts. Burns Trauma. 2017;5(3):1–6.

8. Finlay V, Burrows S, Burmaz M, Yawary H, Lee J, Edgar DW, et al. Increased burn healing time is associated with higher Vancouver scar scale score. Scars Burns Healing. 2017;3:1–10.

9. Brewin M, Homer S. The lived experience and quality of life with burn scarring—the results from a large-scale online survey. Burns. 2018;44:1801–10.

10. Wallace H, Fear M, Crowe M, Martin L, Wood F. Identification of factors predicting scar outcome after burn in adults: a prospective case-control study. Burns. 2017;43:1271–83.

11. Wallace H, Fear M, Crowe M, Martin L, Wood F. Identification of factors predicting scar outcome after burn injury in children: a prospective case-control study. Burns Trauma. 2017;5(1):19.

12. Tyack Z, Ziviani J, Kimble R, Plaza A, Jones A, Cuttle L, et al. Measuring the impact of burn scarring on health-related quality of life: development and preliminary content validation of the Brisbane burn scar impact profile (BBSIP) for children and adults. Burns. 2015;41:1405–19.

13. Best A, Shipchandler T, Cordes S. Midcervical scar satisfaction in thyroidectomy patients. Laryngoscope. 2017;127:1247–52.

14. Juarez M, Ishii L, Nellis J, Bater K, Huynh P, Fung N, et al. Objectively measuring social attention of thyroid neck scars and transoral surgery using eye tracking. Laryngoscope. 2019;129:2789–94.

15. Sethkumar P, Ly D, Tolley N. Scar satisfaction and body image in thyroidectomy patients: prospective study in a tertiary referral Centre. J Laryngol Otol. 2018;132:60–7.

16. Davies C, Brockopp D, Moe K, Wheeler P, Abner J, Lengerich A. Exploring the lived experience of women immediately following mastectomy. Cancer Nurs. 2017;40(5):361–8.

17. Lewis S, Kenny T, Whitfield K, Gomez J. Understanding self-injury recovery: views from individuals with lived experience. J Clin Psychol. 2019;75:2119–39.

18. Lewis S, Mehrabkhani S. Every scar tells a story: insight into people's self-injury scar experiences. Couns Psychol Q. 2016;29(3):296–310.

19. Attoe C, Pounds-Cornish E. Psychosocial adjustment following burns: an integrative literature review. Burns. 2015;41(7):1375–84.

20. Brown B, McKenna S, Siddhi K, McGrouther D, Bayat A. The hidden cost of skin scars: quality of life after skin scarring. J Plast Reconstr Aesthet Surg. 2008;61:1049–58.

21. Everaars K, Welbie M, Hummelink S, Tjin E, de Laat E, Ulrich D. The impact of scars on health-related quality of life after breast surgery: a qualitative exploration. J Cancer Surviv. 2021;15(2):224–33.

22. Simons M, Price N, Kimble R, Tyack Z. Patient experiences of burn scars in adults and children and development of a health-related quality of life conceptual model: a qualitative study. Burns. 2016;42:620–32.

23. Abrams T, Ogletree R, Ratnapradipa d, Neumeister M. Adult survivors' lived experience of burns and post-burn health: a qualitative analysis. Burns. 2016;42:152–62.

24. Martin L, Byrnes M, McGarry S, Rea S, Wood F. Evaluation of the posttraumatic growth inventory after severe burn injury in Western Australia: clinical implications for use. Disabil Rehabil. 2016;10:1–8.

25. Kornhaber R, Wilson A, Abu-Qamar M, McLean L. Coming to terms with it all: adult burn survivors' 'lived experience' of acknowledgement and acceptance during rehabilitation. Burns. 2014;40:589–97.

26. ter Smitten M, de Graaf R, Van Loey N. Prevalence and co-morbidity of psychiatric disorders 1–4 years after burn. Burns. 2011;37:753–61.

27. Zheng H, Wu K, Zhou Y, Fu L. Prevalence and associated factors of posttraumatic stress disorder in burned patients and their family members. Burns. 2020;47:1102.

28. Fauerbach J, McKibben J, Bienvenu J, Magyar-Russell G, Smith M, Holavanahalli R, et al. Psychological distress Postburn injury. Psychosom Med. 2007;69:473–82.

29. Gupta M, Jarosz P, Gupta A. Posttraumatic stress disorder and the dermatology patient. Clin Dermatol. 2017;35:260–6.

30. Duke J, Randall S, Boyd J, Wood F, Fear M, Rea S. A population-based retrospective cohort study to assess the mental health of patients after a non-intentional burn compared with uninjured people. Burns. 2018;44:1417–26.

31. Willebrand M, Andersson G, Ekselius L. Prediction of psychological health after an accidental burn. J Trauma. 2004;57(2):367–74.

32. Kleindienst N, Priebe K, Borgmann E, Cornelisse S, Kruger A, Ebner-Priemer U, et al. Body self-evaluation and physical scars in patients with borderline personality disorder: an observational study. Borderline Personal Disord Emot Dysregulation. 2014;1(2):1–10.

33. Frewen P, Zhu J, Lanius R. Lifetime traumatic stressors and adverse childhood experiences uniquely predict concurrent PTSD, complex PTSD, and dissociative subtype of PTSD symptoms whereas recent adult non-traumatic stressors do not: results from an online survey study. Eur J Psychotraumatol. 2019;10(1):1606625.

34. McGarry S, Burrows S, Ashoorian T, Pallathil T, Ong K, Edgar D, et al. Mental health and itch in burns patients: potential associations. Burns. 2016;42:763–8.

35. Kundu K, Rawat V, Chattopadhyay D. Gender differences in quality of life and psychological impact of facial burn scars in a tertiary care Centre. Burns. 2020;47:1153.

36. Sibbert S, Carrougher G, Pham T, Mandell S, Arbabi S, Stewart B, et al. Burn survivors' perception of recovery after injury: a northwest regional burn model system investigation. Burns. 2020;46(8):1768–74.

37. Palmu R, Partonen T, Suominem K, Saarni S, Vuola J, Isometsä E. Health-related quality of life 6 months after burns among hospitalized patients: predictive importance of mental disorders and burn severity. Burns. 2015;41:742–8.

38. Shepherd L, Tattersall H, Buchanan H. Looking in the mirror for the first time after facial burns: a retrospective mixed method study. Burns. 2014;40:1624–34.

39. Lawrence J, Rosenberg L, Fauerbach JA. Comparing the body esteem of pediatric survivors of burn injury with the body esteem of an age-matched comparison group without burns. Rehabil Psychol. 2007;52(4):370–9.

40. Martin L, Byrnes M, McGarry S, Rea S, Wood F. Social challenges of visible scarring after severe burn: a qualitative analysis. Burns. 2017;43:78–83.

41. Martin L, Byrnes M, McGarry S, Rea S, Wood F. Posttraumatic growth after burn injury in adults: an integrative literature review. Burns. 2016;43:459–70.

42. Cleary M, Kornhaber R, Thapa D, West S. A quantitative systematic review assessing the impact of burn injuries on body image. Body Image. 2020;33:47–65.

43. Ajoudani F, Jasemi M, Lotfi m. Social participation, social support and body image in the first year of rehabilitation in burn survivors: a longitudinal, three-wave cross-lagged panel analysis using structural equation modelling. Burns. 2018;44:1141–50.

44. Connell K, Phillips M, Coates R, Doherty-Poirier M, Wood F. Sexuality, body image and relationships following burns: analysis of BSHS-B outcome measures. Burns. 2014;40:1329–37.

45. Connell K, Coates R, Wood F. Burn injuries Lead to behavioral changes that impact engagement in sexual and social activities in females. Sex Disabil. 2015;33:75–91.

46. Thombs B, Haines J, Bresnick M, Magyar-Russell G, Fauerbach J, Spence R. Depression in burn reconstruction patients: symptom prevalence and association with body image dissatisfaction and physical function. Gen Hosp Psychiatry. 2007;20:14–20.

47. Martin L, Byrnes M, McGarry S, Rea S, Wood F. Quality of life and posttraumatic growth after burn injury. Burns. 2017;43(7):1400–10.

48. Hodder K, Chur-Hansen A, Parker A. A thematic study of the role of social support in the body image of burn survivors. Health Psychol Res. 2014;2(1196):21–4.

49. Bosmans M, Hofland H, De Jong A, Van Loey N. Coping with burns: the role of coping self-efficacy in the recovery from traumatic stress following burn injury. J Behav Med. 2015;38:642–51.

50. Ohrtman E, Shapiro G, Wolfe A, Trinh N, Ni P, Acton A, et al. Sexual activity and romantic relationships after burn injury: a life impact burn recovery evaluation (LIBRE) study. Burns. 2020;46(7):1556–64.

51. Duke J, Randall S, Vetrichevvel T, McGarry S, Boyd J, Rea S, et al. Long-term mental health outcomes after unintentional burns sustained during childhood: a retrospective cohort study. Burns Trauma. 2018;6(32):1–10.

52. Hoogerwerf C, van Baar M, Middlekoop E, Van Loey N. Impact of facial burns: relationship between depressive symptoms, self-esteem and scar severity. Gen Hosp Psychiatry. 2014;36:271–6.

53. Moi A, Gjengedal E. The lived experience of relationships after major burn injury. J Clin Nurs. 2014;23:2323–31.

54. Glover H. Lived experience perspectives. In: King R, Lloyd C, Meehan T, editors. Handbook of psychosocial rehabilitation. Singapore: Blackwell; 2007.

55. Zhai J, Liu X, Wu J, Jiang H. What does posttraumatic growth mean to Chinese burn patients: a phenomenological study. J Burn Care Res. 2010;31:433–40.

56. Tedeschi R, Park C, Calhoun L. Posttraumatic growth: positive changes in the aftermath of crisis. Hoboken: Taylor and Francis; 1998.

57. Joseph S. What doesn't kill us: the new psychology of posttraumatic growth. London: Piatkus; 2011.

58. Baillie S, Sellwood W, Wisely J. Post-traumatic growth in adults following a burn. Burns. 2014;40(6):1089–96.

59. Rosenbach C, Renneberg B. Positive change after severe burn injuries. J Burn Care Res. 2008;29:638–43.

60. Hawkins RMF. A systematic meta-review of hypnosis as an empirically supported treatment for pain. Pain Rev. 2001;8(2):47–73.

61. Hunter T, Medved M, Hiebert-Murphy D, Brockmeier J, Sareen J, Thakrar S, et al. "Put your face to the world": Women's narratives of burn injury. Burns. 2013;39:1588–98.

62. Martin C, Bonas S, Shephers L, Hedges E. The experience of scar management for adults with burns: an interpretative phenomenological analysis. Burns. 2016;42:1311–22.

63. Crofton E, Merdith P, Gray P, O'Reilly S, Strong J. Non-adherence with compression garment wear in adult burns patients: a systematic review and metaethnography. Burns. 2020;46:472–82.

64. Johnson R, Taggart S, Gullick J. Emerging from the trauma bubble: redefining 'normal' after burn injury. Burns. 2016;42:1223–32.

65. Spronk I, Legemate C, Oen IMMH, Van Loey NEE, Polinder S, Van Baar ME. Health related quality of life in adults after burn injuries: a systematic review. PLoS One. 2018;13(5):e0197507.

66. Kvannli L, Finlay V, Edgar D, Wu A, Wood F. Using the burn specific health scale-brief as a measure of quality of life after a burn—what score should clinicians expect? Burns. 2011;37:54–60.

67. Kazis L, Marino M, Ni P, Soley Bori M, Amaya F, Dore E, et al. Development of the Life Impact Burn Recovery Evaluation (LIBRE) profile: assessing burn survivors' social participation. Qual Life Res. 2017;26(10):2851–66.

68. Lawrence J, Heinberg L, Roca R, Munster A, Spence R, Fauerbach J. Development and validation of the satisfaction with appearance scale: assessing body image among burn-injured patients. Psychol Assess. 1988;10(1):64–70.

69. Park C, Zlateva I, Blank T. Self-identity after cancer: "survivor", "victim", "patient", and "person with cancer". J Gen Intern Med. 2009;24(Supplement 2):430–5.

70. Bovend'Erdt T, Botell R, Wade D. Writing SMART rehabilitation goals and achieving goal attainment scaling: a practical guide. Clin Rehabil. 2009;23:352–61.

71. Carver C, Scheier M, Kumari WJ. Assessing coping strategies: a theoretically based approach. J Pers Soc Psychol. 1989;56(2):267–83.

72. Leduc-Cummings I, Milyavskaya M, Peetz J. Goal motivation and the subjective perception of past and future obstacles. Personal Individ Differ. 2017;109:160–75.

73. Mellemkjaer L, Holmich L, Gridley G, Rabkin C, Olsen JH. Risks for skin and other cancers up to 25 years after burn injuries. Epidemiology. 2006;17(6):668–73.

74. Ault P, Plaza A, Paratz J. Scar massage for hypertrophic scarring—a systematic review. Burns. 2018;44:24–38.

75. Douglas H, Luynch J, Harms K, Krop T, Kunath L, van Vreeswijk C, et al. Carbon dioxide laser treatment in burn-related scarring: a prospective randomised controlled trial. J Plast Reconstr Aesthet Surg. 2019;72(6):863–70.

76. Anderson R, Donelan M, Hivnor C, Greeson E, Ross V, Shumaker P, et al. Laser treatment of traumatic scars with an emphasis on ablative fractional laser resurfacing consensus report. JAMA Dermatol. 2014;150(2):187–93.

77. Willows B, Ilyas M, Sharma A. Laser in the management of burn scars. Burns. 2017;43(7):1379–89.

78. Carver C, Scheier M, Weintraub K. Assessing coping strategies: a theoretically based approach, 56, 267-283. J Pers Soc Psychol. 1989;56:267–83.

79. Chao R. Managing stress and maintaining Well-being: social support, problem-focused coping and avoidant coping. J Couns Dev. 2011;89:338–48.

80. Hwang S, Lim E. Factors associated with posttraumatic growth in patients with sever burn by treatment phase. Nurs Open. 2020;7:1–8.

81. Victorson D, Farmer L, Burnett K, Ouellete A, Barocas J. Maladaptive coping strategies and injury-related distress following traumatic physical injury. Rehabil Psychol. 2005;50(4):408–15.

82. Cofini V, Carbonelli A, Cecilia M, Binkin N, di Orio F. Post traumatic stress disorder and coping in a sample of adult survivors of the Italian earthquake. Psychiatry Res. 2015;229:353–8.

83. Brown C, Battista D, Sereika S, Bruehlman R, Dunbar-Jacob J, Thase M. Primary care patients' personal illness models for depression: relationship to coping behavior and functional disability. Gen Hosp Psychiatry. 2007;29:492–500.

84. Duprez C, Christophe V, Rime B, Congard A, Antoine P. Motives for the social sharing on an emotional experience. J Soc Pers Relat. 2015;32(6):757–87.

85. MacLeod R, Shepherd L, Thompson A. Posttraumatic stress symptomatology and appearance distress following burn injury: an interpretative phenomenological analysis. Health Psychol. 2016;35(11):1197–204.

86. Rumsey N, Harcourt D. Body image and disfigurement: issues and interventions. Body Image. 2004;1:83–97.

87. Corry N, Pruzinsky T, Rumsey N. Quality of life and psychosocial adjustment to burn injury: social functioning, body image and health policy perspectives. Int Rev Psychiatry. 2009;21(6):539–48.

88. World Health Organization. Social determinants of health: overview: World Health Organization. 2021. https://www.who.int/health-topics/social-determinants-of-health#tab=tab_1.

89. Backstrom J, Willebrand M, Sjoberg F, Haglund K. Being a family member of a burn survivor—experiences and needs. Burns Open. 2018;2:193–8.

90. Thombs B, Notes L, Lawrence J, Magyar-Russell G, Bresnick M, Fauerbach J. From survival to socialization: a longitudinal study of body image in survivors of severe burn injury. J Psychosom Res. 2008;64:205–12.

91. Delker B, Salton R, McLean K. Giving voice to silence: empowerment and disempowerment in the developmental shift from trauma 'victim' to 'survivor-advocate'. J Trauma Dissociation. 2020;21(2):242–63.

92. Tolley JS, Foroushani PS. What do we know about one-to-one peer support for adults with a burn injury? A scoping review. J Burn Care Res. 2014;35(3):233–42.

93. Davis T, Gorgens K, Shriberg J, Godleski M, Meyer L. Making meaning in a burn peer support group: qualitative analysis of attendee interviews. J Burn Care Res. 2014;35(5):416–25.

94. Kornhaber R, Wilson A, Abu-Qamar M, McLean L, Vandervord J. Inpatient peer support for adult burn survivors—a valuable resource: a phenomenological analysis of the Australian experience. Burns. 2015;41:110–7.

95. Papamikrouli E, van Schie C, Schoenmaker J, Berge A, Gebhardt W. Peer support needs among adults with burns. J Burn Care Res. 2017;38:112–20.

96. Cristall N, Kohja Z, Gawazuik J, Spiwak R, Logsetty S. Narrative discourse of burn injury and recovery on peer support websites: a qualitative analysis. Burns. 2021;47(2):397–401.

Correction to: Lasers and Energy-Based Devices in Scar Therapy: A Practical Use

Hugues Cartier ⓘ, Francois Will, Thierry Fusade, and Hans-Joachim Laubach ⓘ

Correction to:
Chapter 11 in: S. P. Nischwitz et al. (eds.), *Scars*, https://doi.org/10.1007/978-3-031-24137-6_11

In Chap. 11: There are errors in the attribution of the images. The correct attribution has been updated as follows:

1. Figure 28: Correct attribution is image courtesy of Thierry Fusade.
2. Figure 25: Correct attribution is image courtesy of Thierry Fusade.
3. Figure 24: Correct attribution is image courtesy of Thierry Fusade.
4. Figure 23: Correct attribution is image courtesy of Thierry Fusade.
5. Figure 22: Correct attribution is image courtesy of Thierry Fusade.
6. Figure 20: Correct attribution is image courtesy of Thierry Fusade.
7. Figure 19: Correct attribution is image courtesy of Francois Will.
8. Figure 17: Correct attribution is image courtesy of Francois Will.
9. Figure 16: Correct attribution is image courtesy of Francois Will.
10. Figure 46: Correct attribution is image courtesy of Thierry Fusade.

The updated version of this chapter can be found at
https://doi.org/10.1007/978-3-031-24137-6_11

Index

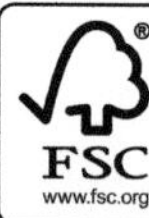